DISASTER MEDICINE

DISASTER MEDICINE

Application for the Immediate Management and
Triage of Civilian and Military Disaster Victims

Senior Editor
Frederick M. Burkle, Jr., M.D., M.P.H.

Associate Editors
Patricia H. Sanner, M.D.
Barry W. Wolcott, M.D.

With an introduction by
Peter Safar, M.D.

MEDICAL EXAMINATION PUBLISHING CO., INC.

Disaster medicine.

    Bibliography: p.
    Includes index.
    1. Disaster medicine. 2. Triage (Medicine)
I. Burkle, Frederick M. II. Sanner, Patricia H.
III. Wolcott, Barry, W. [DNLM: 1. Disasters.
2. Emergencies. 3. Emergency Medical Services
—Organization and administration.] WB 105 D611
RC86. 7. D57 1984 362. 1 83-23803
ISBN 0-87488-186-2

Printed in the United States of America

disclaimer

The opinions and assertions in this publication are those of the
authors and are not to be construed as official or reflecting the
views of the Uniformed Services University, the United States
Air Force, the United States Army, the United States Navy, or
the Military Medical Service at large.

To our patient companions

    Phyllis
    Paul
    Sue Ellen

The medical students at the

    Uniformed Services University
    of the Health Sciences
    Bethesda, Maryland

And

    The dedicated paramedics
    of Maui County, Hawaii

Contents

About the Editors

FREDERICK M. BURKLE, Jr. , M. D. , M. P. H. , received his B. A. degree from Saint Michael's College and his M. D. from the University of Vermont College of Medicine. He completed his internship and residency in Pediatrics at Yale-New Haven Medical Center; received a fellowship in adolescent medicine at Boston Children's Hospital, Harvard Postgraduate School of Medicine; earned a public health degree from the University of California at Berkeley; and completed a residency in psychiatry at Dartmouth-Hitchcock Mental Health Center, Dartmouth Medical School. He practiced pediatrics and adolescent medicine in Connecticut for four years; was formerly Assistant Professor of Pediatrics at the University of Texas Health Science Center, Dallas; and was Director of Inpatient and Emergency Psychiatry, Maui Mental Health Center, Hawaii. He has practiced emergency medicine for five years, most recently at Maui Memorial Hospital, and as Director of Emergency Medical Services, County of Maui, Hawaii; Assistant Clinical Professor of Pediatrics, University of Hawaii; and Visiting Lecturer, Section of Emergency and Operational Medicine, Uniformed Services University.

In 1968-1969, he served as Battalion Surgeon and Triage Officer, Delta Medical Company, as Chief of Pediatrics, Dong Ha Children's Hospital, Third Marine Division, Vietnam, and in 1975, as civilian medical team director for Operation Orphan Lift, Saigon, Vietnam. From 1979 to 1983, he served as Commanding Officer, Naval Reserve, Medical Contingency Response Unit 920, Honolulu, Hawaii.

In 1983, he was appointed Director, Division of Emergency Medical Services, Children's Hospital Medical Center of Akron, Ohio and Associate Professor of Pediatrics, Northeastern Ohio Universities College of Medicine.

MAJOR PATRICIA H. SANNER, M. D. , received her B. S. degree from John Carroll University in Cleveland, Ohio, and her M. D. degree from Baylor College of Houston, Texas, followed by a residency in family practice at the Baylor Center for Medical Education Affiliated Hospitals in Waco, Texas. She then served in the family practice section at Seymour Johnson AFB,

North Carolina, during which time she completed training as
a USAF Flight Surgeon (1980). This was followed by appointment as Assistant Professor of Operational and Emergency
Medicine, Uniformed Services University of the Health Sciences
School of Medicine.

   In 1983, she was appointed Course Director and Faculty,
Battlefield Medicine Course, USAF School of Aerospace Medicine, Brooks AFB, Texas.

COLONEL BARRY W. WOLCOTT, M. D. , received his B. A.
degree from Middlebury College and his M. D. from Johns
Hopkins University School of Medicine. He interned at Walter
Reed Army Medical Center where he also completed a residency in Internal Medicine. Following residency, he was Medical Director of the Intensive Care Unit and Chief of General
Medicine at Brooke Army Medical Center. He became Chief
of Emergency Medicine at that center in 1974, and has concen-
trated in emergency medicine since then. He has served as
consultant in emergency medicine to the Army Surgeon General;
as Director of the Combat Casualty Care Course; as Associate
Professor and Chairman, Section of Operational and Emergency
Medicine, Uniformed Services University; and is presently Chief
of Emergency Medicine at Ft. Lewis, Washington. He is currently president of the University Association for Emergency
Medicine and has served on the initial Residency Review Committee in Emergency Medicine.

Contributors

WILLIAM A. ALTER III, Ph. D. , LTC, Biomedical Science Corps, USAF; Assistant Professor of Physiology, Uniformed Services University of the Health Sciences School of Medicine, Bethesda, Maryland

FREDERICK M. BURKLE, Jr. , M. D. , M. P. H. , Visiting Lecturer, Section of Emergency and Operational Medicine, Uniformed Services University School of Medicine; Captain, Medical Corps, United States Naval Reserve

RANDALL B. CASE, M. D. , Major, Medical Corps, Flight Surgeon, USA; Chief, Emergency Medicine Service, Silas B. Hayes Army Hospital, Fort Ord, California

JAMES J. CONKLIN, M. D. , LTC, Medical Corps, USAF; Deputy Director, Armed Forces Radiobiology Research Institute; Assistant Professor of Radiology, Uniformed Services University of the Health Sciences School of Medicine; Assistant Clinical Professor of Radiology, George Washington University School of Medicine, Washington, D. C.

DENNIS DUGGAN, B. A. , Major, Medical Service Corps, USA; Instructor and Operations Officer, Section of Emergency and Operational Medicine, Uniformed Services University of the Health Sciences School of Medicine, Bethesda, Maryland; 159th Medical Detachment (Helicopter Ambulance), Vietnam 1970-1971.

DAVID V. FELICIANO, M. D. , Assistant Professor of Surgery, Baylor College of Medicine; Director, Surgical Intensive Care Unit, Ben Taub General Hospital, Houston, Texas

EARL W. FERGUSON, M. D. , Ph. D. , LTC, USAF Medical Corps; Associate Professor of Medicine and Physiology, Uniformed Services University of the Health Sciences School of Medicine; Chief of Cardiology, Wilford Hall USAF Medical Center, Lackland AFB, Texas

OSCAR M. JARDON, M.D., Associate Professor, Department
of Orthopedic Surgery, University of Nebraska Medical Center,
Omaha, Nebraska

CRAIG H. LLEWELLYN, M.D., Colonel, Medical Corps, USA;
Commandant, Uniformed Services University of the Health
Sciences School of Medicine; Chairman, Department of Military
Medicine, Uniformed Services University of the Health Sciences
School of Medicine, Bethesda, Maryland

KENNETH L. MATTOX, M.D., Associate Professor of Surgery,
Baylor College of Medicine; Deputy Surgeon-in-Chief and Director,
Emergency Medical Surgical Services, Ben Taub General Hos-
pital, Houston, Texas

ROGER S. MECCA, M.D., Chairman, Department of Anesthesia;
Director, Surgical Intensive Care Unit, Danbury Hospital, Dan-
bury, Connecticut; Former Director, Recovery Services, Co-
Director, Surgical Intensive Care Unit, Staff Anesthesiologist,
Wilford Hall USAF Medical Center, San Antonio, Texas

VALERIY MOYSAENKO, M.D., Chief, General Surgery Service,
Director, Surgery Residency Program, Wright-Patterson AFB,
Ohio; Assistant Clinical Professor of Surgery, Wright State
University School of Medicine, Ohio

ANDRE J. OGNIBENE, M.D., Commanding General (RET),
Brooke Army Medical Center; Hospital Director, San Antonio
State Chest Hospital; Clinical Professor of Medicine, University
of Texas Health Science Center at San Antonio; Consultant in
Medicine, United States Army, Vietnam, 1969

JACK B. PEACOCK, M.D., Associate Professor of Surgery,
Director of Emergency Services, Texas Tech University Health
Sciences Center, El Paso, Texas

RICHARD A. PRATT, M.D., Private Practice of Neurosurgery,
Abilene, Texas; Former Chief of Neurosurgery, Oakland Naval
Hospital, Oakland, California

JAY P. SANFORD, M.D., Professor of Medicine, President
and Dean, Uniformed Services University of the Health Sciences
School of Medicine, Bethesda, Maryland

PATRICIA H. SANNER, M. D. , Major, Medical Corps, USAF;
Assistant Professor, Section of Emergency and Operational
Medicine, Uniformed Services University School of Medicine,
Bethesda, Maryland

DOUGLAS STUTZ, Ph. D. , LTC, MSC, USA, Instructor, Emergency and Operational Medicine, Uniformed Services University
of the Health Sciences School of Medicine, Bethesda, Maryland

JOSEPH W. WAECKERLE, M. D. , Chairman, Department of
Emergency Medicine, Baptist Memorial Hospital, Kansas City,
Missouri; Clinical Associate Professor of Emergency Medicine,
University of Missouri at Kansas City School of Medicine

BARRY W. WOLCOTT, M. D. , Colonel, Medical Corps, USA;
Associate Professor and Former Chairman, Section of Emer-
gency and Operational Medicine, Uniformed Services University
School of Medicine, Bethesda, Maryland

Foreword

This very timely and scholarly text, which deals with disaster from a medical as well as a logistical standpoint, is orchestrated by those experienced in their field and complimented by others whose accolades in their separate fields require no enumeration. All of the contributing authors as well as the editorial staff are nationally and internationally recognized authors in their field of expertise.

Well recognized is the fact that, even in peace time in this country, one-third of those Americans who die do so as a direct result of trauma (National Center for Health Statistics, September 1981). Worse yet, amongst those who die before the age of forty, trauma is the number one cause of death in this country [Boyd, D.R. "Trauma—A Controllable Disease in the 1980s" (Fourth Annual Stone Lecture, American Trauma Society) J Trauma, 20:14-24]. A paradox thus arises. How is it that a nation which trains more physicians than any other, which witnesses more violent crime than any other, but which admittedly has a desparately low level (25%) of "experienced" trauma surgeons among those it considers "trained", achieves preeminence among nations regarding excellence in the care of the trauma victim?

The answer lies in the intellectual endeavors of those whose past experience has gained them the respect of their colleagues in terms of casualty care, whether it be in support of national need associated with combat or other requirements associated with mass disaster at home or abroad.

This text more than adequately addresses those seperate issues which bridge the biomedical disciplines encompassing the broad area we describe as trauma.

To paraphrase a famous "expert in trauma" . . . "The world will little know nor long remember what was said here today but it cannot forget what they did here." Those whose manifold contributions to the care of the trauma victim, having advanced our cognizance of and improved our care of such, deserve special attention. Their dedication to their objective and its outcome arrive high on the list of concerned men and women dedicated to caring for those who, by whatever reasons, are injured.

This treatise addresses amply all of those situations which might arise under most circumstances where trauma is an inciting event. All too often those experiences which past analyses have finalized in fixed recommendations regarding therapy have become indelibly written for succeeding generations. This has been to the disadvantage of those who followed. The latter, as has been written, are victims of the past. As the poet once wrote . . . "Those who cannot remember the past are condemned to repeat it. " (George Santayana, Life of Reason, 1906)

This text should address all of those questions which to date remain unanswered and which require redress. Hopefully their answers will not be a "finished" product of what will ultimately be the answer to trauma management whether on the battlefield, at home, or abroad, but rather an intercession of trauma care management until such time arises when additional science, skills, and experience provide more acceptable alternatives.

Kenneth G. Swan, M.D.

Professor of Surgery
Chief, Section of General Surgery
University of Medicine and Dentistry of New Jersey
Newark, New Jersey

Preface

A disaster may induce many individual or combined stresses: medical, psychosocial, and structural. The intensity of impact on any one of these factors depends on the precipitating event. For example, a 747 aircraft crash, in which there are few or no survivors, is a disaster which does not stress the emergency medical care delivery system, but does stress firefighters, extrication and repair crews, and personnel involved in victim identification. This disaster stresses families of victims but does not create a large homeless population. A sudden terrorist bombing in a busy airport stresses the emergency medical care delivery system as well as those concerned with the control and clearing of structural damage.

Disaster has a variable time dimension. The terrorist bombing example given above may overwhelm the emergency medical care system for a relatively short period, probably less than 24 hours. A natural disaster, such as tornadoes and floods, may yield large numbers of casualties, homeless individuals, and structural damage. This will stress all the emergency services for an extended period of time.

This text, Disaster Medicine, is not meant to be a systems manual for disaster planners. It is directed to an important stress target in disaster care delivery: the primary care provider and his/her immediate staff. These individuals may suddenly find themselves involved in a large scale disaster with a significant number of survivors who require care over a 24-36-hr period.

This book is not a restatement of established procedures in prehospital life support, communications, or transportation. A disaster implies that these established means of problem solving have been overwhelmed or destroyed by the event. Therefore, this text is designed to give the primary care provider some necessary information for planning and practical on-the-scene points for medical care and coping, with suggestions of novel solutions to problems that occur in a disaster. We have drawn on the vast military experience which has been repeatedly required to cope with the disaster of war. In the reality of disaster medicine, there are few differences between military and civilian disaster care.

We hope that the information and ideas in this text will be
helpful to the individual care provider in overcoming the disruption, shortages, and chaos of disaster. Sometimes under
such conditions, one must use imagination and creativity to
make do with existing supplies, but planning is still required.
We feel that this book is a critical link in such anticipatory
planning.

We wish to acknowledge the technical assistance of Sandra
Sillapere, Kathleen Breazile, Print Productions of Maui, and
Charles Matsuda and Mary Ann Ellingson, from Tripler Army
Medical Center, Oahu.

Frederick M. Burkle, Jr., M.D., M.P.H.
Patricia Sanner, M.D.
Barry W. Wolcott, M.D.

Introduction

Our troubled world needs to pay more attention to medical disasters of all kinds and magnitudes because of increasing opportunities to ameliorate their devastating effects on human lives. A "disaster" is defined as an event causing widespread destruction and distress; a "medical disaster" causes, in addition, potentially reversible critical injuries or illnesses in numbers or time frames which overwhelm the community's medical services. In terms of magnitude, there are three categories, each requiring different planning and responses: (1) the multicasualty incident, such as a transportation accident, which should be manageable by the local emergency medical services (EMS) system; (2) the mass disaster, such as a major earthquake, which overwhelms the local EMS system and requires a National Disaster Medical System (NDMS); and (3) the epidemic-endemic disaster, such as the combination of famine, epidemic, terrorism, war, and refugees, as now occurs in some poor, developing countries; this problem needs global economic and political solutions.

Man-made disasters, ranging from errors (technical failures) to the results of mankind's evil side (war), should be preventable. Unfortunately, some of these events will continue to occur. Natural mass disasters, like earthquakes, hurricanes, and floods, are not preventable and will remain relatively unpredictable. How can we maximize human salvage in such events? The opportunities in disasters to reduce crippling and dying before one's time has come have greatly increased with the advent of modern resuscitation and life-support methodologies. "Reanimatology" is the scientific basis, and emergency and critical care medicine (EMS systems) are the delivery arms. Disaster medicine represents major medical, political, and organizational dilemmas. Medical preparedness in disasters requires policy, planning, and a preorganized response system. Each plan must be influenced by estimations of life-saving potentials, since resources will be limited everywhere.

Although the problems are immense, the opportunities are real, as shown by the documented life-saving impact of everyday EMS systems and of military medicine in recent wars. For

civilian medicine, disasters have been confusing topics which
have been approached with defeatism. Disaster medicine in general is not taught to health care professionals. Therefore, this
book, edited and co-authored by Drs. F. M. Burkle, P. H. Sanner,
and B. W. Wolcott, is an important contribution. It is an intro-
ductory text for medical students, physicians, and nonphysician
leaders. Some of them may read or write reports and reviews
on disaster-related topics in the new (first) Journal of Disaster
Medicine[1] and in other pertinent medical publications, and use
this book as a basis for their reports.

The National Red Cross and Red Crescent Societies, linked
worldwide by the League of Red Cross Societies, the World
Health Organization, and other national and international agencies, have made great efforts in recent years to help in mass
disasters. Their main efforts have been directed at public health
oriented measures designed to rehabilitate uninjured survivors.
The World Association for Emergency and Disaster Medicine
(WAED)[2] (formerly the "Club of Mainz," initiated by Rudolf
Frey of Mainz, West Germany in the 1970s) is becoming a
growing worldwide association of physicians and nonphysician
leaders, educators, and researchers who are interested in disaster medicine and are working to enhance worldwide resuscitation (acute medicine) capabilities for disaster victims by working with and through the above existing agencies.

In disaster situations, the main logistic obstacle to resuscitation is obviously the rapidity with which treatment must be
started to be effective — immediate basic life support, and advanced life support no more than six hours later. This writer
recommends two main opportunities to meet this challenge.
First, teaching life-support first aid (LSFA), i. e. , basic
(trauma) life support to the public in all countries to augment
population capabilities in self-help and "buddy" help. The majority of people in the world have not yet acquired LSFA capability. LSFA is easily learned, so that this gap could be quickly
remedied at a very low cost. The League of Red Cross Societies
is embarking on this now. Second, increasing reliance on military medicine for the provision of advanced (trauma) life support

---

[1] Journal of Disaster Medicine, Centrum Publishing, Univer-
sity City Science Center, 3508 Market Street, Suite 230,
Philadelphia, PA 19104
[2] For information on the WAED write: Secretary, Peter Baskett,
M. D. , Frenchay Hospital, Department of Anesthetics, Bristol
BS16 1LE, England

in mass disasters. Civilian advanced life-support EMS systems are developing rapidly in industrialized countries, while most poor developing countries do not even have basic life support on ambulances and have uncertain advanced life support in hospitals. In poor countries without EMS systems, the military could and should help, not only in mass disasters but also in multicasualty incidents.

This book by Burkle, et al., is unique in this regard. It gives the reader some of the authors' first-hand experiences in war medicine and links the lessons learned from military medicine with those of civilian EMS systems. This book is primarily meant for physicians and medical students, few of whom have gained first-hand experience in resuscitating victims of everyday emergencies in their training and practice. Almost none have had early first-hand experience in mass disasters like major earthquakes. Exceptions are military physicians, particularly anesthesiologists and surgeons, with first-hand experience in wars. To remain experienced with acute medicine and trauma surgery in peace time, however, military medical personnel should be involved in everyday civilian trauma care.

In most countries, the military seems to have the only system which is always ready and funded to provide the instant communication, short response time, trained medical personnel, needed equipment and supplies, airlift capability, extrication and rescue technology, and authoritative leadership and organization which are required for the resuscitation of victims of mass disasters. Even international collaboration of military services of several countries should be possible. Involvement of the military in nationwide disaster medicine planning and preparedness would give the armed services a noble role in peace time. The military should participate and perhaps even lead in the planning of each country's national disaster medical system (NDMS), and should be given responsibility and authority for disaster responses which are not promptly and adequately handled by the existing civilian EMS system.

Organizations concerned with disaster medicine must clarify the scope of disaster planning and should mediate between the peace movement, particularly the International Physicians for the Prevention of Nuclear War (IPPNW) — in the United States, the Physicians for Social Responsibility — and the military, which is best for disaster relief actions in war and peace. Most experienced military physicians are pacifists, having personally experienced the horrors of war. In order to clarify the role of disaster medicine and its future planning efforts, the World

Association for Emergency and Disaster Medicine (WAED)[3]
has considered the medical consequences of a major nuclear
war and, in May 1983, made the following recommendations to
all relevant governments and powers and their medical pro-
fessions:

> "(1) that disaster medical preparedness should be con-
> tinued and developed, not only for multicasualty incidents
> and natural mass disasters, but also for conventional
> wars, nuclear accidents, and a single, small nuclear
> bomb explosion (caused by accident, terrorism, or a de-
> ranged leader); (2) that any meaningful disaster medicine
> preparedness for a nuclear holocaust is impossible. Such
> attempts at planning nuclear war medical preparedness
> are misleading and represent an unjustifiable use of med-
> ical and financial resources. However, in the awful event
> of a nuclear holocaust the members would, of course, do
> what they could to relieve pain and suffering; (3) that all
> governments and powers currently in possession of nu-
> clear weapons agree not to assist, in any way, other
> powers at present without nuclear weapons, to obtain
> them in the future; (4) that all governments and powers
> in possession of nuclear weapons take initiatives to re-
> duce and ultimately eliminate their nuclear arsenals
> worldwide. "

Similar recommendations have been made earlier by the World
Health Organization and other national and international medical
groups striving for nuclear disarmament. Each country should
develop its own national disaster medical system which should
not be designed to prepare for nuclear war but, rather, for the
worst imaginable natural disaster, such as a major earthquake.
This would automatically provide a national plan for the protection of civilians in a conventional war.
    This book, through the experiences drawn from military
medicine, stimulates medical students, physicians, and other
health professionals to: (1) acquire life-support expertise
through basic and advanced cardiac and trauma life-support
courses, and through supervised life support of patients in an-
esthesiology, emergency rooms, and trauma surgery, and (2)
acquire knowledge and understanding of everyday EMS systems
and disaster plans of the hospital, community, region, and

---

[3] See note 2.

nation. Physicians should appreciate that they can help give the individual disaster victim a better chance by being better trained and prepared for mass casualty care. Such care would only be as effective as the weakest link in the disaster life-support chain: recognition, detection, self-help, buddy-help, extrication-rescue-resuscitation, triage, stabilization, and evacuation with life support to the most appropriate predetermined definitive care facility, with the least number of intermediate steps of retriaging and restabilizing. Military medicine has demonstrated the efficacy of disaster-oriented planning, organization, and training with simulated victims and scenarios. This book shows that one can effectively prepare and train for mass casualty care.

Peter Safar, M. D.

Director, Resuscitation Research Center, University of Pittsburgh, 3434 Fifth Avenue, Pittsburgh, PA 15260; President, World Association for Emergency and Disaster Medicine (Club of Mainz); Chief Editor, Journal of Disaster Medicine; Consultant, National Disaster Medical Systems Planning (U. S. A.)

notice

The editors, authors, and publisher of this book have made every effort to ensure that all therapeutic modalities that are recommended are in accordance with accepted standards at the time of publication.

The drugs specified within this book may not have specific approval by the Food and Drug Administration in regard to the indications and dosages that are recommended by the editors and authors. The manufacturer's package insert is the best source of current prescribing information.

SECTION 1

THE ORGANIZATION OF DISASTER MEDICINE

Chapter 1

CIVILIAN DISASTERS AND DISASTER PLANNING
Jay P. Sanford, M. D.

DEFINITIONS

Disaster is defined as a grave misfortune or an occurrence inflicting widespread destruction and distress. It is this latter definition which will be used. To be more specific, the term disaster will be applied to a sudden occurrence which results in serious injury or death to 25 or more persons. Another commonly used term is mass casualties. This will be defined as a number of casualties generated more or less simultaneously which exceed the ability to provide usual medical care. Note that this definition does not give a number. The number is determined by a series of variables including number of casualties, types of injuries, and medical personnel and resources available and effectively utilized.

MAGNITUDE OF THE PROBLEM

The frequency of natural disasters is generally not appreciated. In the U. S. in the decade of the 1950's, there were over 3000 natural disasters. The number injured annually in disasters involving 25 or more individuals in the same episode is 13,000-15,000 with approximately 1300 deaths. Disasters thus represent a serious social-medical problem. Studies of past disasters have shown that most deaths and injuries are preventable.

TYPES OF DISASTERS

Planning requires an awareness of the range of disasters which can occur, possible preventive measures, types of injuries, prevention of further casualties after initial impact, and special problems and requirements. The major types of civilian disasters include the following: airplane crashes, avalanches, building collapses, dam collapses, earthquakes, epidemics, explosions, fires, floods, highway accidents, hurricanes, mine disasters, nuclear reactor accidents, panic crushes, railroad wrecks, ship disasters, tornadoes, tidal waves, and volcanic

3

eruptions. The special problems which may be associated with
some of these include the release of toxic chemicals following
highway, railroad, or ship accidents (e. g. , chlorine gas may
be released from tank cars or barges after an accident). Not
all of these are relevant to any given community or region;
however, at least one-half of the list might affect any community.

TYPICAL RESPONSE TO A DISASTER

An understanding of planning requirements will be greatly enhanced by an appreciation of the response of a typical city in
the United States. The events involving the Worcester tornado
in 1953 exemplify many of the problems. Although this represents an experience of 30 years ago, observations drawn from
more recent disasters demonstrate that few, if any, substantive
changes have occurred.

Lessons Gained from the Worcester County Tornado*
John W. Raker, M. D.

"On June 9, 1953, a tornado passed across
Worcester County in the center of Massachusetts. It began in the outlying rural town of Petersham, and at a
rate of 40 miles per hour it passed successively through
the rural towns of Barre and Rutland, the suburban district of Holden, through a narrow upper segment of the
city of Worcester, and then into the suburban area of
Shrewsbury where it broke into two small tornadoes.
Since the tornado passed from rural to suburban to urban and back again into rural areas, and since it passed
through highly congested areas of Worcester, the National Research Council decided that this would be an
interesting tornado disaster to study—one which might
have interesting connotations not only for natural disasters elsewhere, but for possible military disasters.
Accordingly, the Massachusetts General Hospital was
requested to send a team of four persons into the
Worcester area to conduct an inquiry into the medical
handling of this disaster. The team consisted of an administrator, a specialist in public health, an internist,
and a surgeon.

---

*Raker, et al. , Emergency Medical Care in Disaster. A Summary of Recorded Experience, 1956.

STUDY METHODS AND VIEWPOINT

"Mention should be made of the point of view that
the team tried to adopt and the methods that it used.
Such a study is no better than the methods and point of
view. Since the team entered the area about 6 weeks after the disaster, the people had had time to satisfy their
immediate desire to talk about their experiences and had
rid themselves of their worries. They had had time to
construct a pattern of their own behavior and to talk with
other people, and thus had eliminated some of the conflicts in testimony which might have been noted immediately after the disaster. Therefore, one must adopt a
somewhat critical attitude toward the information received. Evidence obtained by interview was checked
against other interviews and other information.

"Wilford Trotter, writing at the time of the World
War II bombing in London, expressed a good way to approach such studies:

"In examining decisions reached under the influence
of panic, we are not to look for blunders and errors of
judgment, for the fruits of ignorance, or the fatuity of
office, but for something at once more subtle and more
characteristic. We are to look for decisions that could
have been reached only by people in whom the faculty of
practical reason was actually impaired. I have expressed belief that we should not be concerned in the
distribution of blame—there is none to distribute. We
have discussed a natural phenomenon and its results.
Decisions bearing the diagnostic marks of having been
affected by panic should be reviewed without mercy or
any regard for the saving of face."

"Comments made here are objective; they are not a
criticism of the city of Worcester, of its doctors, or of
its people.

TORNADO AREA

"In the city of Worcester heavily populated areas
were struck: several large housing projects and many
middle-class family homes. The area in Holden also
contained middle-class family homes and some of the
better-class family homes. The area in Shrewsbury was
similar in nature.

WORCESTER HOSPITALS

"About 2 miles away from the damaged area in
Worcester is the large City Hospital. The City Hospital
has adequate facilities for handling emergency patients.
It has a large emergency ward and is accustomed to having the police ambulances bring casualties to it. On the
south is a slightly smaller hospital called St. Vincent's
which has relatively little accident-room work. On the
east is Memorial Hospital which has highly developed
teaching facilities, but a relatively small emergency
ward setup. To the north, within about a quarter of a
mile of the disaster zone, is Hahneman Hospital, a 100-
bed hospital with a small room occasionally used for accident cases. The small 30-bed Holden District Hospital
was in the process of being enlarged; a new wing under
construction was as yet only walls and floor without
lighting. There is no hospital in Shrewsbury. Shrewsbury
usually sends its casualties directly to Memorial and did
so on this occasion. The casualties from the Lincoln
Street and the Burncoat Street areas began going to
Hahneman, and the casualties of Holden began going to
Holden.

THE TORNADO STRIKES

"The disaster struck Worcester about 5:15 p. m. It
began at Petersham about 4:30 p. m. and ended to the
east of Shrewsbury about 5:35 p. m. There was no effective warning, but there were a number of ineffectual attempts to notify people. The police chief in Barre, for
instance, learning that a couple of houses had been destroyed, called the area state police barracks in Holden.
A state police car was sent to investigate. The police
barracks suddenly lost its own power supply when the
tornado passed within a very short distance of it. A
short time later a passing motorist stopped at the barracks and told the police that many people were injured
in the nearby residential area of Holden. A police patrol
car investigated and radioed back that there was a real
catastrophe. Only then did real notification go out. The
Holden police called Boston State Police. State police in
Boston attempted to notify the Civil Defense headquarters in Worcester. At that moment, the tornado was already passing through Shrewsbury.
"The Hahneman Hospital staff and nurses were at

dinner. Someone looked and saw a man running across
the ambulance yard with a big laceration in his scalp.
Within 10 minutes the place was jammed. They sent out
an emergency radio call for the staff to report and it was
this emergency call which notified most of the medical
personnel of the city that something serious had happened. Without further notification most of the doctors
reported to the hospital.

"In the disaster area, people pulled themselves and
others out of the rubble as best they could. The devastation was extreme. This tornado had a width at its point
of ground contact from 200 yards to perhaps a quarter of
a mile or more. In that very narrow impact zone it lev-
eled almost everything. People who were killed were
mostly in the areas of complete devastation. Many of the
injured were in a state of automatism. Some walked or
ran on broken legs. Others helped other people although
they themselves were bleeding from important lacerations.

"One of the striking things was the intense desire of
everyone to be helpful. Help flowed from the surrounding
regions into every section of this disaster area. Thou-
sands just ran in as best they could; they clambered over
the debris; they surged in and, with little thought of first
aid, pulled people out and bundled them into the nearest
available transportation. Usually the seriously injured
were placed on a ladder or door, carried up over the
rubble, and put in a truck, station wagon, or delivery
car. By 7 p. m. practically no casualties were left in the
disaster zone. Only then were road blocks put on any of
the roads so as to control the removal of casualties.
Practically none of the casualties reached the hospitals
with any evidence of first aid—no tourniquets, no bandages, no splints, practically no first aid.

"The large volume of casualties was carried by volunteer vehicles. One observer commented, "The drivers
seemed obsessed by the idea that speed of evacuation
meant better chance of recovery. " The response of local
volunteers in the control of traffic was simply amazing.
Everyone apparently wanted to control traffic whether
he had any police training or not. It was a terrible problem because everyone wanted to go into the disaster
area; he drove there in his own car and parked at the
nearest point possible. Very soon there was intense con-
gestion of traffic. About 6:30 p. m. the main road to the
city was made open for one-way traffic right through the

heart of Worcester to the City Hospital with policemen
and volunteers at each corner. Down this road, casualties were apparently driven in volunteer wagons and
trucks at speeds from 40 to 60 miles an hour, whizzing
along over railroad tracks in the city center, to arrive
at the City Hospital. Of a number of doctors who went
spontaneously into the disaster zone, only one thought
he saw anyone in clinical shock, although casualties
were there for at least 2 hours after injury; yet the doctors at the receiving points in hospitals reported that
nearly all of the seriously injured arrived in a state of
wound shock.

COMMUNICATIONS

"There was almost immediate failure of the telephone as a means of communication after the tornado
struck. Although few lines were down, calls so jammed
the switchboards that it was impossible to get messages
in or out. Ultimately, each hospital had a mobile radio
unit assigned for the purpose of communications. This,
it is felt, is the best way to establish effective communications in future disasters, and planning should include
some such arrangements. As one would imagine, these
were not well integrated radio circuits. The Holden District State Police Barracks was able to talk to all state
police, both to the west of Worcester and in Shrewsbury.
State police could not talk to Worcester police except by
telephone or by radioing Boston and having Boston telephone Worcester, so practically no messages went
through that way. The Shrewsbury town police had some
cruiser cars in which they could hear the state police
but they could not talk to them, so Shrewsbury was almost isolated. Worcester was in communication with
outside areas only by these few telephone or radio calls
to Boston and elsewhere.

ACTION AT HOSPITALS

"There was very little time for improvisation or
execution of planned arrangements before the disaster
victims arrived. Memorial had no notification of disaster except the sounding of sirens, and Hahneman and
Holden had no notification except the arrival of the injured. About 20 minutes before casualties arrived, City
Hospital was warned by a telephone call from the police;
St. Vincent's had more than an hour's notification.

"The City Hospital had a two-page disaster plan on paper. The superintendent had read it; but no one else at the hospital seemed familiar with it, and most seemed not to know that it existed. In fact, it was not followed because some of the important major points in the plan were ignored as the work began. Some of the hospitals reverted to plans they had developed for military disaster during World War II. At Memorial, a surgeon had been designated as a triage officer in the World War II plan; he came in. At City Hospital, a house staff of about 25 men went to work at once and began to triage at the entrance to the accident ward. At Hahneman, there was no effective triage. Hahneman has four entry points; almost at once patients were coming in through all four. There was no control at any of the entrances, except that one was screened for perhaps 2 hours. Within half an hour the entire area was so packed with cars and with people lying on the lawn and in the corridors, that it was impossible to get anyone in the hospital. Then, and only then, were casualties diverted to the next hospital.

"The situation at Memorial was similar. A high, stone wall completely encircled it except for one entrance point which admitted only one car at a time. The particular wing which serves as the accident room has two entry points, one on either side. Casualties eventually began to come in on both sides. For a long time there was control at only one entrance point to this hospital.

"Dr. Osgood, superintendent of the hospital, described what he termed a "rolling expansion" of the areas involved in the handling of casualties. A few came, the first room was used; a few more, the next room was used. The injured moved down the hospital corridors until they were carried too far from the entry points to reach treatment as the hospital became full. The way Hahneman and Memorial chose to obtain identification of the casualties was to admit everyone—families, friends, everybody. The hospitals were swarming with volunteers, blood donors, and persons looking for injured relatives.

"Holden received about 200 casualties. The chief of staff firmly believed that the hospital should make its contributions to the community as a return for the community's recent support in the construction of the hospital's new wing. Therefore, he felt strongly that each patient who came to the Holden Hospital must be cared for

there. In fact, he went out several times and stopped
people from removing casualties to other hospitals. He
stated, "We think that any hospital which turns a patient
away is very open to criticism. We feel that every casualty must be accepted even if we have to put them on
the roof." Well, they nearly did put them on the roof.
They sent them over into the unfinished wing which had
no lights, no water, and no beds. They spread mattress-
es on the floor and laid their casualties on the mattress-
es. Within an hour or two, it was dark. People went
around in the dark trying to find out who was there, what
the injury was, and also trying to treat the injuries on
the spot. In a number of graphic instances, doctors on
their hands and knees sewed up wounds while a nurse
held a flashlight. They placed litters on sawhorses in a
small operating room, making it into a three-patient
operating room. There was an inadequate supply of
sterile water. Within a very short time, they were out
of sterile water and sterile goods. They immediately
decided that they had two kinds of water: the clean kind
that came out of the tap and the dirty kind that had been
used to wash instruments. Instruments were passed
from hand to hand and washed in tap water between operations. There was no further attempt at sterility.

"The dead totaled 94, and of these 88 were killed
outright. During the first 48 hours, 490 persons were
admitted to some 17 hospitals. Memorial had the most,
about 168. Hahneman and Holden each had 55 admissions. City Hospital had 103, and St. Vincent's had about
27. The number of minor injuries treated in the hospitals is variously estimated, but it must have been at
least 900. A total of about 1,500 were injured; this
means that this tornado would be called a limited disaster. If there had been many more injured to handle, the
medical facilities would have been horribly overwhelmed.

TYPES OF INJURIES

"Most of the serious casualties suffered fractures
and head injuries. Most of the 88 deaths resulted from
head injuries—persons flung through the air or struck
by flying objects. The force of the tornado was such that
several persons had their skulls broken open in a small
rent and had the soft tissues of the brain sucked right
out by the vacuum created by the storm. Among the living, there were 77 who had skull fractures and head

injuries; about 180 other fractures, most of long bones; 28 eye injuries; 9 kidney contusions; 6 ruptured spleens; 5 burns; and 147 major lacerations. The reason for the small number of burns was that the public works employees quickly pulled the electric power switches, and no one suffered electrocution. There were no known explosions from leaking gas mains.

"One hundred sixty-seven units of blood, 101 units of plasma, and about 54 units of plasma volume expanders were used in the first 24 hours. There were on hand about 66 units of blood and 126 units of plasma. From outside sources 159 units of blood, and 1,014 units of plasma were obtained. The amount of blood and plasma used (something much less than one unit of blood or plasma per injured patient) was probably not ideal for the severity of the injuries. There was little plasma volume expander on hand. The doctors had little previous experience with it, so they did not use it very much. Blood and plasma were available and more could have been obtained if there had been a real demand.

"In the first 24 hours, they drew 1,120 units of blood. All excess personnel were set to work drawing blood, and the hospitals exhausted their supply of sterile containers, needles, etc. Finally, those who came from miles away in response to calls for blood donors had to be turned away. There was a good bit of bitterness about that. This blood was so taken that the next day they were not certain of all of the typing. Some blood was hemolyzed, and there was not adequate refrigeration to store it. Apparently, not a single unit of this blood was used for a casualty of the tornado. All of it was converted into gamma globulin—the only way in which it could be salvaged.

SURGICAL THERAPY AND RESULTS

"In the 24 hours after the tornado, there were 14 neurosurgical operations. There are two neurosurgeons in Worcester, both of whom have had military experience. One was called by Hahneman and told that a man with a severe head injury was in the hospital. Within a minute or two, he was told that several more were coming. He said, "I am going to the City Hospital. Send the neurosurgical casualties there." He instructed his associate to go to Hahneman and pick out the neurosurgical casualties, tag them, place them in some form of transportation, and send them to City Hospital. The associate was then to go to Memorial and spend the rest of the night working on neurosurgical patients there. This was done very smoothly and efficiently. It was entirely the idea of the neurosurgeons themselves and no part of any prior official planning. At City, one neurosurgeon and the house staff handled about 11 major neurosurgical injuries during the first 24 hours, and the second neurosurgeon handled about three at Memorial during the same time. All of these patients were operated upon with full attention to asepsis in the operating room, in the way these neurosurgeons were accustomed to work on the occasional injuries which they received from the main Worcester Turnpike to New York. All of these patients lived, with the exception of one man nearly moribund upon arrival. None developed any sepsis and, on the whole, it was a very heartening record.

"There were about 15 orthopedic operations during the first night, mostly on long bone open fractures. They were variously handled by the various men, and it is difficult to determine the results. Approximately 30 long bone fractures have had some kind of fixation procedure done over the course of time. Of the rest of the 1,500 injuries, both major and minor lacerations, it appears that all except 23 were handled by debridement and primary suture using the nearest material at hand. Some of these debridements were carried out under circumstances such as those described at Holden.

"This tornado apparently was especially dirty, even for tornadoes. It passed over two lakes, sucked up water and dust, and impregnated all wounds with blown-in mud. The force was such that the sides of automobiles were tattooed by this flying matter, and its removal required a powerful burnishing machine. Wounds were similarly contaminated. Of course, anesthesia was required in most of these patients. Many operations were done under local anesthesia, and that may be one of the reasons that they were inadequately debrided. At the City Hospital, for example, a receiving line organization was developed in one of the dining rooms. The patient with a minor laceration entered, was washed, and usually had a tetanus shot and a shot of penicillin. Then someone tried to infiltrate the area with a local anesthetic; and finally, the surgeon saw the patient, cleaned the wound and sutured it primarily. That is the way most of the minor injuries were handled.

"The operations performed at City and Memorial corresponded in numbers to a usual operating schedule on a busy day. Therefore, those hospitals were able to handle the volume of anesthesias. At St. Vincent's, which received only 27 casualties, only one major case required the use of the operating room. The rest of the operations were done in the emergency ward under local anesthesia. The only reason any patients reached St. Vincent's is that the City ambulance entrance finally became jammed. St. Vincent's probably could have handled four or five times as many patients as it received.

"Most of the hospitals gave tetanus antitoxin indiscriminately, but a few also gave tetanus toxoid to appropriate persons. There were no serious anaphylactic reactions to the antitoxin, although there were some minor instances of serum sickness after about 10 days.

"Some of these wounds apparently had to be redebrided. Several hospitals told a story of a patient with a long bone fracture in a cast who appeared from another hospital and was sent to bed without having the cast opened. The patient developed fever on the second or third day. The cast was opened and there was the fracture not set; an open fracture with dirt and leaves in it. This may have occurred several times. There were only 123 major lacerations treated by debridement with planned delayed closure. These were done by four or five surgeons with extensive military experience, who carried on much as they would have with military injured.

"Only three instances of probable Clostridial myositis were found; and none of these patients died. One additional patient had a gas-forming infection in the soft tissues, but Clostridia were never isolated from it. In estimates of the incidence of other kinds of sepsis there was wide variation. Some surgeons reported practically no sepsis, maybe one case in ten. In contrast to this, the house staffs of the same hospitals, who followed the patients in the outpatient departments, said they never saw such poorly healing wounds. Some of the family physicians said that almost universally those wounds sutured in the Worcester hospital became infected. It is a fact that on July 27, approximately 6 or 7 weeks after the catastrophe, the District Nursing Association of Worcester still was following about 600 patients for septic wounds. There is very little doubt but that there was a higher incidence of sepsis than would have been obtained if these casualties had been handled by debridement and delayed closure.

EMOTIONAL REACTIONS

"The injured were apathetic, automatic in responses. Even the children who were injured are said to have been completely quiet—no laughter, no play, nothing. The people who were frantically looking for relatives were extremely disturbed, and some of them had to be handled as hysterical patients on the night of the disaster and during the next several days.

"About 100 children from a damaged low income housing area were separated from their parents and sent to nearby summer camps. Within a day or two, the experienced summer-camp operators were in serious trouble. The children were having nightmares, and they were having enuresis. When darkness fell, they ran around screaming. Whenever any kind of cloud formed in the sky, they screamed, "Here is the icecream-cone cloud coming back again. "

"On the other hand, in another damaged housing project of a somewhat better class financially, families were taken in by neighbors in parts of the project which were not destroyed. An experimental project of discussion and controlled play was conducted so that mothers and children were together for at least an hour or two of this play time. They talked it out, really. Over the course of about a month, the tenor of the conversations changed from preoccupation with the tornado back to consideration of more normal topics. There were practically no unusual psychiatric disturbances in this group.

"A doctor from the Worcester State Hospital happened to live in one of the disaster areas, and his reaction was interesting because he was able to think about his own reactions in an objective way. He said, "I went in that area, and I did things that I cannot understand. " Seeing a child bleeding from an arm wound, he picked up an electric cord to which was attached an iron and put that on as a tourniquet, leaving the iron still attached. The child went along swinging the iron from the end of the tourniquet.

"The medical administrator of one hospital said, "One of the things that I don't understand is that I never thought of evacuating the hospital. We didn't evacuate a single patient from our hospital until the next morning,

when we suddenly realized that we were going to be
benefited by getting rid of the patients already in the
hospital. "

CONCLUSIONS

"This was believed to be a fairly typical response
in a city of 200,000 to a disaster of this magnitude.
Worcester did no worse or no better than would another
area of our country. This must be taken into account in
planning for the future. Although a large-scale military
disaster might produce a general exodus of panic-
stricken populace, it seems apparent that planning can
rely on the wholehearted and encouraging individual response of persons remaining in or around the disaster
area. This response is expressed in two ways: it is a
mental attitude, such that the individual is willing to
subordinate his own interest to those of other individuals
and to those of the group at large, at least initially; and
it is an active physical participation in helping others.
This volunteer response is spontaneous and completely
undisciplined. In future planning, it must be assumed
that this response is to be controlled and channeled in
proper directions. If proper guidance is provided in the
immediate response, the public can be counted upon to
be cooperative and favorable.
"Events of the Worcester County tornado demonstrate a striking lack of central organization and planning, and a lack of responsible central authority with
power to implement actions agreed to be in the best in-
terests of the entire area involved. This lack of organization and planning is evident in many ways. It is evident in the lack of communication between the disaster
zone and contiguous areas, between the hospitals, and
between the hospitals and other agencies. Telephone
communication proved to be inadequate. The police
cruiser cars and other public vehicles equipped with
two-way radio entered the tornado zone early. They are
a potential source of adequate communication between
any future disaster area and its surrounding regions.
Cruiser cars or mobile radio units stationed near a
hospital in several instances were the only means of
communication. In future disasters, such units could
serve a similar function, assuming always that radio
circuits have been established in advance.
"Lack of central organization was evident in the

uncontrolled evacuation of casualties from the stricken areas, and in inadequate first aid rendered by the volunteer evacuation personnel. These defects existed partly because no arrangements had been made for providing adequate first aid in the event of disaster and partly because of the spontaneous mass reaction which brought so many lay volunteers to the disaster zone. Concern for the injured moved the lay rescuers to take hasty action. No attempt was made to establish a system of triage. Doctors who went into the area were without adequate equipment, and except in the places where police cruiser cars were working with first aid equipment and doctors, which did happen in Shrewsbury in several instances, no effective first aid was available in the disaster area until most of the injured had been removed.

"Lack of organization and lack of control over transportation were evident. The city manager had sent one of the department heads home at 2 p. m. because he was ill. About 4 p. m. just before the tornado hit, a big windstorm felled some trees near his property. He called the city manager and asked to have the trees removed. The head of the Department of Public Works had finished dinner at 4 p. m. (why, I have no idea) and decided to go in his own vehicle which is equipped with a three-way radio connecting it with all other vehicles of the public works department—bulldozers and what-not. He arrived within 3 minutes after the tornado had gone through. He was in an ideal situation; he immediately called the bulldozers. They all arrived quite early in the game and were able to get in before the tremendous traffic jams occurred. That would probably not happen again in several disasters.

"In most of the other areas, the first vehicles to arrive (other than the caterpillars and the trucks, and the people with the chain saws, all of whom arrived very quickly) were the police cruiser cars. In Holden, it was the state police; in Worcester and Shrewsbury, it was the city police. These are the potential sources of control. If evacuation is to be controlled it must be controlled by people who will be on duty 24 hours a day, who would be expected to be on hand at the time, who have communications available, and who have authority. The policeman not only has the recognized authority, but he has a uniform to back it up. If they had been given instructions from some better organized central source and had sealed off the area and told people not to remove casualties, there would have been adequate medical personnel help in the area fairly soon; and, if supplies arrived in some way, this would be a fairly good way of handling a future disaster. Our thought is that this is not a gloomy outlook. With planning, something can be done about it.

"There was a lack of coordination between the agencies involved in the various phases of disaster management. Civil Defense plans had been designed for action in the event of enemy air attack. There was some indecision among Civil Defense personnel as to whether or not the organization was to function in this nonmilitary disaster. The American Red Cross could not be mobilized as an effective force for emergency medical care in the immediate crisis; but when the officers of the national organization appeared and began to function, the American Red Cross served as a highly effective welfare agency. This occurred about 48 hours after the tornado. Before each of the agencies discovered for itself the role it should play during and subsequent to the disaster, there was considerable argument and some display of emotion.

"The personality and ability of the heads of the agencies which are to have responsibility for disaster management are of major importance to the success of the effort. If the authority of a central agency is not made evident, its directives might be ignored in the time of stress. If the organizational ability of its head is not unusually high, confusion will exist and no plan can be executed in orderly fashion. In Worcester and in several surrounding towns, the heads of certain key agencies normally were in posts subservient to those of officials whom they were expected to command in times of crisis. This arrangement inevitably contributed to the lack of central control over the various organizations.

"It seems apparent that the hospital administrative and medical staff personnel were unprepared for disaster. Lack of preparedness and lack of well organized disaster plans was [sic] evident by the lack of proper utilization, in many instances, of inexperienced and inadequate personnel. It was evident in the lack of adequate control over the incoming patients at the portals of entry into the hospitals and in the failure to exclude interfering persons who entered the receiving areas. It

was evident in the lack of satisfactory triage and identification of casualties as they entered the hospitals. It
was evident in the failure to keep adequate records of
the treatment given the injured and in the fact that not
even one hospital developed an adequate tagging system.
Finally, in certain hospitals, it was evident in the lack
of planning for emergency needs and for standby equipment to function in the event of failure of outside sources
of supply.

"Medical decisions made by the medical staffs were
influenced by mental attitudes induced by disaster conditions. Notable exceptions to this general statement
are the carefully planned management of the severely
injured neurosurgical patients by the two neurosurgeons
previously cited, and the careful handling of serious
soft-tissue injuries by several experienced surgeons.
The most striking example of the influence of emotion
upon the thinking of medical personnel was the decision
of most of the physicians to treat major and minor lacerations by debridement and primary closure, even under these disaster conditions. There is little doubt that
the incidence of sepsis in the wounds so managed was
greater than it would have been if they had been handled
by debridement and delayed suture. It is worth noting
that the incidence of invasive sepsis, particularly of
Clostridial myositis, was encouragingly low. This low
incidence is probably related to the universal use of antibiotics. There was no tetanus because everyone received some type of tetanus prophylaxis.

"Amounts of whole blood and plasma used during
the early treatment of the injured seem surprisingly
small when the severe nature of many of the injuries is
considered. It would be difficult to prove that any patients suffered or died unnecessarily because of inadequate blood replacement, but it is likely that a more
liberal use of whole blood might have been indicated.

"There is an attitude among doctors and administrators in civilian hospitals which opposes the suggestion that assignment of patients should be made by any
central authority which might be in a position to consider the general medical needs of the entire area involved in the disaster and to render medical decisions
based upon its evaluation of the needs. This over confidence [sic] in the independence of one's own hospital
varies in its expression from extreme belligerence to a
guarded willingness to consider the recommendations of

central authority. It was present among most of the
physicians and administrators encountered in this survey, and it must be reckoned as an attitude of mind
which will need consideration in future planning.

"One final thing, this type of study does not provide
the answers; it merely raises questions which must be
answered. It is recognized that a disaster of catastrophic
proportions might cause failure of any plan based upon
the active voluntary cooperation of nonmilitary agencies.
It might then be necessary to declare martial law and to
exercise military control over some or all civilian hospitals and disaster relief agencies. (It was not done
here. The National Guard was activated, but only to protect property.) However, even in such extreme circumstances, civilian agencies would have to assume responsibility for medical care and for relief activities
during the first few hours after the impact of disaster.
Even after military control began, they would still be
helpful and would be expected to function as normally as
possible.

"The efforts which may be made in any part of our
country to prepare for the medical care of disaster casualties will not be wasted even if disasters are never
encountered. It is hoped that the lessons to be learned
and the experience gained in the Worcester County tornado of 1953 may aid these efforts."

PRINCIPLES OF DISASTER MANAGEMENT

1. Prevent the occurrence of disaster.
2. Minimize the number of casualties.
3. Prevent further casualties.
4. Rescue.
5. Provide first aid.
6. Evacuate the injured.
7. Provide definitive medical care.
8. Facilitate reconstruction-recovery.

While most of these principles are self-evident, we think that
some specific illustrations may be helpful to the reader. To
minimize the number of casualties, for example, evacuation of
populated areas in advance of a hurricane has become standard
practice. Preventing further casualties can involve control of
observers, e.g., in the Texas City disaster of 1947, most of
the 561 deaths occurred among the curious sightseers who came
to the dock to watch. Further casualties can also be prevented

as they were in Worcester, when the first firemen arrived on
the scene within a few minutes after the tornado struck. They
saw the injured; they also saw piles of flammable lumber from
destroyed homes and at least six fires starting. The firemen
did not rush to give first aid to the victims, instead they put
the fires out and kept them out. This action probably prevented
a conflagration which would have killed many more people than
the tornado did.

BASIC AREAS OF DISASTER PLANNING

ORGANIZATION

Planning and organization are essential if chaos is to be kept to
a minimum. Medical considerations constitute an important aspect of the problem; however, medical planning and activities
can function only in concert with all other phases of emergency
operations. Health planners tend to forget that they are not
skilled in most phases of emergency operations.

Table 1-1 is a prototype table for organization of disaster
medical services; this one was developed by the state of Texas.
The state of Texas is subdivided into 17 disaster relief districts or subdistricts which correspond to the districts of the
State Department of Public Safety. This subdivision was utilized
since it provided the best communications between areas of the
state, and communication is the keystone to disaster management. Each of the 17 districts has an organizational structure
similar to that at the state level.

The provisions of medical care for a metropolitan area will
likely cross arbitrary district lines, hence a plan designated as
the Zone Support Concept was developed for the provision of
health services following a disaster which exceeded the medical
resources within a metropolitan area. An example of such a
zone support plan is illustrated in Figure 1-1.

Each of the surrounding communities, which has a medical
capability consisting of either personnel and/or resources, will
develop plans to provide support for the metropolitan area and
to integrate these plans with more distant medical resources.
Concurrently, the metropolitan area will develop plans to provide support for a surrounding community should a disaster,
which exceeds its indigenous resources, occur there.

LEADERSHIP

In any attempt to bring order and efficiency out of disaster,
sound leadership is necessary.

Table 1-1.   Organization of Disaster Medical Services

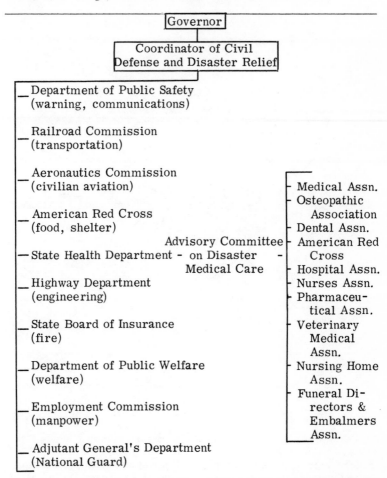

Community Leadership

It should be emphasized again that medical problems represent
only one aspect of disaster management. The higher levels of
leadership in a disaster should ideally be held by persons who
already have authority recognized under existing law, e.g., the
mayor, sheriff, police chief, fire chief, and National Guard
commander. Activation of a community's disaster plan should
be the responsibility of such higher levels of leadership.

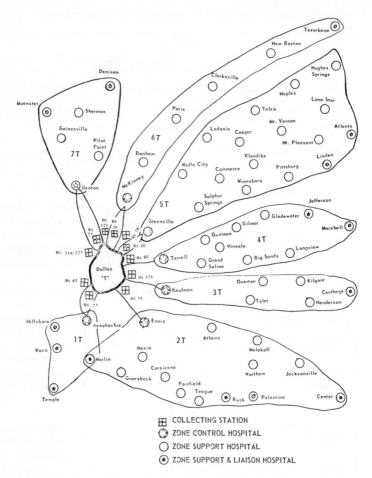

COLLECTING STATION
ZONE CONTROL HOSPITAL
ZONE SUPPORT HOSPITAL
ZONE SUPPORT & LIAISON HOSPITAL

Figure 1-1. Zone support plan. (Reproduced with permission from Committee on Emergency Medical Services, Dallas Medical Journal 54:587-593, 1968).

Medical Leadership

The establishment of health-medical leadership requires greater planning and poses more problems than are encountered in many other areas. Since most of the medical resources in a community are independent and privately based, e. g. , physicians, nurses, hospitals, and medical supply and distribution activities, an established organizational structure and chain-of-command does not exist.

Selection of designated medical leaders should include consideration of a number of attributes including the following:

1. Professional respect and recognition both by medical colleagues and by the higher levels of leadership.
2. An interest in disaster planning and a willingness to commit time and energy to planning, coordination, and training.
3. An understanding of the principles of organization.
4. The ability to delegate authority.
5. The ability to communicate clearly, effectively, and speedily.
6. Prior military experience (may provide a useful background).

In planning and selection of medical leaders, an order of succession, with predesignated alternates, should be established.

Leadership should be open-minded. The most qualified person either on the scene or in a hospital takes charge initially. In the hospital, this may be the senior resident or senior staff physician in the hospital at the time of the disaster. As more qualified or predesignated leaders reach the scene, a turnover of leadership is required.

Leaders should be provided with readily recognizable leadership symbols, such as an armband, a hard hat with name/title, etc. An excellent example of a leadership symbol is a nurse's white cap.

Emergent Leaders

Individuals who are predesignated and trained for leadership roles are far more likely to function effectively in a disaster. However, some individuals may not. In most disaster situations, if organized leadership is lacking or ineffective, leaders will emerge.

Staff Organization

Within a community and within a hospital, a staffing plan must be developed. The organization should include at least the elements shown in Table 1-2.

The Medical Disaster Director, Chief of Professional Services, and Executive Officer should be located in an area which will function as the command center. Clerical support is essential. These individuals should not be personally involved in

Table 1-2.   Staff Organization

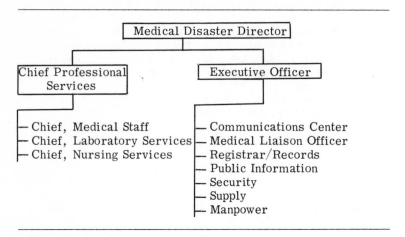

hands on patient care.   The functions of the other staff positions
are self-evident except perhaps for the Medical Liaison Officer
(MLO). MLO duties include keeping in communivation with the
disaster scene and with other hospitals, and keeping abreast of
medical resources in his own hospital as well as in others.

TRAFFIC CONTROL

Convergence, which is the movement of persons into the impact
area from the periphery, is one of the major obstacles to efficient first aid, rescue, and evacuation operations. The following
situation is an example of convergence: At 4:30 p. m. , May 11,
1953, a tornado struck the business district of Waco, Texas,
killing 114 people and injuring over 600 more. By 5:00 p. m.
nearly 10,000 people were standing at one large intersection
for no constructive reason.
      Convergers have been classified into five major groups: (1)
returnees, (2) the anxious, (3) helpers, (4) the curious, and (5)
the exploiters. In the past, the major problem has been serious
underestimation of the extent of convergence. A major requirement for traffic control is speed in implementation since within
10 minutes roads to the impact area may be clogged.

Medical Facilities

To a lesser extent, hospitals experience the same convergence
behavior, primarily the anxious, the helpers and the news
media. Coordination between the hospitals and police should

establish road blocks at one to two blocks distant from hospital access roads to assure ingress and egress of ambulances and vehicles carrying casualties and authorized medical personnel. Traffic flow patterns should assure that patients are unloaded in a manner which does not require backing in or out or even turning around. A one-way pass-through traffic pattern should be used, employing the usual access since habit will bring casualties in that way.

Security should be established at all entrances to the hospital, with patients being admitted through one, personnel through one other. Internal security should assure that the families of casualties are not allowed free access to hospital areas. Families should be guided into a large waiting area. Also, internal security should assure that all hospital personnel not actually working in an area be sent to a manpower holding area. Hospital personnel tend to converge to the emergency room or triage area just as lay people converge.

Identification

The establishment of traffic control measures requires that key medical personnel be issued an emergency assignment which contains positive identification (a photograph). This card must be recognized by the police. When considering key personnel, do not overlook the need for clerks to tag patients and orderlies to move patients. Because of turnover in personnel, cards need to be updated regularly.

COMMUNICATIONS

In virtually all disasters, lack of communication, hence lack of coordination, has stood out as one of the problems. There is lack of communication from the impact area to hospitals, between hospitals, and within hospitals. Most hospitals do not have a dedicated hospital radio frequency. Many of those which have radio communications do not have equipment in the police, fire department, or Civil Defense frequencies. In planning for a metropolitan area, one hospital should be identified as the communications base hospital. This hospital should have equipment which will enable voice communication with police, fire, ambulance, and Civil Defense services. The base hospital should be tied to all other hospitals with a dedicated interhospital radio network. The medical liason officer should report to the communications center at the base hospital to facilitate coordination of patient flow.

Notification

An important aspect of communications is notification of key
hospital personnel. A call roster should be maintained at the
hospital switchboard. Such a roster should include a limited
number of key personnel and alternates if the primary individuals cannot be reached. Notification of other personnel, usually necessary only during nights or weekends, should depend
upon calls being made by personnel from their homes, since
hospital exchanges will be overloaded. When notified, individuals should know where to report. In the preparation of staff
rosters, coordination between hospitals is essential since many
senior physicians are on the staff of several hospitals. Hospital
A has to know that Hospital B plans to use Dr. Smith as triage
officer and not count on him to head a surgical team in Hospital
A.

Telephone Communication

In most disasters, the flood of incoming calls has jammed all
switchboards so that outgoing calls become impossible. Every
hospital should have at least one unlisted telephone, preferable
in the office of the administrator, which is independent of its
switchboard. This number should be known to higher authorities
and to other hospital administrators. Another alternative is to
use pay phones. Most hospitals have pay telephones throughout
the building. These do not go through the switchboard, hence
they usually provide multiple potential lines. Planning should
include (1) identification of such phones, (2) assignment of hospital personnel to these phones to assure that they are used for
essential communication, (3) assignment of specific phones for
special functions, e. g. , to central supply, (4) stockpiling of
coins, dimes, nickels, or quarters in bags in the business office which can be issued for use by assignees.

Public Information Office

The prompt activation of a public information office is essential.
Information regarding casualties must be transmitted promptly
from triage and other areas to this office. This office should
also be responsible for the prompt transmission of specific information to local authorities, usually the American Red Cross.
Anxious relatives and friends who live in other areas will often
call the American Red Cross.

RESCUE AND FIRST AID

In the area of rescue operations, the importance of preventing further casualties cannot be overemphasized.

EVACUATION

Planning for evacuation usually involves considerations of transportation of casualties from the disaster area to medical care facilities.

Evacuation of Patients from Hospitals

With larger disasters, an important prerequisite to the avail- ability of hospital beds is a plan to discharge or relocate pa- tients who can safely be moved. When a disaster is declared to exist (i. e. , key personnel are notified), an individual(s) should have been predesignated as responsible for assessing all pa- tients to determine who can be moved and whether they are am- bulatory or litter bound. Assessment should include patients' name, unit number, diagnosis, physician, ward, and room num- ber. The individual should be in the hospital and not have to be called in; therefore he or she may be a senior house staff physician or a nursing supervisor. Such information should be transmitted to the command center, but it is of little value to the center unless plans have been formulated as to what to do with these patients; they cannot just be sent home and you do not want to increase traffic by calling family or taxi cabs. An area should be identified in which such patients can be housed under nursing supervision for some hours. Such an area may be in the clinic or in an adjacent teaching or professional building. It is essential to control such transfers and to have records of who was transferred to what location. Without these records, pa- tients may be lost for days.

HOSPITAL CAPABILITIES AND PLANNING

Experience in past disasters has shown that the average hospi- tal is seldom able to handle the load of emergency cases follow- ing a moderate disaster. For example, in 1955 a bridge col- lapsed in a town of 7000; about 30 workmen were injured. Even with the evacuation of the more seriously injured to a large city 200 miles away, and the importation of surgical teams, the last patient was not operated on for 72 hrs. The reasons for this difficulty include confusion, lack of planning, and lack of emergency training. Based upon military experience, a

surgical team with a well-trained surgeon and trained assistants
should be able to perform seven lifesaving operations on severely wounded persons in a 12-hr day. Thus, a 200 bed hospital
with eight operating rooms, theoretically should be able to care
for 56 seriously injured disaster casualties within a 12-hr time
span. Unless there is considerable preplanning, this does not,
however, mean that this hospital can handle 150 casualties in
36 hrs. Instruments and supplies are likely to be limiting factors. For planning purposes, the ability of an average civilian
hospital to provide emergency surgical care to seriously injured casualties in a 12-hr period is:

the number of operating rooms x 7 x 1/4.

This hospital will more likely be able to handle 24 serious casualties in 12 hr or 42 within 36 hr. The preplanning will have to
include the rescheduling of operative teams. The same eight
teams cannot function for 36 hrs. If it is possible to identify
16 teams, the second shift of 8 teams should be held in reserve
to provide relief 12 hrs later, at which time the original group
rests and are then themselves placed in a reserve status.

Disaster Care Areas

Usual space allocations for various hospital functions will be
inadequate; hence alternative spaces have to be identified and
known to all hospital personnel. Corridors should not be used
as care areas.

    1. Triage Area. This should not be the usual emergency
room but rather a large area near a readily accessible entrance
(without stairs) which is or can be well lighted. The triage offi-
cer(s) has to be able to survey a large number of casualties
quickly while going from individual to individual. This area may
be a clinic waiting area or an auditorium.
    2. Shock Treatment Area. This should be close to triage
and if possible to the blood bank.
    3. Minor Surgery Area. The usual emergency room may
function in this capacity.
    4. Minor Medicine Area. This area should be away from
the triage area.
    5. Mortuary Area.

Electrical Power

Electrical outages occur in many disasters. Every hospital
should have emergency generators which will provide the power

necessary to light and run equipment in critical areas. Outlets
on emergency power should be readily identifiable; the use of
red face plates is one effective method.

Elevators

Hospital employees should be assigned to run any automatic
elevators during such times.

Patient Accession Movement

Planning must include preparation and stockpiling of patient
identification tags and treatment records. These must be at-
tachable to the patient. Standard hospital records are inadequate
under disaster circumstances. Lists must be made of all patients admitted to an area and when a patient is moved to another area, this move must be noted on the list. For example,
if a patient is moved from triage to shock treatment, the records
in triage should show this move and should also include the time.
If the patient is then sent to x-ray, this should also be recorded
with the time to be certain that patients are not lost.

Patient Care

Evaluation and care should be provided by teams, appropriate
to personnel available and to types of casualties being seen.
Records should be completed by clerical personnel rather than
by physicians and nurses.

Supplies

Depending upon the type of disaster, anticipated number and
types of casualties, the chief of central supply, director of the
blood bank, etc. , should be requested to provide a rapid inven-
tory of required items which are apt to be in limited supply.
The transition from reusable equipment to disposable equipment compounds the problems since most hospitals maintain
relatively little stock. In many areas, even distributors are
dependent upon almost daily deliveries to maintain stocks.
There are many items to be considered; therefore, lists should
be prepared in advance by walking various types of casualties
through the required procedures. How much tetanus toxoid is
stocked or available?

TRAINING AND TESTING

The best of disaster planning will be for naught if the plans are
not tested periodically by involving all participating individuals.

Such exercises provide training and the opportunity to identify and correct deficiencies.   Field Marshall Foch succinctly summarized disaster planning by stating, "No study is possible on the battlefield; one does there simply what one can in order to apply what one knows.   Therefore, in order to do evan a little, one already has to know a great deal and know it well."

SUGGESTED READING

American Hospital Association. Principles of Disaster Planning for Hospitals, G-87-56. Chicago, 1963.

American Hospital Association. Readings in Disaster Planning for Hospitals, G-88-56. Chicago, 1956.

American National Red Cross. Disaster Manual. ARC 209, Washington, D. C. , 1955.

Fritz, C E, and Mathewson, J H: Convergence Behavior in Disasters. National Academy of Sciences. National Research Council. Publication No. 476. Washington, D. C. , 1957.

Garb, S, and Eng, E: Disaster Handbook. New York, Springer Publishing Co. , 1964.

Public Health Service. Hospital Planning for National Disaster. Publication No. 1071-G-1. Washington, D. C. , U. S. Government Printing Office, 1968.

Raker, J W, Wallace, A F C, and Rayner, J F: Emergency Medical Care in Disaster. A Summary of Recorded Experience. National Academy of Sciences, National Research Council. Publication No. 457. Washington, D. C. , 1956.

Chapter 2

EMERGENCY MEDICAL SERVICES RESPONSE TO
DISASTER PLANNING
Joseph F. Waeckerle, M.D.

Disasters are occurring at an increasing rate in the United
States. In order for the medical community to successfully
deal with them, the special organization and mobilization of a
rescue system, i.e., disaster planning, is required.
    The goal of disaster planning is to "insure efficient utiliza-
tion of local health resources so that they will not be overwhelmed during the initial disaster relief period."[1] Although
the Joint Commission on Accreditation requires that each hospital seeking accreditation in the United States have a disaster
plan that is tested at least twice yearly, there are no requirements for community medical disaster plans to meet the goals
stated by the United States Public Health Service.

MODELS OF DISASTER RESPONSE

There are two models of disaster response; the "Civil Defense
Model" and the "Emergency Medical Services Model."[2] Disaster planning may be based upon either one of the two models
which may exist simultaneously or separately in a community.
If the plans coexist, duplication of services may lead to confusion as to which plan should be primary at the time of a disaster
causing manpower shortages and wasted medical resources.
    The Civil Defense Model of disaster response is derived
from the experience of military and civil defense planners. The
model is based upon the need to mobilize a large number of
volunteers to the site of a disaster to provide first aid. The
organization and direction of these volunteers is provided by the
local civil defense office. This model calls for the use of
"field medical units" composed of volunteers recruited from the
community under the direction of a civil defense-designated

Contents of this chapter first appeared in: Orr SM and Waeckerle
JF: Disaster Planning. Curr Topics III Emerg Med, Med Coll
of PA, 2(16), 1983.

medical officer. Hospitals, under the civil defense model, are
left to mobilize their own staffs and prepare to receive casualties autonomously. The local civil defense organization serves
to coordinate the efforts of the field medical "team" and the
hospital "team."

The Civil Defense Plan is based upon a time frame of days
for disaster response activation. It presumes a predisaster
alert to allow for the notification and recruitment of volunteers,
mobilization of medical supplies, and the establishment of reliable communications. The military-civil defense approach
to disaster management relies upon a "scoop-and-run" philosophy which allows only very limited first aid skills to be applied
at the scene. It places the swift delivery of victims to a hospital
as the number one priority. Under the Civil Defense Model of
disaster management, triage, field stabilization, and advanced
life support are not emphasized.

The Emergency Medical Services Model of disaster management places a greater burden on the hospital in the management
of medical resources, both internally and at the scene. Overall
supervision for the Emergency Medical Services Model of operations is provided by the "base hospital." This model of disaster management relies upon the "escalation of everyday response" of the already functioning local emergency medical services system to handle disaster casualties.[3] By doing so, this
model utilizes the preexisting organization, communications,
and command structure of the local emergency medical services
system with only slight modifications in accordance with the
nature of the disaster. Triage, field stabilization, and advanced
life support take precedence over the rapid transport of disaster
victims. Figures one and two outline the basic components of
each system of disaster management.

This is the more generally accepted plan in the United States
due to the development of cummunity emergency medical services systems. The following disucssion will be based on the
Emergency Medical Services Model.

THE DISASTER PLAN

The disaster plan should be basic, simple, and well rehearsed,
incorporating all of the emergency medical system including the
prehospital phase, the interhospital communication system, the
intrahospital teams, and the community. The public health
director, or whoever in the community has the authority to institute and enforce such a plan, should involve the police, fire,
civil defense and community authorities in the design and implementation of the plan. The plan must identify leaders ensuring
that they are intelligent, well trained, highly respected and con-

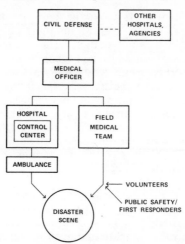

Figure 2-1. Organizational relationships—Civil defense model
of disaster response. (Modified from Melton JR, Riner RM:
Revising the rural hospital disaster plan: A role for the EMS
system in managing the multiple casualty incident. Ann Emerg
Med 10:39-44, 1981).

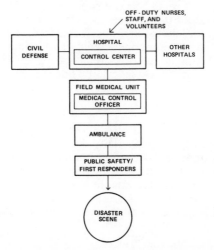

Figure 2-2. Organizational relationships—EMS model of response to the mass casualty incident. (Modified from Melton JR,
Riner RM: Revising the rural hospital disaster plan: A role for
the EMS system in managing the multiple casualty incident. Ann
Emerg Med 10:39-44, 1981.)

fident decision makers. It should be kept simple, so that the personal initiative of such leaders and their ability to adapt to the various situations is not stifled. The disaster plan delineates the divisions of authority and labor which may occur naturally, but preferably occur due to it. This will allow specialists to perform in their specific area, such as: paramedics in charge of the rescue triage; physicians in charge of the casualty clearing station and disposition of patients; fire department and structural engineers in control of the rescue situation; and police in control of the crowds, etc.

CENTRAL COMMUNICATIONS

An adequate communication system is essential during a disaster. It must be centrally located, easily accessible to all personnel, and reliable/dependable. The system can utilize existing "hardlines" as well as radio signals and even messengers to establish communications with the rescue site; the ambulances; the various hospitals; and, if at all possible, the police, fire, civil defense, and other accessory personnel. There must be contact with the ambulances so that their location and disposition is known at all times. In some instances, the on-site communications system, if directed by the public health director or other person in charge of the rescue operation, may function as a command post and dispatch ambulances from the disaster site to the hospitals. In other instances, the command post may be a predesignated base hospital communicating with the disaster site and coordinating the prehospital and hospital systems.

SUPPLIES

The disaster plan must anticipate needed supplies for any situation and, equally as important, devise a scheme whereby they are organized and delivered in an appropriate fashion. One suggestion is to deliver all supplies to the casualty clearing station and bring them forward to the rescue triage site as needed. Initially, this may require the stripping of ambulances and then restocking at the hopsital upon delivery of patients.

PERSONNEL

All personnel involved in a disaster situation must be knowledgeable regarding the disaster plan, well trained to perform and carry out their duties during the implementation of the plan, and always aware of the designated authorities at the site. They must be readily identifiable to all others involved, either by uniform or other identification. Also, all personnel involved

in the disaster must be informed of any hazardous situations
they might encounter during the disaster. The disaster personnel should be divided into teams. These teams have specific
assigned duties, and practice and train together to carry out
such duties. They might also be crosstrained with another
team in case they are needed.

INITIAL RESPONDER TEAM

The initial responders at the site usually are the fire department, police, and lay people who have stayed to volunteer their
services. Paramedics will soon arrive at the scene. It is the
duty of the paramedics, in this initial period, to perform an
immediate survey and accurately assess the situation, the environment in which it has occurred, the number of patients and
their accessibility, and anticipated needs. They then must
concisely advise the central dispatch of their assessment and
their recommendations. The fire department's responsibility
is to ascertain whether there is further danger, due to structural instability, electric, gas or other hazards, and to control
any fires which have occurred. The police that arrive at the
scene must control the crowds, secure perimeter, and ensure
the safety of all the other initial responders. The police must
also control the volunteers with regard to the private transportation of injured victims. It is essential that all patients be kept
in the system and dispatched to the appropriate medical treatment centers, rather than being taken to various hospitals by
private vehicles without guidance. The plan must protect patients by allowing proper evaluation and treatment at the scene.
Triaging must occur; overloading of nearest hospitals must
not occur!

RESCUE TRIAGE TEAMS

The rescue triage teams consist of paramedics, fire personnel,
volunteers, and possibly a physician who is team leader in certain situations. The numbers needed are proportional to the size
of the area and the number of victims. Their duty is to triage
each patient in accordance with preestablished guidelines. Once
each patient is triaged, basic stabilization and treatment occur
in a quick and efficient fashion. The patients are then evacuated
according to the priorities established by triage. If there are
appropriate numbers of rescuers on the rescue triage team, it
is best to have a paramedic, a fire person, and a volunteer assigned to each salvageable individual so they receive the utmost
in care. During the initial rescue triage work, especially with

many victims or trapped victims, the teams may need to make difficult decisions with regard to who should be treated and evacuated first and who should be left unattended. In these instances, an on-site medical director who is specifically trained to evaluate and organize the disaster rescue and triage would be most appropriate in making such decisions.

Some authors have recommended coding or tagging each triaged individual, then evacuating them according to their code prioritization. The inherent difficulty with this system is that it takes a certain amount of time to do this—time that rescue teams may not have. Still, in mass casualty situations, if the rescue personnel tag quickly and correctly, it will greatly help subsequent medical personnel.

CASUALTY CLEARING STATION TEAMS

The clearing station is the end point for all victims at the disaster site. It is established in a safe place as close to the disaster site as possible, hopefully with easy access to the site and to ambulances which carry patients to the hospitals via cleared traffic lanes. There is a Medical Director who should be the most highly trained and experienced physician available. There are also a number of other physicians, if needed, each working with a nurse, paramedic, fire person, and police or volunteer. These teams provide further triage treatment and stabilization prior to disposition to the appropriate hospital. The amount of treatment that the teams provide is related to the accessibility and availability of the various hospitals which will ultimately receive patients. In some instances, the casualty clearing station will need to perform heroic lifesaving measures and in other instances will provide only continued first aid prior to disposition to the hospital. The expected types of injuries the victims have suffered will determine how advanced the casualty clearing station supplies and personnel need be.

EMERGENCY DEPARTMENT TEAMS

Each hospital involved in a disaster plan must have preestablished teams in their emergency department to receive all victims. The expertise and specialization of these teams will, in part, be determined by the type of victims the hospital receives. The personnel will usually be divided into teams ready to take the patients directly to surgery, teams prepared to take the patients to the intensive care unit to provide further care, and teams prepared to treat in the emergency department. It must be pointed out that care to the regular patients in the hospital must not suffer at any time because of lack of personnel. It is also

obvious that the hospitals must be categorized in the rescue
plan so that the type of patient, severity of injuries, and patient
load each hospital is able to handle are known to the dispatch
personnel.

SECURITY TEAMS

Security teams are usually law enforcement personnel because
they are easily recognized, well structured, and impowered and
armed by law. The security forces must control crowds;
control looting; control and inform the press, media, and relatives; and, if present, control further terrorist activity. It is
essential that the victims and workers, both of whom are under
tremendous pressure in carrying out their responsibilities do not
have to work in a hazardous environment. Also, they must keep
the site accessible and traffic lanes open.
   The identification of victims and their belongings and the
notification of family and friends is a distasteful but essential
part of the rescue plan. The security teams should establish
a temporary morgue site at or near the casualty clearing station
or set up a separate transportation system to deliver the dead
to the city or county morgue.
   Certain other suggestions gleaned from previous disaster
response experiences must be made at this time with regard to
the "team approach." It is essential that there be a communication system, not only among the various teams, but between
team members. Such communication is required to insure coordination of efforts in an efficient manner. It is also highly
advisable to identify personnel by clothing, such as a vest or
coat, etc. In large rescue operations where a great deal of
confusion exists, badges and small items of identification make
it difficult to readily identify other personnel involved and their
functions. By using clothing—vests, jackets, or jumpsuits that
are coordinated by teams—the rapid identification of team members and their function is more easily done. Moveover, it is
essential that all personnel involved in the rescue operations be
protected at all times. This may require certain clothing or
may require the security forces to protect them. It also requires that the fire department insure that the environment in
which they work is safe, such as, no faulty electric lines, no
gas leaks, etc. The personnel involved in the rescue also need
food, water, and rest, which they will be reluctant to ask for due
to the situation. It is advisable that the authority figures at the
site enforce rest, food, and water breaks for the rescue personnel.

RECORD KEEPING

Record keeping during the disaster is difficult but should be as
accurate and complete as possible. The difficulty is to decide
when and where such record keeping should be done. One sug-s
gestion is to have brief records started at the casualty clearing
station and to further develop the records on all individuals
during their trip in the ambulance to the various hospitals.

POSTDISASTER ACTIONS

After the disaster has occurred, group critiques and after-action
reports should be taken from all teams. A supervisory committee should then carefully review such critiques and reports
so that all involved can have a positive learning experience from
the disaster. This would ensure that any mistakes made would
not occur in future disaster situations. Also, group sessions
with mental health personnel, not only for the victims but also
for the rescuers, is advisable. This could range from a de-
briefing session to intense therapy for some individuals. A
public relations team to interface with the press and other news
media might also be helpful after the disaster has occurred. Most
personnel who have worked in the disaster are physically, men-
tally, and emotionally drained, and might find it very difficult
to interface with the media for a period of time after the disaster.
    Overall, the speed of the response is not as crucial to the
effective operation as is the coordination of the response by
trained and experienced personnel.

CONCLUSION

A disaster is a sudden, serious, man-made or natural disruption to life, threatening or causing injuries to a number of
people, in excess of those which the system can normally handle.
Such a situation requires special organization and mobilization
of the emergency medical services rescue system. In any disaster, emergency medical personnel must provide the maximum
benifits to the greatest number of victims. This can be done
with a well defined and often rehearsed contingency plan. It is
too late to organize a response once a disaster occurs.
    Today and the future hold many promises but also many
problems. With technologic advancement comes technologic
accidents; with socioeconomic and political change comes
dissatisfaction, terrorism and war; with living comes natural
calamities.

It is our responsibility as health care providers and cival officials to be prepared at all times for any catastrophe. We must continually strive for this end.

REFERENCES

1. United States Department of Health, Education and Welfare Service: The role of medicine for emergency preparedness. Emerg Health Series 5, 1968.
2. Melton RT and Riner RM: Revising the rural hospital disaster plan: A role for the EMS system in managing the multiple casualty incident. Ann Emerg Med 10: 39-44, 1981.
3. Holloway RD, Steliga JF and Ryan RT: The EMS system and disaster planning: Some observations. JACEP 7:60-61, 1978,

Chapter 3

ORGANIZATION OF MILITARY MEDICAL UNITS
Dennis Duggan, B. A.

I. INTRODUCTION

Few physicians ever imagine they will be called on to function in a combat environment. If this situation should occur, however, they would quickly discover that combat is the most confusing and chaotic endeavor known to man. Most natural disasters are local in nature, and medical support is provided by teams and organizations which enter the area during periods of relative safety. Untouched and fixed facilities serve as their base of support. The practice of battlefield medicine requires medical personnel to share the risk and danger with their patients because they are both in war zones which cover large areas of land, sea, and air.

This chapter provides a brief overview of the systems established by the military to triage, treat, and evacuate casualties during an air/land battle. Many of the medical lessons learned in the Vietnam War are now essential concepts used in civilian Emergency Medicine Systems (EMS). These military concepts and systems have direct application during community disasters.

II. TREATMENT AND EVACUATION AT THE FRONT

On the battlefield, enemy activity and careless accidents produce numerous trauma victims who are treated at one, or possibly all, levels of care. Within minutes after being injured, a service man receives first aid from his buddies or a medic. Medic, corpsman, and aidman are terms used by the military services to describe an individual who is trained to provide medical care similar to the basic civilian emergency medical technician (EMT). This person accompanies the combat troops and carries limited medical equipment and supplies in a small pack. The medic quickly moves the casualty to an aid station manually, by litter, or by jeep ambulance. The aid station is a treatment site and collection point for vehicle or helicopter evacuation; it is usually within range of enemy rifle fire.

The casualty officially becomes a patient in the military medical system upon arrival at the aid station. If he has not had a field medical card attached to him prior to arrival, he is tagged here. The field medical card is a small card which is attached to the patient and identifies him, his injury, and the treatment rendered. It is the battlefield medical record.

Depending on service, the senior care provider at the aid station is a physician assistant (PA) or senior medic. Care is provided in the open, under a small tent, or in an armored truck vehicle. Human and material medical resources are extremely limited. Since this first medical treatment facility is very close to the front, it must remain highly mobile.

Before proceeding to the type of care provided at the aid station, we must discuss a principle governing patient disposition in combat. Combat leaders cannot afford to lose experienced personnel during a critical engagement. Therefore, patients are returned to duty as far forward as possible. On the battlefield, a surprising number of patients who would be hospitalized in peacetime are returned to duty. Even though this principle conflicts with the normal standards of care, military medical personnel learn that their own survival is dependent on the combat skills of their patients. From a management point of view, proper use of this principle diminishes the requirements for evacuation resources. The senior person at the aid station functions in a medical milieu where tactical considerations must influence medical decisions.

At the aid station, only essential emergency procedures are performed; these include airway management, hemorrhage control, IV fluid resuscitation, bandaging, and splinting. Drug administration is limited. Since physicians rarely function at this level, their roles are limited to the training and supervision of medics for these forward units.

When the decision is made to evacuate a patient from the aid station, another principle of battlefield medical operation is employed. The receiving medical facility sends transportation forward to pick up the patient. Only in unusual circumstances would there be an exception to this procedure. Depending on the tactical situation, nonmedical vehicles and aircraft (tanks, trucks, boats, trains, etc.) may be used for patient transport.

The rapid helicopter evacuation from the scene of action directly to a hospital, as practiced in the Vietnam War, was highly dependent on United States air superiority. This could be the exception in future conflicts. Peacetime use of helicopter evacuation is, of course, not limited by air combat, but helicopter operations are always limited by weather conditions, ground/air communication systems and availability of landing sites (see Chapter 8).

III. THE PHYSICIAN'S ROLE AT THE CLEARING STATION

Physicians at the remaining levels of battlefield medical operations have an assignment which is dependent on both their medical specialties and the needs of the service. The clearing station or its equivalent is the next level of care. It is established
a few kilometers behind the front lines, still within range of
enemy artillery fire. Clearing stations are staffed with five or
six Medical Corps officers, one or more Dental Corps officers,
a Medical Service Corps officer, and at least 50 medics and
medical technicians of various skills. A surgeon or internist
commands the unit with the majority of the patient management
being conducted by general medical officers (GMOs). A physician triage officer examines all patients on entry to this treatment facility and establishes priorities of treatment and evacuation. Emergency care is continued at this level where surgeons and nonsurgeons will perform basic surgical procedures
(e. g. , venous cutdowns, limited gunshot wound debridement,
chest tube insertion, cricothyroidotomy). GMOs must be prepared to stabilize patients for up to 12 hrs. To allow for rapid
movement, this level has limited holding capability. It lacks the
24-hr nursing care staff found at higher levels.
    The clearing station is usually a tent facility. All unit equip-
ment is portable and there are sufficient vehicles with this unit
to move the entire facility at one time. This unit has limited
laboratory, x-ray, and operating room capability. Water, ra-
tions and fuel are coordinated through a common supply system
and the physician medical unit commander competes with combat commanders for these vital resources. Medical resupply is
usually established within a dedicated system operated for and
by medical personnel. Provision of whole blood is dependent on
tactical and strategic considerations.

IV. FORWARD HOSPITALS

The next level of care is provided at semifixed facilities. At
this level the medical unit resembles a civilian hospital in organization and function. In fact, the word, hospital, appears in
the names of these units: Mobile Army Surgical Hospital, Combat Support Hospital, Evacuation Hospital, Field Hospital, Hospital Company, and Air Transportable Hospital. These organizations are located a few kilometers behind the clearing stations
and generally are out of range of enemy artillery. Usually,
these hospitals are also tent facilities, but they are not required to be completely mobile as are the clearing station.
Staffing may include up to 100 people, including physicians,

dentists, nurses, medics, medical technicians, and administrative personnel. After triage, the care provided includes resuscitation, initial wound surgery, and postoperative treatment. A forward field hospital usually maintains 200-400 beds.

V. MANAGEMENT OF EVACUATION RESOURCES

Evacuation policy establishes the maximum number of hospital days that a patient may be held at a specific level. The evacuation policy is based on several factors: planned combat operations, number of fixed and rotary wing evacuation aircraft, current number of beds in the war zone, projected replacement personnel, and the expected time to recovery and return to duty for each surgical procedure. Medical care providers and administrators balance patient needs against medical resources.

The coordination and control of patient movement through military medical treatment facilities is called medical regulating. The medical regulators identify the number, type, and location of patients awaiting evacuation as well as the beds available. Since transportation must be coordinated to ensure timely movement, the medical regulating personnel must continually move patients from the forward type hospital to more rearward facilities.

VI. REAR AREA FACILITIES

The next level of care, which is still located within range of enemy fighter/bombers, is the most complex. These units are staffed with medical and surgical specialists similar to community general hospitals; they are established in abandoned buildings, hospital barracks, hotels, warehouses, or schools. Definitive care and rehabilitation of patients are the major goals of these facilities. If evacuation is required from this level, it will be to a medical center in the United States for complex reconstructive surgery or other long-term treatment.

VII. SUMMARY

The battlefield medical treatment system is summarized schematically in Figure 3-1.

The practice of battlefield medicine requires the health care provider to provide the best possible care with a minimum of human and material resources. Success in time of crisis, whether in the military or civilian community, is dependent on several key factors:

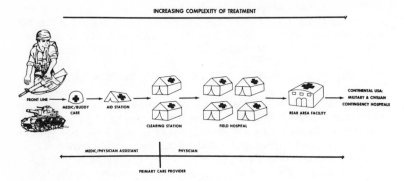

Figure 3-1. Battlefield medical treatment system showing the increasing complexity of treatment.

  Respect for authority
  Teamwork
  Priorly established, simple, workable plans and procedures
     providing for the maximum use of human and material re-
     sources
  Community-wide training which includes disaster exercises

SUGGESTED READING

American Academy of Orthopedic Surgeons. <u>Emergency Care and Transportation of the Sick and Injured</u>. 3rd Ed. Chicago, George Banta Co. , Inc. , 1981.

Erskine, J F, et al. : <u>Medical Operations in Combat</u>. Department of Military Medicine and History, Bethesda, Md. , Uniformed Services University of the Health Sciences, 1981.

Lam, David M: <u>Aeromedical Evacuation: A Handbook for Physicians.</u> Ft. Sam Houston, Texas, U. S. Army Health Services Command, 1979.

Neel, Spurgeon (Major General, USA): <u>Medical Support of the U. S. Army in Vietnam, 1965-1970</u>. Washington, D. C. , U. S. Government Printing Office, 1973.

United States Department of Defense: <u>Emergency War Surgery— NATO Handbook.</u> 1st Revision. Washington, D. C. , Government Printing Office, 1975.

Chapter 4

TRIAGE
Frederick M. Burkle, Jr. , M.D. , M.P.H.

I. TRIAGE

Triage is a French word meaning to pick out or sort. It was first introduced into the English language during World War I as a military process of classifying casualties. The modern definition has two major components: (1) sorting of victims according to severity of injury or illness, and (2) assigning priorities of treatment.

The civilian definition of triage over the years has become somewhat clouded. Triage in a modified form is carried out daily and automatically in physicians' offices, clinics, and emergency rooms, primarily by nursing personnel. An office physician may be interrupted from a scheduled consulting appointment to evaluate briefly and treat an unexpected asthmatic patient. Patient rescheduling or delays are common daily occurrences. Emphasis, however, is on efficient and excellent care to ALL patients.

A triage situation is defined as a temporary prioritizing of critical care. For example, one emergency medicine physician who has a limited nursing staff in a rural hospital and is faced with two critically injured patients will be in a triage situation until on call assistance arrives. Triage situations are often anticipated and planned for in hospitals and emergency care systems. The triage situation can be nullified immediately with the addition of as few as one or two health care professionals to the scene.

This chapter addresses mass civilian or military disasters where triage is performed under circumstances of stress when the number of patients exceeds the normal capabilities and resources for a prolonged period of time.

Triage is the first of three principles of mass casualty care:

1. Triage
2. Evacuation (see Chapter 8)
3. Standard procedures (see Chapter 6, and addendum this chapter)

II. BASIC REQUIREMENTS FOR ANY TRIAGE

A. Preplanning
B. Full use of all available personnel
C. Forward movement with continuing triage at each medical echelon
D. Simplicity
E. Full acceptance by all personnel of the following principles of triage:[1]
   1. Salvage of life takes precedence over salvage of limb
   2. Principal threats to life are asphyxia, hemorrhage, and shock leading to cardiac arrest
F. Designation of qualified triage officer(s) whose orders are to be followed by all other personnel

III. TRIAGE OFFICERS

On-site triage of mass casualties, both civilian and military requires a clearly designated area of command (command post) and commander (triage officer).

In field civilian disasters attended by ambulance crews, the senior paramedic or medical intensive care technician (MICT) from the first ambulance to arrive assumes command. The field triage officer wears a reflective vest with the initials, TO, clearly visible, front and back. In military field situations, the senior medic or corpsman assumes this role.

Rarely do physicians or teams of physician and nurses need to be dispatched to the scene of a major disaster. In British experience, if a team is sent, the firemen and ambulance crews are often overawed by the presence of the hospital team, and may be inhibited from doing their work properly. In Belfast, which has 20 years of experience in civilian disasters, sending teams is a rarity. [2]

All community disaster plans should include a designated triage officer at the entry point to the hospital. The in-house emergency room physician assumes the triage officer role until relieved by the designated triage officer. Several alternate triage officers should receive training in anticipation of the possibility that the senior designated triage officer is unavailable.

The choice of triage officer is critical. Unfortunately, numerous disaster plans call for the senior surgeon to be triage officer-in-charge. At the time of the disaster, this surgeon may already be in surgery and unable to respond rapidly, or he/she may be compelled to accompany the first surgical case to the operating room. This could leave a critical void. Surgical experience is important in making proper clinical judgments.

However, a well-rounded emergency physician, general physician, or general surgeon, who would not be called upon to function in another role, could make an ideal triage officer.

In military disasters at the field hospital level, general medical officers (GMOs), trained in triage, initial trauma assessment, resuscitation, and communication, assume this role. Rear echelon hospital triage officers are senior experienced surgeons who are often assisted by an anesthesiologist and an orthopedic surgeon. [3]

Triage may be completed within 30 min or continue for several hours or days; this requires sophisticated, well-coordinated planning, and relief time for fatigued triage officers and their assistants.

In-hospital triage officers are usually chiefs of individual departments (e. g. , laboratory, radiology, surgery, and ICU). They screen requests and prevent interdepartment bottlenecks. They constantly communicate department status to the designated triage officer-in-charge.

Desirable characteristics of triage officer-in-charge are:

1. Surgically experienced
2. Easily recognized and respected by medical staff
3. Good judgment and leadership qualities
4. Unflappable under stress: ability to practice suppression and handle unpopular criticism
5. Decisive
6. Knowledgeable: familiar with resources, staff skills and limitations, equipment, and evacuation potential
7. Sense of humor (This important quality assists in maintaining leadership and staff relaxation at a time of considerable stress.)
8. Imaginative and creative: ability to make decisive and creative decisions under stress, especially when resources and equipment dwindle over a period of time (e. g. , using leg elevation with ACE wraps in lieu of expended MAST suits; hose showering rather than individual soaks for numerous heat casualties)
9. Availability: closeness to hospital. (All essential personnel should be available within 5-15 min of summons.)
10. Anticipate type of casualties: ability to plan from anticipated categories of patients (e. g. , aircraft disaster: multiple injuries and burns; hotel fire: smoke inhalation, burns, psychological stress; earthquake: crush injuries)

The full extent of the disaster may not be fully known for several hours. Triage officers must maintain control of a situation which is often unpredictable. Few cases are sorted improperly where trained triage officers exist. The parameters of patient flow, patient care, and rapid recognition of priorities require the continued attention of the triage officer.

IV. TRIAGE ASSESSMENT

With increased organization of emergency medical services (personnel, training, advanced equipment) and the application of these advancements to both civilian and military disasters, it is commonplace for rear echelon hospitals to be faced with a high number of severe, but temporarily stabilized, casualties. In prior wars or disasters, many of these patients would not have left the battlefield or disaster site alive.

In the Korean War it was suggested that the higher mortality associated with delayed, as compared with immediate, care was related mainly to five factors:[4]

1. Delay in correcting blood volume deficits
2. Delay in correcting mechanical defects
3. Increased morbidity associated with infection
4. Increased tissue destruction
5. Delay in closing secondary wounds

These findings were translated into military medic training and into current EMS programs nationwide. Emphasis in the field is placed on the following:[5]

1. Rapid correction of shock (the physician's main enemy)
2. Rapid institution of the principles of wound cleanliness
3. Rapid correction of mechanical defects
4. Application of first aid measures which reduce further tissue destruction

In addition, qualified data from recent disasters and military conflicts have assisted medical planners and triage officers in placing critical emphasis on the following:

1. Attention to saving limbs for possible reanastomosis
2. Triage to dialysis units in crush injuries
3. Continued intensive nursing care at all levels with controlled and orderly evacuation techniques at every echelon[3]

Triage officers must never lose sight of the critical ABC's of Advanced Cardiac Life Support (ACLS) and the necessary

application of initial trauma assessment guidelines recommended by the Advanced Trauma Life Support (ATLS) course of the
American College of Surgeons. [6,7]
　　Guidelines for triage assessment have become popularized
in numerous indexes of injury severity (IPCAR, Injury Severity
Score, ER Triage Model, Hospital Trauma Index, Triage Index,
Anatomic Index of Injury Severity). [8-14] Although valuable review and study guides, these systems have little practical application to the scene of mass disaster triage. There is no substitute for good judgment, sound experience, and attention to the
principles of triage.
　　Ongoing reevaluation and reassessment is inherently done
by a well-trained triage officer. Certain intuitive measurements
are automatically performed.

TRIAGE SENSITIVITY

How well the triage senses or detects the patients actually requiring care (e. g. , if casualties in the field or hospital are left
untreated for hours, this would reflect a weak triage sensitivity). [5,15,16]

TRIAGE SPECIFICITY

How well the triage avoids the inclusion of nonemergency cases
(e. g. , ability of the triage to prevent inclusion in the immediate
Care Area of those either lightly injured and in no need of care
and of those beyond help and/or resources). [5,15,16]
　　Additional quantified data will assist disaster planners in
prioritizing medical personnel and assist triage officers in em-
phasizing or deemphasizing priority of care options in various
diagnostic categories. Several standardized rates prove helpful
in this assessment:[3]

Rate of total mortality:	$\dfrac{\text{number of casualties who died}}{\text{total number of casualties}}$
Rate of killed:	$\dfrac{\substack{\text{number of casualties who} \\ \text{died in the field before being} \\ \text{seen by medical personnel}}}{\text{total number of casualties}}$
Rate of those who died of wounds:	$\dfrac{\substack{\text{number of casualties who died} \\ \text{after being attended by surgeon}}}{\substack{\text{total number of live, injured} \\ \text{soldiers}}}$

V. CIVILIAN OR COMMUNITY DISASTER: TRIAGE

A. TRIAGE SITES

A minimum of three triage sites exist in any civilian disaster situation[17] (Figure 4-1):

    Triage Site 1: Field (scene of disaster)
    Triage Site 2: Hospital or emergency room entry
    Triage Site 3: In-hospital triage
    1. Immediate care or resuscitation area
    2. Delayed treatment area
    3. Ambulatory treatment area
    4. Expectant treatment area
    5. Radiology department
    6. Laboratory
    7. Surgery
    8. ICU, acute care wards
    9. Predischarge or evacuation area

At triage sites 1 and 2, casualties are examined rapidly, sorted, moved forward to a resuscitation area, and evacuated. At triage site 3, definitive care or evaluation is performed, and casualties are moved forward to a ward or holding unit before eventual discharge or evacuation.

B. PITFALLS TO SUCCESSFUL TRIAGE

1. Never move a casualty backward, e. g. , x-ray studies ordered in the Immediate Care Area will be performed on the way to the operating room. Patient never returns to the Immediate Care Area once discharged.
2. Never hold a priority patient for further treatment: a bottleneck effect will rapidly occur. This applies to all triage sites.
3. Triage officers do not stop to treat patients.
4. Patients are never moved before triage. Exceptions to this rule are as follows:
    a) Darkness (which prevents proper sorting)
    b) Bad weather
    c) Continued risk of injury (e. g. , risk of aircraft fire, landslide, or building collapse)
    d) Availability of nearby proper facility (e. g. , large, dry, well-lit gymnasium)
    e) Militarily insecure position

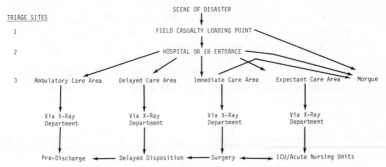

Figure 4-1. Triage sites. (Reproduced with permission: Yates, D. W.: British Journal of Hospital Medicine, Oct., 1979.)

5. In the hospital phase (Triage Site 2) physicians and administrators may have difficulty shifting gears requiring the practice of triage:
   a) Traditional patient-physician relationships do not exist in disaster medicine.
   b) Full resources cannot be given to everyone, but administrators may take the tenacious position that under no circumstances will any patient be turned away from the hospital. [18]
   c) Staff physicians and administrators who are normally in a leadership role may refuse to follow the dictates of the designated triage officer-in-charge. Obedience without understanding is a futile exercise.

C. TRIAGE: CLASSIFICATION AND SITE PROCEDURES

Triage is an ongoing process that is constantly reevaluated and reassessed. The basic principles are the same whether the casualties are traumatic, from infectious epidemics, or from radiation injury or burns. Triage classification is worthless unless it is able to distinguish those patients at the extremes of care. Patients classified in the extremes should not enter or burden the system needlessly (i. e., the minimally ill who will get well anyway, and those who will die in spite of treatment).

D. TRIAGE SITE 1

1. Primary Survey

When casualties are viewed for the first time in a field situation, the process of triage begins with a primary survey. [1] This is an immediate and automatic process performed by the

designated triage officer in the field (usually the senior and
most experienced ambulance crew paramedic). The primary
survey is rapid, taking several seconds at most to complete.
Classifying allows the triage officer to prioritize for rapid
treatment. The simplest form of classification must be utilized,
e. g. , lightly injured, seriously injured, critically injured, or
hopelessly injured.

a) Lightly Injured: Injuries are not disabling. Little or no
professional treatment is required. They must be treated
and quickly returned to normal activities or required to
assist in the treatment of others.

b) Seriously Injured: Injuries requiring time and adequate
definitive care but are of no immediate urgency. Treatment may be delayed without risk to loss of life, e. g. ,
chest injuries without respiratory failure; penetrating
wounds of chest or abdomen with controlled hemorrhage.

c) Critically Injured: Patients who require rapid care to
save a life. Those in danger of death from asphyxia,
hemorrhage, or shock, e. g. , patients with airway obstruction, sucking chest wounds, or exsanguinating
hemorrhage.

d) Hopelessly Injured: Patients whose prognosis is poor and
who would not withstand evacuation. These patients receive nothing more than relief of pain and suffering.
Time, effort, and supplies must not be spent on this
group to the detriment of the first three categories.

2. Triage Rounds

The first round of triage begins immediately. Those patients in
the critically ill classification require first priority care as
shown in Table 4-1). Attention to the ABCs (airway, breathing,
and circulation) in the simplest and most direct manner are
performed by paramedics assigned by the triage officer. Procedures utilize several seconds of time. The triage officer re-
surveys those patients placed on the second, third, and fourth
priority groups but does not stop to treat patients.
    The second round of triage begins automatically by the tri-
age officer. Paramedics are performing basic or advanced life
support procedures unless assigned elsewhere by the triage officer. The continuous survey by the triage officer confirms that
procedures are carried out on the first priority group before
assigning procedures to the second priority group (e. g. , O_2,
MAST suit).
    Preplanning, prior disaster drills, and paramedic skills

Table 4-1. Priorities of Treatment of Triage*

Priority Group	Problem	Treatment			
		1st Round Triage	2nd Round Triage	3rd Round Triage	4th Round Triage
First	Airway obstruction	Airway opened manually	Endotracheal intubation; cricothyrotomy		
	Sucking chest wound	Sealed manually	Sealed with occlusive dressing; O_2	Chest tube with Heimlich valve	
	Apnea	Mouth-to-mouth ventilation	Bag-valve-mask with O_2	Continue artificial ventilation	
	Cardiac arrest	External cardiac compressions (ECC)	Continue ECC; start IV; O_2	Drugs; defibrillation	

Table 4-1. Priorities of Treatment of Triage (cont'd)

Priority Group	Problem	Treatment			
		1st Round Triage	2nd Round Triage	3rd Round Triage	4th Round Triage
First (cont'd)	Exsanguinating hemorrhage	Manual control of bleeding; MAST	IV infusions; O₂		
Second	Tension pneumothorax		O₂	Chest tube with Heimlich valve	
	Pericardial tamponade		O₂; ECC	Evacuate blood from pericardium	
	Impending shock		O₂; MAST	IV infusions	
	Massive hemothorax		O₂	Chest tube	

Third	Head injury	Secure airway	Stabilize cervical spine
	Evisceration	IV; cover viscera	
	Open fractures	Dress wounds	Splint
	Spinal injuries	Immobilize	
Fourth	Lesser fractures, wounds		Splint; dress wounds

*Reproduced with permission: Caroline, N. L.: Emergency Care in the Streets. Boston: Little, Brown & Co., Inc., 1979.

will determine the efficient flow of care from one priority and triage round to another. The triage officer's supervision, leadership, and clinical judgment is of critical importance in the efficiency of this process.

Triage rounds may be completed from several seconds to 15-30 min depending on the number and severity of first and second priority patients.

3. Communication with Base Hospital

The triage officer may choose to communicate at any time with the base hospital physician. Usually this occurs during or after completion of the third round of triage. Initial communication includes:

    a) Nature of the disaster.
    b) Exact location.
    c) Approximate number injured.
    d) Special circumstances of the disaster (e. g. , trapped patients, risk of fire, excess elderly, or pediatric caudalities).
    e) Additional equipment required in the field.
    f) Unit serving as command post (usually first ambulance to arrive) and name of triage officer.

4. Tagging in the Field

Tagging is critical to continuity of care. Several varieties of triage tags exist. The most useful are those which are easy to read and also give clear instructions (Figures 4-2 and 4-3A, B, C).

Triage tag information should include:

    a) Patient identification by name or number. Alphabet identification may be confused with patient's initials and should never be used.
    b) Sex.
    c) Injuries. Main problems only, using accepted abbreviations (i. e. , cpd fx of femur, mult lac).
    d) Any procedures or medications provided.
    e) Paramedic's name. This is essential to medical documentation, disaster care critique, and tracing of circumstances leading to patient identification.
    f) Ambulance number.
    g) Tags should be attached to the large toe. If toe is not available, attach to the wrist. Never attach to clothing or shoelaces.

1. NAME (Last-First-Middle initial) / NOM, PRENOMS
2. SERVICE NUMBER / NUMERO MATRICULE
3. GRADE / GRADE
4. NATION / NATION (e.g. Etats Unis)
5. FORCE / ARMEE
6. BRANCH AND TRADE / ARME (e.g. Infanterie)
7. UNIT / UNITE
8. SERVICE (Yrs) / DUREE DES SERVICES (e.g. 2 6/12)
9. AGE / AGE
10. RACE / RACE
11. RELIGION / RELIGION
12. FACILITY WHERE TAGGED / LIEU D'ETABLISSEMENT DE LA FICHE
13. DATE AND HOUR TAGGED / DATE ET HEURE D'ETABLISSEMENT DE LA FICHE
14. DIAGNOSIS (Including cause) / DIAGNOSTIC (Cause comprise)
15. LINE OF DUTY / EN RELATION AVEC LE SERVICE

NATURE OF CASUALTY OR ILLNESS
NATURE DE LA BLESSURE OU MALADIE

DISABILITY / INCAPACITE	ENEMY ACTION / DU FAIT DE L'ENNEMI	
16. INJURY / BLESSURE	YES / OUI	NO / NON
17. SICK / MALADIE	YES / OUI	NO / NON

18. DATE & HOUR INJURED / DATE ET HEURE DE LA BLESSURE
19. WHAT WAS HE DOING WHEN INJURED / QUE FAISAIT-IL LORSQU'IL FUT BLESSE
20. TREATMENT GIVEN (For antibiotics specify which and give dose, hour and date) / TRAITEMENT EFFECTUE (Si des antibiotiques ont été donnés, précisez leur nature, la dose, l'heure et la date)
21. TOURNIQUET (Yes or No; Time & date applied) / MISE EN PLACE D'UN GARROT (Oui ou Non; heure et date)

TREATMENT / TRAITEMENT EFFECTUE	a. DOSE / DOSE	b. HOUR AND DATE / HEURE - DATE
22. MORPHINE- 1st / MORPHINE- 1ere		
23. MORPHINE- 2nd / MORPHINE- 2eme		
24. MORPHINE- 3rd / MORPHINE- 3eme		
25. TETANUS TOXOID / VACCIN ANTITETANIQUE		
26. A.T. SERUM/SERUM ANTITETANIQUE		

27. DISPOSITION-DISPOSAL / DESTINATION DONNEE AU BLESSE
28. HOUR AND DATE / HEURE ET DATE
29. MEDICAL OFFICER (Signature & Grade) / SIGNATURE ET GRADE DU MEDECIN

DD FORM 1380, 1 JUN 62

U. S. FIELD MEDICAL CARD/FICHE MEDICALE DE L'AVANT ETATS-UNIS

FRONT

30. a. ABSOLUTION / CONFESSION
b. HOLY COMMUNION / SAINTE COMMUNION
c. EXTREME UNCTION / EXTREME ONCTION
d. OTHER MINISTRATIONS / AUTRES MINISTERES
e. CHAPLAIN (Signature) / SIGNATURE DE L'AUMONIER

31. DIET / REGIME ALIMENTAIRE
REGULAR / NORMAL
LIQUID / LIQUIDE
NOTHING BY MOUTH / RIEN PAR VOIE ORALE

32. REMARKS / REMARQUES

☆ U. S. GOVERNMENT PRINTING OFFICE: 1967—245— 357

BACK

Figure 4-2. Military triage tag. (Reprinted with permission, Washington, D. C., U. S. Government Printing Office, 1967—245-357.)

5. Evacuation Priorities

The field paramedic is faced with two priorities: priority of care and priority of evacuation. A patient stabilized after requiring immediate airway opening may require a less immediate priority of evacuation as shown in Table 4-2. Color-coded

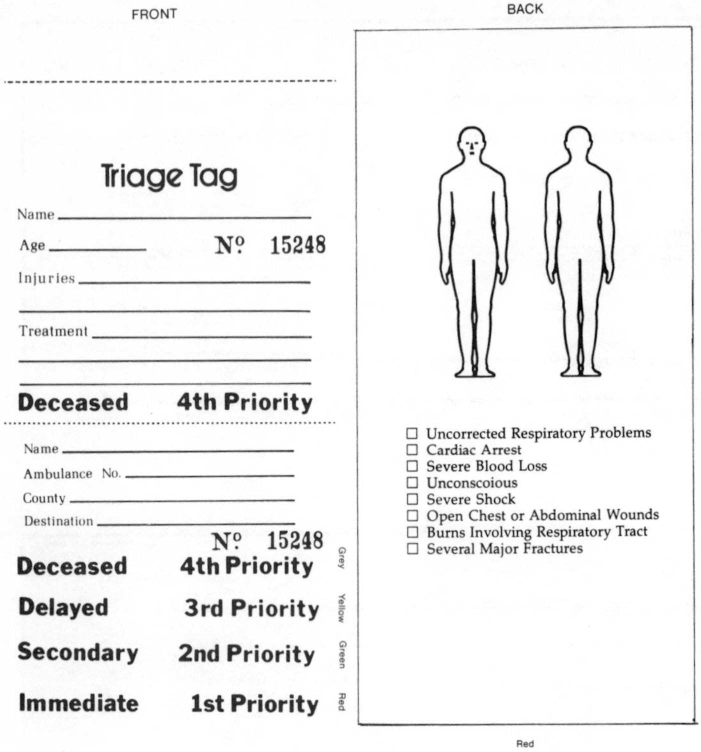

FRONT   BACK

Triage Tag

Name _____

Age _____   Nº 15248

Injuries _____

Treatment _____
_____
_____

Deceased   4th Priority

Name _____

Ambulance No. _____

County _____

Destination _____

Nº 15248

Deceased   4th Priority   Grey

Delayed   3rd Priority   Yellow

Secondary   2nd Priority   Green

Immediate   1st Priority   Red

☐ Uncorrected Respiratory Problems
☐ Cardiac Arrest
☐ Severe Blood Loss
☐ Unconscoious
☐ Severe Shock
☐ Open Chest or Abdominal Wounds
☐ Burns Involving Respiratory Tract
☐ Several Major Fractures

Red

Figure 4-3A. Civilian triage tags.

tagging is commonly used (Figure 4-3). Inappropriate color codes are detached leaving the appropriate evacuation color code at the bottom of the tag. Internationally recognized codes now correspond to the color sequence in traffic signals: red, yellow, green.

A field triage plan utilizing color codes was developed for Montgomery County, Maryland[32] as follows:

METHOD OF REMOVAL

A. Nonentrapped patients: Removed first
    1. Red
    2. Yellow
    3. Green
B. Entrapped patients
    1. Red
    2. Yellow
    3. Green

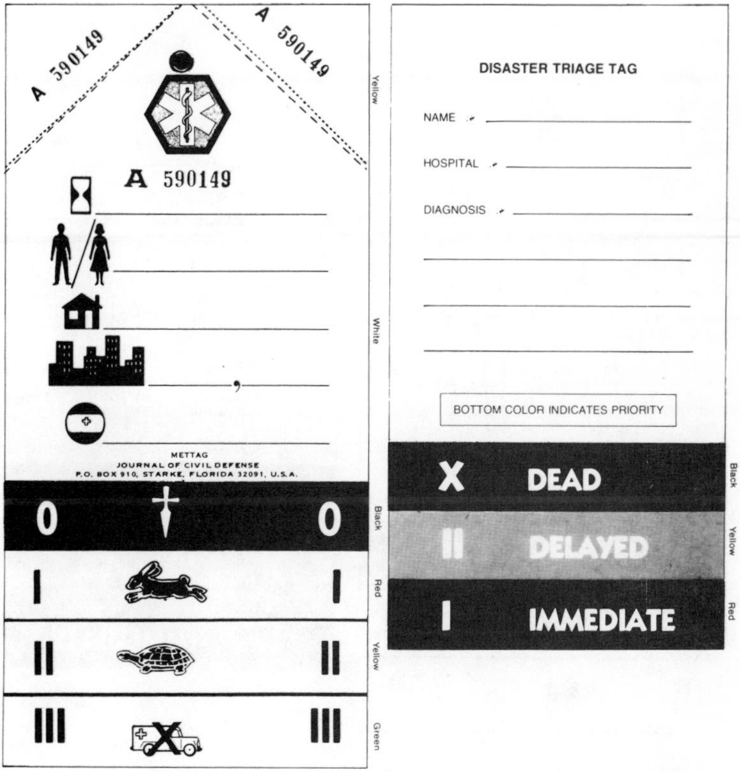

Figure 4-3B. Civilian disaster triage tags. (Reprinted with permission from METTAG, P.O. Box 910, Starke, Florida 32901, U.S.A.)

4. Nonentrapped gray
5. Entrapped gray

RED TAG

A. Uncorrected respiratory problems
B. Cardiac arrest*

*Never provide CPR in those situations where a casualty is a doubtful survivor or while others more salvageable are allowed to deteriorate.

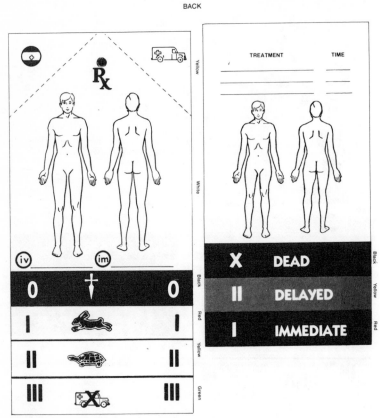

Figure 4-3C. Civilian disaster triage tags. (Reprinted with permission from Honolulu County Medical Society, HMA Disaster Committee, Honolulu, U. S. A.)

C.   Severe blood loss (2 pints or more)
D.   Unconscious
E.   Open chest or abdominal wounds
F.   Several major fractures
G.   Severe shock
H.   Burns (complicated by respiratory tract injury)

Table 4-2. Field Priorities

Patient	Priority of Care	Priority of Transportation
1. Dyspnea, stridor, UNC	1	3
2. Abrasions, mod. hysterical	5	5
3. Bleeding profusely from neck laceration	2	1
4. Grossly deformed FX leg, FX mandible, and blood loss	4	4
5. Elderly PT, FX arm, substantial pain, dyspnea	3	2

*Reproduced with permission: Hughes, J. H.: Triage. Postgraduate Medicine. Vol. 60, No. 4, Oct., 1976.

YELLOW TAG

A. Severe burns
B. Moderate blood loss (1-2 pints)
C. Back injuries with or without spinal cord damage
D. Conscious with serious head injuries

GREEN TAG

A. Minor fractures
B. Other minor injuries
C. Minor burns
D. Obviously mortal wounds in which death appears reasonably certain

GRAY TAG

A. Without pulse or respiration for 20 min
B. Injuries make CPR effort impossible

Where tags are not available, a system using crosses marked on the forehead with indelible pens is acceptable[19] (Figure 4-4).

6. Fatal Injuries

Fatalities should be immediately identified and labeled "deceased." Time and personnel are often wasted reconfirming

System used for marking foreheads according
to severity of injury:

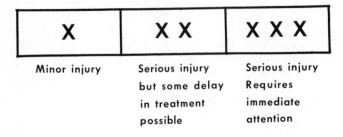

X	X X	X X X
Minor injury	Serious injury but some delay in treatment possible	Serious injury Requires immediate attention

Figure 4-4. Rapid triage identification method. (Reproduced
with permission: Moorgate tube train disaster. Br Med J, Vol.
3, 1975.)

death. Portable monitor paddles to confirm heartbeat are easily passed from one casualty to another.[17] The remains, with
all personal effects, are covered appropriately with sheet or
body bag and removed as soon as possible to designated morgue
or mortuary. The remains may be placed in a polythene tube
bag with 200 cc of 4% formaldehyde injected intraperitoneally
and an additional 200 cc placed in the bag itself. Decomposition
will be delayed by this process for up to two weeks.[20] Identification of the deceased may take equally as long in large disasters where severe burns or disfigurement occurs.

7. Community Physician's Obligation in the Field

Invariably, physicians or other health professionals will be
present or will arrive quickly at the scene of a disaster. Paramedics will be following standardized triage and treatment protocols which have been developed by local EMS agencies. Health
care providers should not interfere or intervene in this process.
Accepted guidelines for these professionals are as follows:

  a) Identify yourself to the person in charge, i.e., the tri-
     age officer. Briefly state your qualifications for care
     (e.g., "I am an internist.").
  b) Ask how you can assist and accept assignment willingly
     unless you do not possess such skills.
  c) Stay away from nonfamiliar procedures, e.g., extrica-
     tion.

E. TRIAGE SITE 2

1. Prior disaster planning will have designated the hospital an-
trum, emergency room, or other suitable entrance as Triage
Site 2.

The designated triage officer and assistants remain in this
area until completion of triage tasks.

The triage tags are rapidly reviewed by the triage officer.
Examination of the ABC status is made and further resuscitation is provided. Tasks are assigned to assistants by the triage
officer. The triage officer does not stop to treat patients. A
similar primary survey is undertaken as new loads of casualties arrive. If field triage has proceeded well, the hospital triage officer will make contact with the most critical patients in
the first evacuation to the hospital. Attention, however, is
given to every casualty. Patient status may shift rapidly. Mis-
diagnosis in the heat of field triage is common, and ABC stabilization is never certain. Retagging and alteration in treatment
priorities will, therefore, occur. Triage tagging is accurate
approximately 70% of the time. The new tag is placed over the
original tag, which is never removed.

The triage officer allocates a nurse, medical student, paramedic, or student nurse to each patient.

2. The triage officer must be kept informed of all data critical
to the triage decision-making:

> Type of disaster
> Number injured
> Distance in time from hospital
> Special circumstances, e. g. , severe weather, elementary
> school bus accident
> Number of health care providers available for assistance:
> physicians and specialty
> Laboratory and blood bank availability
> Surgical teams availability
> Presence in the hospital of department chiefs and disaster
> team members
> Evacuation capabilities
> Available acute care beds
> Simplified diagrams of triage flow of patients
> Easy access to communication system both internal and ex-
> ternal
> Available runners and clerical assistants

3. At Triage Site 2, all patients are assigned to one of four
treatment categories:21

Ambulatory treatment
Immediate treatment
Delayed treatment
Expectant treatment

F. TRIAGE SITE 3

1. Designated Areas

Areas are designated for each treatment category. The principle of categorization is the length of time needed to carry out treatment, not the severity of the injury or illness.

Triage is a continuous process to be repeated in all areas of the hospital. Patients are constantly being changed from one treatment category to another as justified by shifting circumstances of available resources.

a) Immediate Treatment Area (ITA): Usually resuscitation area of established emergency room. Larger institutions may have separately designated acute burn, shock, and fracture treatment areas.

Qualifications	Examples[21]
(1) Minor injuries requiring brief treatment not appropriate to ambulatory treatment area (2) Severe injuries that require brief lifesaving procedures	Easily correctable airway defects; hemorrhage from easily accessible areas, incomplete amputations of extremities: burns 15-40% of BSA; open fractures of major bones, uncomplicated major soft tissue wounds

Disposition

(1) Surgery
(2) ICU
(3) CCU
(4) Acute care wards
(5) 1-4 often via x-ray

b) Ambulatory Treatment Area (ATA): Patients are treated and discharged to provide space for other casualties.

Qualifications	Examples[21]
Injuries or illnesses not requiring immediate hospitalization	Select third degree burns of less than 15% BSA; lacerations of soft tissue requiring only cleansing and dressing; fractures that permit ambulation; patients exposed to radioactive contamination

c) Delayed Treatment Area (DTA):

Qualifications	Examples[21]
(1) Casualties where some delay in treatment will have little effect on final result (2) Patients with serious or multiple injuries needing time-consuming intensive care	Closed lower extremity fractures; severe eye injuries; fractures of pelvis and spine

Disposition

(1) Patients receive supervised IV stabilization with frequent vital signs
(2) Patients triaged to ICA as openings occur

d) Expectant Treatment Area (ETA):

Qualifications	Examples[21]
Casualties with a poor prognosis	Severe multiple injuries requiring more care than resources available; less severe injuries but with poor prognosis from age or other debilitating illness; massive radiation exposure

Disposition

(1) Receive supervisory custodial care
(2) Analgesics and sedation as required for pain

2. Laboratory

Triage Officer: Chief of laboratory services or experienced chief technician.

Expectations:

a) Extended laboratory services are required for 2-5 days before many casualties are stabilized and evacuated.
b) Laboratory triage office must report all blood and colloid availability to the triage officer-in-charge.
c) Laboratory should be prepared to provide the following:[22]

immediate availability of low titer "O" whole blood
5-min capability for group and type specific whole blood
20 min for 4 units or less of fully cross-matched blood[22]

d) Contingency plans to organize a community "walking blood bank" must be anticipated and put into effect.
e) Limit and streamline lab requests. Results must be simplified in anticipation of those values most critical to clinical decisions.

Normal Request $\longrightarrow$ translated to $\longrightarrow$ Actual Need

Normal Request	Actual Need
CBC	Hct, Hgb
Electrolytes	Sodium, potassium
Urinalysis	Specific gravity, presence of blood
Urine function tests	BUN
Glucose	Finger dextrostix
Arterial blood gases	Adequate ventilation; PCO$_2$

Pitfalls:

Large blood volume request will cause a bottleneck. Limit requests for crossmatches to 2-4 units at any one time.

3. Radiology Department

Triage Officer: Senior radiologist

Expectations:

a) X-ray examinations should be discouraged. [17] A baro-
meter of good disaster management is an underutilized x-ray
department. Treat all suspected fractures as fractures. No x-
rays will be done before resuscitation. Known compound fractures require x-rays only after surgical correction.

b) Examination requests should be streamlined to those
views most critical to necessary clinical management. Suspected hemothorax should receive a lateral decubitus view
alone. [23] This view will identify as little as 15 cc of fluid in the
chest. Routine AP and lateral views are not necessary to the
clinical decision to vent the hemothorax.

c) Military-type canvas litters serve as splints; x-rays are
easily taken through canvas portion preventing unnecessary patient movement. [24]

Pitfalls:

a) Requests for x-ray examination may come from various
sources and thereby confuse priorities. Be attentive to requests
from the immediate care area. Requests from ambulatory, delayed, and expectant care areas should receive strict scrutiny
and decisive refusal.

b) Physicians, either out of anxiety over a complex
multiple-injured case or during a lull in the care of stabilized
patients, tend to react by hasty and often inappropriate order-
ing of x-ray examinations.

4. Surgery Department

Triage Officer: Senior surgeon or designate

Expectations:

a) Triage critical and serious cases around available surgeons, surgical nursing teams, and anesthetists/anesthesiolo-
gists.

b) Critical unstable cases requiring brief but definitive
surgical correction come first.

c) Serious stabilized cases must have their vital signs,
fluids, and blood closely monitored by critical care nurses or
nonsurgical physicians. Any evidence of instability must be

communicated to the surgical triage officer. Many abdominal
wounds awaiting surgery can be successfully stabilized for 3-4
hrs on crystalloids alone.

d) Specialty surgeons (ophthalmologist, urologist, obstetri-
cian-gynecologist, plastic surgeons, etc.) are utilized by the
surgical triage officer to close major surgical wounds in order
to allow general, thoracic, and orthopedic surgeons to work on
the next priority case.

Pitfalls:

a) Inattentiveness to the priority of delayed secondary closure in many disaster or battlefield wounds.

b) Surgeons may not be familiar with the characteristics of
devitalized muscle and the requirements for debridement.

c) Contaminated or poorly debrided smaller wounds treated
by physicians in the Ambulatory Care Area may return with
wound infections. Few minor wounds necessitate immediate
closure. 25 Proper early debridement, wound immobilization,
extensive drainage, and delayed closure in 5-7 days are the
fundamental principles.

d) Allowing low priority surgical cases to arrive in surgery
to be operated on immediately, without attention to the possibility that more severe cases requiring immediate definitive surgical intervention are at that moment being stabilized in the
Immediate Care or Resuscitation Areas.

5. Acute Nursing Units

Triage Officer: Nursing supervisor or director of nursing.

Expectations:

a) Discharge or transfer noncritical patients to home or
alternate care facility. In any major hospital nationwide, at
least 50 patients can be safely discharged to home on an immediate basis. Hospitals vary from 30-60% clearance ability of
noncritical patients.

b) Staff critical care units with appropriate nursing personnel. Practical nurses, nursing students, medical students,
paramedics, or experienced community volunteers may be utilized to staff noncritical nursing units or to supplement nursing
requirements on acute care units.

c) Disaster plans should be reviewed to determine the
feasibility of utilizing one ward or block beds on individual
wards for disaster victims. Utilizing one ward may provide for

more efficient staffing and critical care, especially where
nursing staff is limited in number. [26]

Pitfalls:

Acute care beds must be planned for up to 5 days. Staff fatigue, exhaustion, and equipment limitations may necessitate
early triage to another facility. Inattention to this may lead to
delayed morbidity and mortality of otherwise properly cared
for victims.

6. Medical Department

Internists and pediatricians provide critical responsibilities to
triage in the following areas:[27]

    a) Fluid and electrolyte consultation
       (1) Early recognition and treatment of crush-related
          hyperkalemia and renal impairment.
       (2) Nutritional and electrolyte requirements of victims
          of prolonged entrapment.
       (3) Dialysis requirements associated with severe trauma.
    b) Infectious disease consultation
       (1) Treatment of sepsis secondary to complications of
          trauma and contaminated wounds.
       (2) Anticipation of outbreaks of communicable disease
          associated with postdisaster phase.
    c) Radiation, chemical, and environmental casualty care
       consultation
       (1) Evaluation, treatment, and follow-up of casualties in
          these areas fall primarily to the internist, pediatri-
          cian, or generalist.
       (2) Consultation with military, federal, state, or univer-
          sity experts in these areas of care must be obtained
          early in the course of disaster care.

7. Predischarge Areas for Ambulatory Patients

The predischarge area should be a quiet, easily accessible
gathering area removed from the original triage entry point.
Triage tags, records, and identification procedures are completed and collected. All patients should be:

    a) Instructed in the management of their condition.
    b) Provided with a brief description of the treatment.
    c) Provided with a brief description of their condition and
       information for follow-up.

VI. COMMUNITY PHYSICIAN'S OBLIGATION
TO IN-HOSPITAL TRIAGE

A. Identify your presence to triage officer-in-charge.
B. Accept assignment.
C. Know standard procedures (see Chapter 5).
D. Resist temptation to change from locally accepted stan-
dard procedures.
E. Examine minor cases and discharge them rapidly.
(There is a tendency for medical staff to stand by and
await the "really big cases. ")

VII. MILITARY TRIAGE

The objective of mass casualty triage is to accomplish the
greatest good for the greatest number in the shortest time. In
the stark reality of combat, the major objective of battlefield
triage is to determine who can be returned to the front immediately, treat them, and move them back to duty. Quick treatment
and evacuation of the more seriously injured is an important but
a secondary objective.

The process conducted on the battlefield where medical
facilities are limited involves the unpleasant but necessary military decision to evacuate first those with the best chance of
survival and leave for later evacuation those who have no chance
of survival.

An improvement in survival of casualties was seen when
triage principles were applied in the Korean War. Further improvement in survival rates of casualties was noted during
combat activities in Vietnam where sophisticated triage and
evacuation practices were performed. [5, 28, 29] Table 4-3 illustrates this improvement.

Table 4-3. Time of Wound to Definitive Care[28]

WWI	12-18 hrs
WWII	6-12 hrs
Korean War	2-4 hrs
Vietnam War	1-2 hrs*

*Nine out of 10 consecutive laparotomies performed were
started within 70 min of the wound.

Mortality rates have dropped significantly since World War
II. This decrease is shown in Table 4-4. [28]

Table 4-4. Mortality

WWII	4. 7%
Korean War	2. 0%
Vietnam War	1. 0%

     Contributing factors to the 1% mortality rate in the Vietnam War include: immediate helicopter evacuation, well equipped and staffed hospitals, rapid triage and treatment, and limitation of enemy weaponry. [29]

     Casualties are sorted at every medical installation in the chain of evacuation and hospitalization (Figure 4-5).

A. FIELD SITUATION[30]

The corpsman in the field is prepared to sort and treat casualties rapidly and efficiently.

    1. Corpsman maintains a position in the immediate proximity of the front lines.

    2. The casualty is first removed from the direct line of fire. Corpsman must have knowledge of

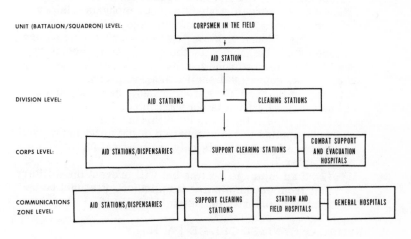

TYPICAL MILITARY FIELD TRIAGE OPTIONS
AND SUPPORT FACILITIES AT
LEVELS OF THEATER OPERATIONS

Figure 4-5. Medical operations in combat. (Reproduced with permission: Department of Defense, Washington, D. C.)

    a) field of fire
    b) type or ordnance encountered
    c) protective features of the terrain
3. A corpsman never exposes himself recklessly to reach a casualty.
4. The squad or platoon leader provides protective fire coverage.
5. When the casualty has been removed to an area of relative safety, first aid measures are carried out.
6. The responsibility of the initial sorting of casualties falls to the first corpsman who attends to the casualty. Decision must be made as to:
    a) Need for evacuation
    b) Urgency of evacuation
    c) Advisability of returning the soldier to duty
7. Battlefield triage involves three categories of casualties. The corpsman's evaluation is essential in assisting the military commander on the scene who will pass through air request channels for MED-EVAC assistance if necessary.
    a) _Emergency_: Critical wound, illness, or injury; immediate evacuation is a matter of life or death.
    b) _Priority_: Serious wound, illness, or injury. Requires early hospitalization but not immediate evacuation, e.g. , minor multiple wounds; muscle damage which is less than major; thoracic wounds without asphyxia; dislocation and lesser fractures; and injuries of the eyes.
    c) _Routine_: Wound, illness, or injury of a minor nature. These should be handled by the corpsman immediately and the soldier returned to duty, e.g. , minor cuts, abrasions, superficial shell fragments, sprains and strains, mild headaches, toothaches, diarrhea, and constipation. Evacuation is not warranted.
        (1) Routine category is used through air channels when applied to the evacuation of the deceased as well as transfer of patients between medical facilities (see Chapter 7).
        (2) If an injury is routine but will prevent the military unit from accomplishing its mission, it should be upgraded to priority to hasten MED-EVAC.

B. INITIAL ORGANIZED TRIAGE FACILITY

These may be mobile aid stations close to the battle area or, somewhat more removed, casualty clearing stations. These areas are used when evacuation is primarily performed by foot or limited military vehicles.

These open facilities may be manned by one clinically experienced medical officer, veterinarians, dentists or nurses, and eight corpsmen. [33] Tri-Service (Army, Navy, Air Force) Combat Casualty Care Courses (C-4) presently provide all military health care professionals with instruction in emergency resuscitation and triage procedures.

Nonphysician health professionals are critical in manning these facilities under battlefield priorities.

Evacuation to second echelon triage facilities or field hospitals is performed by armored personnel carriers.

Helicopters may evacuate casualties from field or initial triage facilities. Where field helicopter MED-EVAC is utilized, the initial triage facility is usually overflown and bypassed in favor of the second echelon triage facility.

C. SECOND ECHELON TRIAGE FACILITY

Usually no more than 20-30 minutes from the initial triage facility by vehicle. This facility may represent a casualty-receiving hospital ship where coastal evacuation by helicopter is an organized entity. These facilities are manned by organized teams of general medical officers, anesthetists or anesthesiologists, general and orthopedic surgeons; several specialty surgeons if the facility warrants this; and nurses, corpsmen and nonmedical support personnel who assist in supply, evacuation, and recordkeeping duties.

Many of the principles and objectives discussed under Section V (Civilian or Community Disaster Triage) are applicable to Military Triage. The efficiency of sorting which was discussed under triage rounds is critical to any echelon level (Figures 4-6 to 4-10).

VIII. MEDICO-LEGAL ASPECTS OF TRIAGE IN CIVILIAN DISASTERS

A. Assessment of liability will take into consideration the various circumstances surrounding the disaster situation. Major factors include:

1. Availability of physicians to treat disaster victims
2. Reasonableness of the triage procedure

Paramount to this is the presence in the community of a specific disaster plan; the presence of trained triage officers who act in the reasonable fashion expected of their duties; and the provision of services by health care professionals working

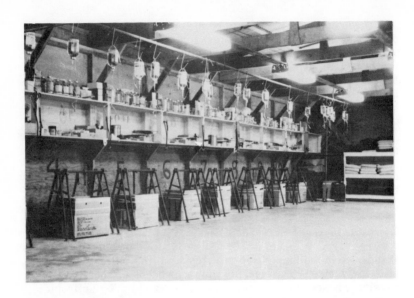

Figure 4-6. Triage bunker, Delta Medical Company, 3rd Division, Vietnam, 1968. Separate numbered stations were manned by one physician and two to three corpsmen. Hung IVs will remain sterile for 2-3 days.

to the best of their abilities with the resources available to them.

ADDENDUM TO CHAPTER 4 (TRIAGE)

STANDARD OPERATING PROCEDURES FOR TRIAGE PERSONNEL

Primary care providers may find themselves assigned to treat, evaluate, and monitor trauma victims in various stages of shock. Providers will be asked to stabilize these victims and maintain stabilization until resources (i. e. , operating room or evacuation) for definitive treatment become available. Providers may find themselves sitting on a potential time bomb of a patient. The waiting period may seem endless. The provider must monitor the stabilization and notify the Triage Officer immediately if it appears stabilization can no longer be maintained. It will be the responsibility of the Triage Officer to either upgrade the victim to an immediate place in the operating room, recommend an alternate stabilization method (i. e. , auto transfusion) or possibly reroute the victim to the Expectant Treatment Area.

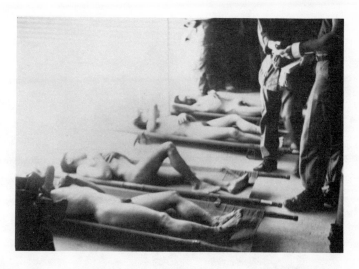

Figure 4-7. Soldiers triaged and tagged during military conflicts (Vietnam, 1968). Conditions warranted that casualties be
stripped to allow for full view of all injuries. This is more
critical where casualties are unable to provide information due
to injury or language barriers.

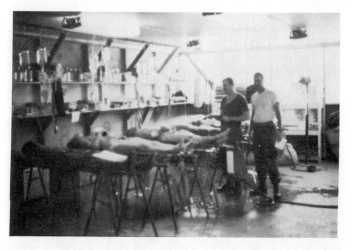

Figure 4-8. Treatment of heat casualties expedited by common
showering by means of hose. Unfortunately, personal privacies
are often compromised by the demands of disaster care (Vietnam, 1968).

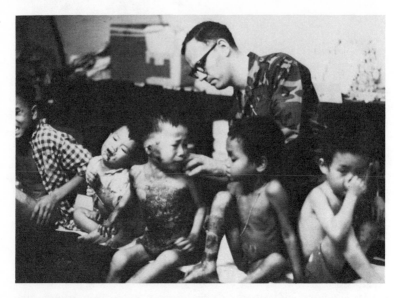

Figure 4-9. Assembly line approach to common injuries.
Minor burns in these children were triaged, efficiently managed, and discharged (Vietnam, 1968).

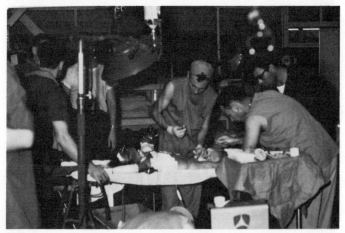

Figure 4-10. Pediatric trauma casualty (Vietnam, 1968). Full
utilization of all resources and personnel are critical to disaster medicine. Paramedic (corpsmen) personnel predominate
this scene.

The anxiety and confusion of the disaster situation will not allow for review of basic trauma resuscitation. Primary care providers can be handed a simplified list of guidelines to stabilization when they arrive at the hospital. Do not assume knowledge of trauma stabilization by the majority of physicians, especially those in nonsurgically oriented specialties. These guidelines assume the victim has either been resuscitated or has received preliminary stabilization of the ABCs in the Immediate Care Area.

CLINICAL SHOCK*

Stage 1: Responsive

1. Establish IV route: at least two large bore IV's with normal saline or Ringer's lactate.
2. Monitor VS: BP, pulse, capillary refill, EKG monitor if available.
3. P.E. and history (especially chest).
4. Laboratory: type and crossmatch (no more than 2-4 units at a time).

   hematocrit
   blood gases
   urinalysis

5. Splint fractures.
6. Foley catheter, nasogastric tube, O_2 per mask, peritoneal lavage by consult with surgeon.
7. X-ray studies: simplified (i.e., lateral decubitus of chest to rule out hemothorax).

Stage 2: After vital signs are stabilized:

1. Continue intravenous fluids.
2. Continue to monitor and record VS.
3. P.E. more complete.
4. Lab: T+C, Hct, blood gases, urinalysis as necessary.
5. Splint fractures.
6. X-rays: other diagnostic studies if indicated prior to definitive care.

Stage 3: Preparations for Transportation

1. Stable vital signs.
2. Assured airways.
3. Secure intravenous routes.
4. Nasogastric tube.
5. Foley catheter.
6. Trained personnel.
7. Resuscitation equipment.

---

*Modified from Larkin, J. , and Moylan, J. : Priorities in management of trauma victims. Crit Care Med 3(5):192-195, 1975.

REFERENCES

1. Caroline, N. D. : <u>Emergency Care in the Streets</u>. Boston, Little, Brown & Co. , 1979.
2. Rutherford, W. H. : Experience in the Accident and Emergency Department of the Royal Victoria Hospital with patients from civil disturbances in Belfast, 1969-1972, with a review of disasters in the United Kingdom, 1951-1971. Injury 4(3):189-199, 1973.
3. Noggan, L. : Medical planning for disaster in Israel. Injury 7(4):279-285, 1976.
4. Howard, J. M. , and DeBakey, M. E. : The Cost of Delayed Medical Care. Symposium on Management of Mass Casualties. Medical Field Service School, Fort Sam Houston, Texas, 1962.
5. Hughes, J. H. : Community Medicine. Triage—a new look at an old French concept, Postgrad Med 60(4):223-227, 1976.
6. McIntyre, M. D. , and Lewis, A. J. (ed): <u>Textbook of Advanced Cardiac Life Support</u>, American Heart Association, 1981.
7. American College of Surgeons Committee on Trauma: Advanced Trauma Life Support. 1980.
8. Buckingham, R. E. : The IPCAR score: A method for evaluation of the emergency patient. J Indiana State Med Assoc 67:21, 1974.
9. Baker, S. P. , et al. : The Injury Severity Score: A method of describing patients with multiple injuries and evaluating emergency care. J Trauma 14:187, 1974.
10. Vayda, E. , et al. : An emergency department triage model based on presenting complaints. Can J Public Health 64: 246, 1973.

11. Stoner, H. B. , et al. : Measuring the severity of injury.
    Br Med J 2:1247-1249, 1977.
12. American College of Surgeons: Hospital Trauma Index.
    The Bulletin, 1980.
13. Champion, H. R. , et al. : Assessment of injury severity:
    The triage Index. Crit Care Med 8(4):201-208, 1980.
14. Champion, H. R. , et al. : An anatomic index of injury
    severity. J Trauma 20(3):197-202, 1980.
15. Gibson, G. : Evaluative criteria for emergency ambulance
    systems. Soc Sci Med 7:425, 1973.
16. Thurner, R. R. , and Remein, Q. M. : Principles and Pro-
    cedures in the Evaluation of Screening for Disease.
    Washington, D. C. , Public Health Monograph 67, U. S.
    Government Printing Office, 1967.
17. Yates, D. W. : Major disasters: Surgical triage. Br J
    Hosp Med 323-328, 1979.
18. Brown, R. K. : Disaster medicine. What is it? Can it be
    taught? JAMA 197(13):133-136, 1966.
19. Medical Staff, Three London Hospitals: Moorgate tube
    train disaster. Br Med J 3:727-731, 1975.
20. Hart, R. J. , et al. : The Summerland disaster. Br Med J
    1:256-259, 1975.
21. Division of Emergency Health Services: The Treatment of
    Mass Civilian Casualties in a National Emergency. Public
    Health Service, Publication 1071-C-5, Washington, D. C. ,
    U. S. Government Printing Office, 1970.
22. Monagham, W. P. , et al. : Laboratory Briefing, U. S. S.
    Sanctuary (AH-17). Unpublished document.
23. Swan, K. G. , and Swan, R. C. : Gunshot Wounds, Patho-
    physiology and Management. Littleton, Mass. , PSG Pub-
    lishing Co. , Inc. , 1980.
24. Whittaker, R. , et al. : Earthquake disaster in Nicaragua.
    J Trauma, 14(1):37-43, 1974.
25. Whyte, A. G. : Disaster wound treatment (Letter to the
    Editor). Br Med J 4:43-44, 1975.
26. Caro, D. , and Irving, M. : The Old Bailey bomb explosion.
    Lancet 1:1433-1435, 1973.
27. King, E. G. : The Moorgate disaster: Lessons for the in-
    ternist (Editorial). Ann Intern Med 84(3):333-334, 1976.
28. Maughon, J. S. : An inquiry into the nature of wounds re-
    sulting in killed in action in Viet Nam. Milit Med 135:8-13,
    1970.
29. Eiseman, B. : Combat casualty management in Vietnam.
    J Trauma 7(1):53-63, 1967.
30. United States Navy: Handbook of the Hospital Corps. Sec-
    tion 12, Fleet Marine Support, NAVMED, P5004.

31. American Medical Association: Guidelines regarding disaster plan for a community hospital: Personal communication. Feb. , 1981.
32. Based on Triage Plan developed originally for Montgomery County, Maryland. Unpublished document.
33. Chipman, M. , et al. : Triage of mass casualties: Concepts for coping with mixed battlefield injuries. Milit Med 145(2): 99-100, 1980.

Chapter 5

INITIAL ASSESSMENT OF DISASTER VICTIMS
Barry W. Wolcott, M.D.

I. INTRODUCTION

This chapter is based on several assumptions about the setting
in which you are working as a physician.

A. The nature of the disaster is known.
B. Stage 1 and Stage 2 triage, as discussed in Chapter 4,
   have occurred.
C. Prehospital care, if it took place at all, was of variable
   quality.
D. Your goal is to stabilize individual patients so they will
   live to reach the next level of care; thus, during this initial assessment, you must detect both obvious and subtle threats to the patient's life.

Working in such a setting will be physically and emotionally
demanding. To keep these stresses from producing errors of
thought and technique, your initial evaluation must conform to
certain basic principles:

1. This will be the patient's first complete examination. It
will easily detect the patient's obvious injuries; it must also
be sufficiently detailed to detect remediable subtle defects.
Too detailed examinations are wasteful, for there is no
reason to expend resources searching for problems which
cannot be ameliorated even if detected.
2. The basic initial assessment sequence should be the
same regardless of injury type. In the chaos of a disaster,
you will be hard-pressed to adhere to a single assessment
sequence. Customizing each assessment will place patients
at risk of omission or commission errors.
3. Your skills limit treatment of detected life threats. * You
must also limit treatment to that which will stabilize the

_____
*This book assumes health care provider familiarity with skills
of Advanced Cardiac and Advanced Trauma Life Support (ACLS,
ATLS).

patients long enough for them to reach the next level of
care. Adherence to this principle is essential even if your
personal skills and local resources would permit more
definitive care. In the disaster setting, care for one patient
beyond minimum essential stabilization is directly at the
expense of the next patient awaiting care.

II. INITIAL ASSESSMENT

With these assumptions and principles in mind, you should proceed with an initial assessment (Figure 5-1) of the patient as
follows:

A. OPENING OF ASSESSMENT

While touching the patient, communicate some identification,
instructions, and reassurance: "I'm doctor _____. You are
at _____ hospital. It appears you are _____ (badly burned,
very sick, etc.). We know what to do for you, and you must
cooperate so we can do it. We need you to be quiet unless we
talk to you and to lie quietly unless we ask you to move. We
may hurt you, but we will tell you what we are doing."
   Rationale: This introduction takes about 10 valuable seconds, but it will calm the patient and decrease his interference
with your care, thus saving time. Do not use obviously false
reassurance (i.e., "Nothing is wrong.", "Don't worry.", etc.).
Such comments label you as either a fool or a liar; either label
will increase, not decrease, the patient's anxiety.

B. AIRWAY ASSESSMENT

   1. Ask: "What is your name?"
   Rationale: If the patient can talk, his airway is probably
adequate.
   2. If the patient cannot talk but is making respiratory efforts and you feel no air flow, search for common, easily
reversible causes of airway obstruction:

   a. Chin lift
   b. Jaw lift
   c. Finger sweep

   Rationale: Common things are common; simple things
are easy to remedy.
   3. If the airway is still obstructed, consider performing
the following:

THE INITIAL ASSESSMENT

AIRWAY
Talking?
Respiratory Efforts?
Moving Air?
Reversible Problems?

CIRCULATION
Adequate Cardiac Output?
Hemorrhage?
Pericardial Tamponade?
Myocardial Dysfunction?
Peripheral Resistance
  Adequate?

BREATHING
Volume Adequate?
Reversible Problems?

DELIVERY OF O$_2$
Adequate?
Reversible Problems?

M AND N COME IN THE MIDDLE

MINIMUM DATA BASE
Patient Says?
Wallet?
ID Tag?
Friends?
Rescue Workers?

NAKED
What's Wrong on the
  Other Side?

DISASTERS HAVE NO "Z'S" – JUST MORE PATIENTS

RECTAL - VAGINAL EXAM
Tears?
Blood?
Sphincter?

VISION
Acuity?
Foreign Bodies?

STABILIZE C-SPINE

WRAP UP QUESTIONS
What Happened?
What's Wrong?
How Bad is It?

TEETH
Missing?
Jaw Stable?
Severe Bleeding?

XTREMITIES
Symetrical?
Deformities?
Range of Motion?

URETHRA
Intact in Males?
No Meatal Blood?

YOUR DECISION
Discharge?
Treat?
Evacuate?

NEXT PATIENT PLEASE

Figure 5-1. Questioning the ABCs.

    a. Chest/abdominal thrusts
    b. Tracheal intubation (keeping cervical spine in align-
        ment)
    c. Esophageal obturator airway insertion (contraindi-
        cated in a conscious patient or when there is blood or
        debris in the mouth)
    d. Cricothyrotomy
    e. Jet insufflation via needle cricothyrotomy

Rationale: This list exhausts reasonable measures to
reverse or bypass an obstructed airway in a disaster setting.
Each has specific contraindications which you must learn in
advance. You must consider each method, and then select the
least dangerous for a given patient, rather than routinely use a
particular method to secure an airway.
    4. If these maneuvers do not relieve the obstruction, at-
       tempt positive pressure ventilation.
    Rationale: Failure of earlier efforts indicates probable
sublaryngeal obstruction. Positive pressure ventilation may
drive an obstruction distally into a single lung, thus allowing
ventilation via the remaining lung; otherwise the patient will
die.
    5. Consider early endotracheal intubation with a cuffed
       tube in patients with

    a. Thermal burns of the face
    b. Chemical inhalation injuries
    c. Direct anterior neck trauma (blunt or penetrating)

Rationale: Airway edema leading to obstruction may follow those injuries. During a disaster, postresuscitation observation will be suboptimal; many of the patients will require
prolonged transport. Risking intubation initially may be preferable to risking unobserved airway obstruction later.

C. BREATHING ASSESSMENT

    1. Look at the patient and ask yourself if he is moving
"enough" air with each breath.
    Rationale: Although this requires judgment of tidal vol-
ume adequacy rather than its exact measurement, your evaluation can be sufficiently accurate. Assess adequacy of breathing
by observing the chest movements and the degree of respiratory
effort, and by cupping your hands in front of the nose/mouth to
feel the breath. During disasters, management decisions cannot await more accurate measurements (i. e. , ABGs). If tidal

volume is insufficient, you must control the airway as discussed above since reduced tidal volume can result from partial
airway obstruction. Relieving the obstruction can correct the
hypoventilation.

2. If controlling the airway does not reverse the hypoventilation, insert an endotracheal tube and control ventilation
with

    a) A hand-powered bag ventilator (e. g. , Ambubag$^{®}$)
    b) An oxygen-powered resuscitator (e. g. , Marion valve
       ventilator$^{®}$)
    c) A volume or pressure-regulated ventilator (e. g. ,
       MA-1)
    d) A high pressure O_2 tube fed directly from wall or
       tank outlet. This will require alternately opening/
       closing a side port on the delivery line or opening and
       closing an in-line valve so as not to overinflate the
       patient's lungs.

Rationale: In the best of circumstances, bag-mask ventilation is difficult for the novice to perform effectively; it is
totally out of place for the novice in the disaster setting. Even
mouth-to-mouth ventilation is superior. All other methods of
assisted ventilation require control of the airway with a cuffed
endotracheal tube. Subsequent different ventilation techniques
will depend primarily on what is available to the physician
rather than any absolute physiologic advantage. The key is to
intervene quickly once hypoventilation is diagnosed.

3. Once hypoventilation has been mechanically reversed,
begin a search for reversible causes of hypoventilation.

    a. Pneumothorax (either simple or tension)
    b. Flail chest
    c. Painful rib fractures
    d. Hemothorax

Rationale: These four problems are often clinically obvious; at other times they fail to announce their presence. In
the disaster setting, treatment for pneumothorax and/or hemothorax should be based on the presence of hypoventilation,
which is not due to upper airway obstruction, and a clinical
setting in which they are possible. Delay for chest x-ray confirmation is not appropriate. Suspect flail chest or chest wall
splinting secondary to rib fracture-induced pain when AP or
lateral rib cage compression produces a severe pain response
or detectable chest wall deformation. Chest wall stabilization

and/or intercostal nerve block can decrease interference with air exchange.

In this setting, hypoventilation, secondary to spinal cord injury or head injury, is not reversible. However, if you suspect spinal cord injury, C-spine stabilization or cervical traction may prevent further neurologic damage.

D. CIRCULATION EVALUATION

1. Assess the adequacy of the patient's cardiac output by palpating the radial, femoral, and carotid arteries. Compare the patient's capillary filling time to your own.

Rationale: The presence of a palpable radial pulse indicates a BP of over 80 mmHg; a palpable femoral pulse indicates a BP of over 70 mmHg; a palpable carotid pulse indicates a BP of over 60 mmHg. The capillary filling time gives a reliable indication of microcirculation adequacy. Therefore, low cardiac output states can be clinically detected with equipment which is literally at the physician's fingertips.

2. If the cardiac output is inadequate, consider the following causes:

a) Hemorrhage (either internal or external)

Rationale: External hemorrhage of major proportion, especially in dependent body areas, can be overlooked unless you see the entire patient. Fortunately, external hemorrhage can usually be controlled with direct pressure, occasionally assisted with ligatures. You can easily overlook internal hemorrhage unless you carefully seek it out. In the trauma victim with inadequate cardiac output and no signs of external hemorrhage, consider the possibility of hemorrhage into the pleural spaces, peritoneum, retroperitoneum, pelvic area, or leg compartments. Chest tube evacuation of the pleura may help control hemorrhage by allowing lung expansion; pneumatic trousers (military antishock trousers [MAST]) can decrease peritoneal, retroperitoneal, pelvic, or thigh hemorrhage.

b) Pericardial tamponade

Rationale: The occurrence of hypotension refractory to combined hemorrhage control and volume repletion suggests this diagnosis—especially in patients with penetrating chest or abdominal wounds, or in patients with severe, direct blunt chest trauma. In the hypovolemic patient, tamponade can even be present in the absence of distended neck veins and/or narrowed pulse pressure. Transthoracic pericardial aspiration can rapidly reverse the effect of tamponade on cardiac output.

c) Myocardial dysfunction

Rationale: Myocardial contusion secondary to direct chest wall trauma will produce a decrease in cardiac output. A decreased cardiac output also follows myocardial infarction or exposure to direct myocardial depressants. This diagnosis is important because patients with low cardiac output secondary to myocardial depression may be made worse by fluid administration and/or MAST.

d) Decreased peripheral vascular resistance (PVR)

Rationale: Inhaled or ingested toxic agents, toxic products of tissue breakdown, and toxic products of infectious agents can all produce major reductions in PVR. Effective treatment includes use of vasoconstrictors, volume expanders, and/or MAST.

e) Arrhythmias. Some patients will have cardiac arrhythmias; you can detect them by palpating the pulse. They are only important if they cause a significant reduction in cardiac output.

Rationale: Either brady- or tachy-arrhythmias can significantly reduce cardiac output. In patients with already compromised cardiac output, loss of atrial contraction with atrial fibrillation/flutter can produce clinically significant decrease in cardiac output. Even during a disaster, rapid evaluation of arrhythmias by EKG will be relatively easy, due to the almost universal presence of battery operated portable cardiac monitor/defibrillators. Similarly, arrhythmia treatment, in accordance with ACLS protocols, will be possible using drugs kept in omnipresent "crash carts."

After consideration of these aspects of a patient's condition and correction of detected abnormalities, the patient should live through the remainder of your initial assessment. However, without the remainder of that assessment, he may not live for long. The second phase of the initial assessment examination detects more subtle abnormalities which, if not reversed, will kill the patient during evacuation or while awaiting definitive care.

E. OXYGENATION EVALUATION

Observe the patient for signs of ineffective delivery of oxygen
to tissues (i. e. , cyanosis or otherwise unexplained mental
confusion/agitation). If they are present, consider the following
treatable causes:

1. Ineffective breathing (see C above)
2. Inhaled poisons of O_2 transport mechanisms, such as
    carbon monoxide and freon (which displace O_2 from
    hemoglobin), or cyanide (a poison of mitochondrial en-
    zymes)
3. Preexisting lung disease

Rationale: If this diagnosis is not considered specifically, it will be missed; missed with it will be the opportunity to
treat with oxygen, which is the only potentially available therapy.

F. GENERAL SECONDARY EXAMINATION

1. Begin by completely stripping the patient.

Rationale: This is the quickest way to find all the problems (conversely, not stripping the patient is the quickest way
to miss them). Patient modesty can be preserved if the purpose
of the disrobing is explained, and if the patient is properly
draped when moved to a holding area (patients are able to suspend modesty during emergency medical evaluation; however,
it suddenly reappears when that evaluation concludes).

2. Collect, write down, and attach to the patient a minimum
    data base derived from the patient's statements, state-
    ments of people accompanying the patient, statements of
    rescue workers, ID tags, and contents of the patient's
    purse/wallet. This should include:

    a. Demographics (name, age, sex, race)
    b. Medications normally taken
    c. Chronic problems normally under physician's care
    d. Prior major surgical procedures
    e. Medication allergies
    f. Time of last food/drink
    g. The patient's answer to the question, "What else
        should I know about you?"

Rationale: This information will be important regardless of the nature of the disaster; each part of it is designed to detect aspects of the patient's predisaster status, which will influence, or be influenced by, their injury or illness.

G. FOCUSED SECONDARY EXAMINATION

1. The remainder of the examination must discover remedial defects which would otherwise remain hidden and quietly kill the patient. You must perform it with a clear view of the disaster's character; thus it is not in a preordained format.

Rationale: Each disaster is different, and the predictable consequences of one may only rarely occur in another (i. e. , inhalation injuries are rare following tornadoes; major trauma is not a common accompaniment of infectious epidemics). Still, when working during a disaster, you must keep in mind that there can be mixed medical components in victims of all disasters (e. g. , heart attacks following tornadoes, inhalation injuries following chemical tank ruptures during earthquakes, motor vehicle accident injuries in refugees fleeing damaged nuclear power plants).

2. You should literally conduct your focused secondary examination from head to toe, paying particular attention to commonly forgotten items—items forgotten to the patient's detriment.

a) Determine visual acuity.

Rationale: Injuries which decrease visual acuity have an urgency similar to those which threaten limbs.

b) Search eyes of unconscious patients for contact lenses or foreign bodies.

Rationale: Their presence can destroy an eye in less than 24 hrs.

c) Search for midface fractures.

Rationale: These injuries frequently have concomitant cribiform plate fractures which contraindicate nasogastric or nasotracheal intubation.

d) Stabilize the cervical spine in patients whose injury patterns or findings increase the likelihood of C-spine injury.

    (1) Face/head injuries
    (2) Acceleration/deceleration injuries
    (3) Patients with neck pain and altered neurological findings in arms/legs/anus

Rationale: This stabilization may be required for a long period if x-ray facilities are not available or are overloaded.

e) Perform a rectal (and, in females, a digital pelvic) exam.

Rationale: This will detect subtle, but deadly, injuries to the urethra or rectum as well as detect lower cord injuries.

f) Check the stability of the pelvis.

Rationale: This will detect pelvic fractures which, when present, have large associated retroperitoneal hemorrhages that require treatment.

g) Examine the range of motion and neurovascular integrity of the arms and legs.

Rationale: Displaced fractures can often be sufficiently reduced (without x-rays) to reverse arterial or nervous compromise. If they are not detected and relieved, they lead to amputation.

h) Perform peritoneal lavage only if detecting or ruling out intraperitoneal hemorrhage or bowel perforation will alter your therapy or evacuation plans.

Rationale: During disasters, in the absence of surgical capability or rapid evacuation capability, the knowledge derived from a peritoneal lavage frequently does not change management, but it does consume time, supplies, and personnel.

i) Do not insert a Foley catheter into males without checking prostatic integrity by digital rectal exam and observing for blood at meatus.

Rationale: Attempting to catheterize a patient with a ruptured prostatic urethra or disruption of the uretheral wall will produce new injuries. You can detect prostatic urethral

Eyes	Open	Spontaneously........ 4
		To verbal command 3
		To pain................ 2
	No Response. 1
Best Motor Response	To verbal command	Obeys................. 6
	To painful stimulus*	Localizes pain......... 5
		Flexion-withdrawal 4
		Flexion-abnormal...... 3 (Decorticate rigity)
		Extension .... 2 (Decerebrate rigidity)
		No response 1
Best Verbal Response**		Oriented and converses............ 5
		Disoriented and converses............ 4
		Inappropriate words 3
		Incomprehensible sounds................ 2
		No response 1
TOTAL		3-15

*Apply knuckle to sternum, observe arms
**Arouse patient with painful stimulus if necessary

Figure 5-2. Glasgow coma score.

rupture by digital rectal examination; blood at meatus points to wall disruption.

    j) Use the Glasgow Coma Scale (Figure 5-2) to measure

patient's neurological function.

Rationale: This examination is easily and reproducibly carried out by the next people in an evacuation chain. Thus, changes in a patient's condition are more easily detected than if only adjectives (e. g. , confused) are used (see Chapter 25 for score significance).

k) Examine the skin for burns or discolorations.

Rationale: Such injuries to the skin point to other injuries.

l) Examine the teeth and upper and lower jaws.

Rationale: Fractured/avulsed teeth can get into the airway. Also, oral injuries can produce airway obstruction from blood clots or later swelling. Jaw (upper or lower) fractures can lead to airway compromise from later swelling or from the tongue's falling posteriorly.

H. WRAP UP OF THE INITIAL EXAMINATION

1. You can now query the patient as follows:

   a) "Tell me briefly what happened. "
   b) "What is wrong with you?"
   c) "How ill/injured are you?" "Why do you think so?"

Rationale: Osler was correct; patients frequently can tell you what is wrong with them. If they don't know, you are no farther ahead. However, if they do tell you what is wrong, give their impression strong consideration.

2. At this point you should be able to answer the following questions:

   a) Is it safe to discharge this patient?
   b) Does this patient require observation? If so, what is to be observed?
   c) Does this patient require (available) care now, or should he be evacuated to receive care elsewhere?

Answering these questions concludes the initial evaluation.

III. SUMMARY

If pressed into service during disasters, you must rapidly examine large numbers of patients, discovering and treating both obvious and subtle life/limb threats. As in other aspects of medical function during disasters, you will be better able to aid your patients if you have earlier contemplated how you plan to act. By carrying out a structured examination as discussed in this chapter, you will miss little of significance. At the same time, you will not waste effort and thus delay care to other patients who need you. Once practiced, the examination is easy to perform; if it is not practiced, it will not aid you or your patients when you need it.

BIBLIOGRAPHY

Committee on Trauma, American College of Surgeons: Advanced Trauma Life Support Course, 1981.

United States Department of Defense: Emergency War Surgery. Washington, D. C. , U. S. Government Printing Office, 1975.

Chapter 6

STANDARD PROCEDURES IN CASUALTY CARE
Barry W. Wolcott, M. D.

I. WHAT ARE STANDARD OPERATING PROCEDURES (SOPs)?

Standard Operating Procedures are preplanned ways to react to
given situation; they answer the question, "What do I/we do
if. . . ?" SOPs may be as simple as "the first person finding
evidence of a fire will sound the alarm"; likewise they may be
as complex as a statewide disaster plan. SOPs are valuable because they direct your response to elements of a disaster in
the following three ways:

    1. Preplanned SOPs mean you need not plan for disaster
management during the stress of the disaster.
    2. SOPs represent the best thoughts of experts who will
probably not be present when the disaster occurs.
    3. Other disaster workers can predict your actions without
talking to you since they know that the SOPs will be guiding
your responses.

    Numerous SOPs governing medical responses to disasters
already exist. These include SOPs which meet the requirements
of the Joint Commission for Accreditation of Hospitals (JCAH)
for hospital-wide disaster response planning, city-county civil
defense plans, EMS area disaster plans, and similar plans for
military installations, airports, nuclear power plants, etc.
Unfortunately these SOPs may be of little use to an individual
thrust suddenly into a disaster as a provider rather than as a
planner/organizer. This is because of the common deficiencies
of these disaster response SOPs (Figure 6-1).

    1. SOPs assume the disaster will occur when all func   ial
areas are fully equipped and staffed. Therefore, they ar   ۽-
quently unworkable during a disaster that occurs at an ١   ıl
time, e. g. , 2 a. m. on Sunday.
    2. SOPs are too complex to be followed during the stress
of a disaster by people who are unfamiliar with them. The authors of the SOPs forget that most people never plan for disasters nor read plans for disaster operations written by someone
else.

94

GOOD SOP's

1. Sparing of Resources
2. Outlining Simple Solutions
3. Maximizing Use of Shortcuts
4. Demanding Only Pre-Existing Motor Skills
5. Focusing on a Few Crucial Issues

BAD SOP's

1. Assuming Normal Staffing Patterns
2. Detailing Complex Solutions
3. Continuing the Normal Bureaucracy
4. Requiring New Motor Skills
5. Addressing the Trivial

Figure 6-1. Characteristics of good and bad SOPs.

3. SOPs require that all administrative safeguards taken during normal operations continue during disaster response. While this appears desirable to planners during normal operations, such patently ridiculous requirements as "a complete admission process will occur for each treated patient" quickly bring all aspects of the SOPs into disrepute—and disuse.

4. SOPs anticipate that, during a disaster, people will learn new, complex, manual procedures by reading about them (e. g. , "Emergency Thoracotomy SOP for the Novice"). During the Vietnam War, nonsurgically trained physicians did indeed become adept at debridement, cutdowns, and chest tube insertions. They learned these skills by working with surgeons, not by reading SOPs; and it took weeks for them to become truly competent.

5. SOPs spend many pages addressing trivial or uncommon problems. (Few workers really care how the hospital plans to deal with requests for vegetarian diets during a disaster.)

All the above deficiencies seem to indicate the hopelessness of designing effective disaster situation SOPs for individual practitioners. In fact, they mean that useful SOPS must have specific characteristics:

1. They must be resource-sparing and be implementable
by the least trained/experienced person who could be involved.
2. They must be simple and be presented in an easy to read
and follow format.
3. They must recognize and encourage use of appropriate
shortcuts during the disaster.
4. They must require no new motor skills of the worker.
5. They must address common problems whose solution
will contribute meaningfully to the disaster control effort.

Some useful disaster SOPs are described below.

II. SOPs FOR CARE OF NONURGENT ILL/INJURED PATIENTS

During the postdisaster period, especially if it is prolonged,
medical workers will be confronted with many people suffering
from minor ailments or injuries. Even in war, military medical workers care for patients with colds, headaches, and blisters. A well-functioning triage system can detect, among these
patients, the small minority at significant risk of serious illness (e. g. , the meningitis among the headaches). Such a system can also direct the symptomatic therapy of these nonurgent
conditions with minimal physician involvement. A triage system
of this sort should work in conjunction with the physician-
operated triage system evaluating the obviously urgently injured and ill. To spare medical assets and to return workers to
disaster relief, such a system must be implemented early in
the course of the disaster response. Two such triage systems
have particular merit in the disaster setting. One is described
by Vickery et al. in the book, Take Care of Yourself;[1] the
other is outlined in the Army Medical Department publication,
Algorithm Directed Troop Medical Care. [2] Both are useful systems which a provider can easily adapt to serve as a disaster
SOP (Figure 6-2).

III. SOPs FOR TRIAGE OF TRAUMA VICTIMS

Numerous studies have tested scoring systems purported to
predict survival of trauma victims. These systems are based
on clinical parameters which can be easily and reliably gathered
by rescue workers. Clinical trials show:

1. Such scoring systems do reproducibly distinguish groups
    of patients with differing probabilities of survival.

NAUSEA / VOMITING / DIARRHEA
TRIAGE ALGORITHM

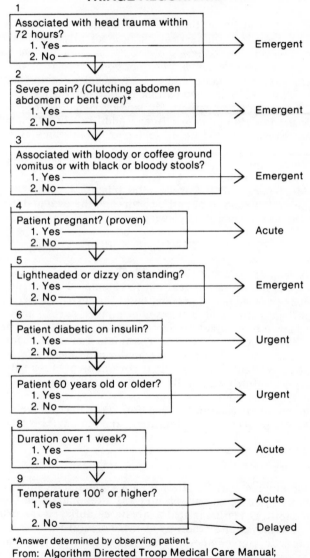

*Answer determined by observing patient.

From: Algorithm Directed Troop Medical Care Manual;
US Army Health Services Command, Ft. Sam Houston,
TX 78234. Attn. DSC-PA

Figure 6-2. Minor illness injury triage.

2. The relative predictive value is independent of the soph-
    istication of the medical care given. *

The clinical utility of these scoring scales is limited in normal medical settings where everything medically possible is
done for everyone and where knowing that a given patient has
only a 30% chance of survival does not commonly alter therapy.
However, during a disaster, knowing how salvageable one patient is compared to another patient will directly affect care.
Easy to learn scoring systems, if used by rescue workers, will
simplify the job of the triage officer. Additionally, when used
by rescue workers in the field, such scoring systems allow:

1. More rapid and precise communication with hospital-
    based physicians.
2. More sophisticated prehospital triage.
3. Selective routing of patients through the evacuation sys-
    tem based upon injury severity.

IV. SOPs FOR TRIAGE OF BURN PATIENTS

There is something about the individual burned patient which
stresses and deranges medical care systems. The degree of
this stress is often out of proportion to the threat of the injury
to the patient's life, and appears due in large part to an unusually high degree of medical worker identification with the burn
victim. Frequently, workers overestimate the urgency for burn
center treatment. In the rush to transfer, they may overlook
more life-threatening needs of that person or of other patients.
Workers sometimes wastefully transfer fatally burned patients
because they underestimate the severity of injury and overestimate the potential benefits of transfer. Both errors are costly
to individual patients, their families, and society. However,

---

*All such studies analyze clinical data collected on each patient
  in terms of individual patient survival after maximum therapy
  at that facility. Mathematical analysis establishes the probability of survival after therapy at that hospital for a group of
  patients with a given score. One would expect that the more
  sophisticated the care available, the higher the survival; indeed that is the case. However, independent of the medical
  sophistication of the treating institution, patients with different
  scores still have predictably different relative probabilities of
  survival (i. e. , it is always better to be a 15 than a 2).

BURN INDEX

		Score
Sex	Female	0
	Male	1
Age	0-20 Years	5
	21-40 Years	4
	41-60 Years	3
	61-80 Years	2
	81-100 Years	1
Inhalation Injury		1
Full Thickness Burn		1
Total Body Surface Burn	1-10%	10
	11-20%	9
	21-30%	8
	31-40%	7
	41-50%	6
	51-60%	5
	61-70%	4
	71-80%	3
	81-90%	2
	91-100%	1
TOTAL		

Total Burn Score	Threat to Life	Probability of Survival
12-13	Very Low	.99
10-11	Moderate	.98
8-9	Moderately Severe	.8-.9
6-7	Serious	.5-.7
4-5	Severe	.2-.4
2-3	Maximum	≤.10

Figure 6-3.   A triage scoring system for burn victims.

since in many disaster settings, burn victims will be common, health workers must have a method of dealing with such patients which minimizes disruption of overall patient care. Workers at the University of Virginia (Figure 6-3) have developed a burn severity scoring system which functions like the previously discussed trauma severity scoring system. [4] Such a system allows rescue workers and triage officers to sort burn victims rapidly into groups of differing potential survival rates and then to decide on treatment and evacuation plans. It seems reasonable to postulate that by allowing rescue workers to rely on expert opinion as outlined by the burn severity score, such a structured system would reduce the emotional stress burn patients place on the members of triage teams.

V. SOPs FOR TRAUMA VICTIM MANAGEMENT (Figure 6-4)

The initial management of the trauma victim is discussed elsewhere in this book. Since certain motor skills are involved, such management cannot be reduced to a clinically useful SOP. However, once the patient's initial management is complete, and the observation/reevaluation period begins, problem-specific SOPs, which meet the guidelines discussed earlier in this chapter, can be very useful to a physician who normally does not care for such patients. An excellent collection of such SOPs is in The Shock Trauma Manual. [4]

VI. COMMON PROBLEMS ARE COMMON

As noted earlier, few physicians get involved in disaster planning. However, readers of this book may desire to become more involved. What follows is a discussion of common problems that occur in the initial phase of disaster relief. These are problems you may face personally to which you could devote some planning time when developing SOPs for your own use.

A. COMMUNICATIONS

1. If the telephone service remains in operation, most incoming lines to physicians' offices and hospital information/paging desks will be jammed by information seekers. Suggestion:

   a) Have a pay station in the area and keep sufficient coins for 400 phone calls secured nearby.
   b) Keep a list of the "unlisted" numbers of wards/labs/offices you may wish to call. The public will be unable to jam numbers not listed in the phone book.
   c) Pocket pager systems may remain operative and will allow one way communication.

2. If phone communication is interrupted, most people will attempt to use CB or police/fire/EMS radio nets. These will probably become overloaded early. Instead:

Retroperitoneal Hemorrhage Algorithm
(EXAMPLE)

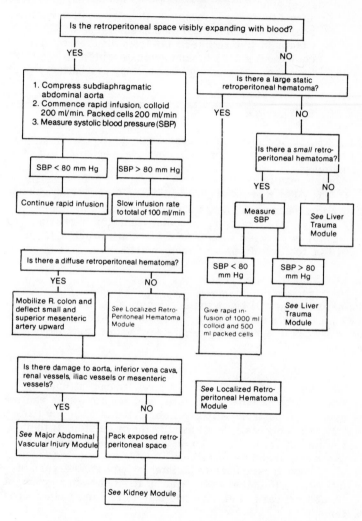

Figure 6-4   Trauma management algorithms.

a) Use runners with messages written on your prescription blanks. This will identify the notes as originating from your facility (see example for components of an adequate written message). Require written replies because memories fail during emergencies.

b) Obtain hard wire intercoms from local electronic equipment stores to communicate within your facility; they are easily and quickly set up, are battery operated, and work well.

B. CROWD CONTROL

Police will be occupied elsewhere. Your medical facility needs will probably have to be controlled by local nonpolice workers. <u>Suggestions</u>:

1. Establish and mark approach lanes for arriving and departing rescue vehicles, walking wounded, and others.
2. Put an intelligent, resourceful volunteer in charge, and let him/her come to you only if there are problems; you will be too busy to be a policeman also.

C. NEWS MEDIA CONTROL

The news media will be on the scene almost as soon as you are. News media personnel must be channeled so that their activity and questions do not markedly interfere with patient care. <u>Suggestions</u>:

1. Operate on the principle: Unless it is preventing me from helping the most people I possibly can, it isn't worth worrying about now. In general, you and the media can co-exist. If reporters truly are interfering in <u>what you personally are doing,</u> tell them; usually they will stop. If they don't stop, treat them like disruptive patients—with an overwhelming show of force.
2. If reporters appear to be interfering with the work of others, let the others worry about it. Remember, your job is medical care. Let someone else worry about other problems.

D. WATER SUPPLY

The water distribution system may fail early on; leaks/heavy usage may so lower pressure that running water is not available. <u>Suggestions</u>:

1. Send a runner to the nearest supermarket to pick up distilled/bottled water. If necessary, give the supermarket owner a receipt for the purchase so he/she may be reimbursed later.
2. Inquire about local springs/reservoirs/streams/wells/ swimming pools as water sources.
3. Use motor homes as water carriers and pumpers (most have 50 gallon storage and water pumps).

NOTE: Be careful people do not carry drinking water in containers which were used earlier to carry petroleum products. Drinking from such containers will produce a secondary mass casualty problem.

E. ELECTRICAL SUPPLIES

Frequently disasters cause loss of power distribution. Emergency power generators must preferentially power hospital elevators, ORs, ICUs, etc. Usually there is little power for the triage area. Suggestions: Many recreation vehicles have 1100-3600 watt generator capacity with 1-2 days of gasoline on board the vehicle; one or two of these generators can be used to power a very sophisticated triage/initial assessment area.

F. SUTURE MATERIAL WILL BE AT A PREMIUM

Lacerations are common problems in any disaster. They are treatable and people want something done for them. Unfortunately, treating them can rapidly use up all the available suture supplies at a time when resupply is impossible. Suggestions:

1. Use delayed primary closure on all wounds. Not only does this save suture, but it is also good medicine in this environment.
2. Use tape closures if primary closure is deemed appropriate.

G. BANDAGING AND SPLINTING MATERIAL WILL BE IN SHORT SUPPLY

For the same reasons described above, bandaging and splinting material will become scarce. Suggestions:

1. Alternate bandaging material includes sanitary napkins (from neighborhood supermarkets), cloth (from fabric stores), masking and duct tape (from hardware stores), and sheets and towels (from department stores).

2. Alternative splinting supplies include chainlink fencing, disassembled wooden fences, and wood from lumber yards.
3. Doors and shutters can serve as makeshift backboards.

VII. SUMMARY

Prior planning can help; however, it must realistically assess the setting in which disaster response will occur as well as the natural tendency of most people to worry about that possible future event. Health workers should be certain they think their own actions in their own small area in advance before they embark on large scale plans for others to follow. Problems should be identified before health officials consider solutions which they can personally implement.

REFERENCES

1. Vickery, D. M. , and Fries, J. F. : Take Care of Yourself. Philippines, Addison-Wesley Pub. Co. , 1976.
2. U. S. Army Health Service Command (DCSPER): Algorithm Directed Troop Medical Care. Triage Manual (Training Manual). Fort Sam Houston, Texas.
3. Champion, H. R. , and Sacco, W. J. : Trauma Risk Assessment: Review of Severity Scales. Emergency Medicine Annual. Norwalk, Conn. , Appleton-Century-Croft, 1983.
4. Gill, W. , and Long, W. B. : Shock Trauma Manual. Baltimore, Williams & Wilkins Co. , 1979.

Chapter 7

COMMUNICATIONS
Patricia H. Sanner, M.D.

I. INTRODUCTION

Communication is a vital aspect of any contingency medical operation. Poor communications may be the most significant obstruction to effective rescue and medical treatment during a natural or manmade disaster. One must coordinate all conventional modes of communications for use during a disaster and plan an emergency communications network in the event that all or most of the conventional means are damaged or destroyed. Prior areawide or regional planning is mandatory and should address the following questions:

A. Who needs to talk to whom?
B. What information is needed?
C. What methods of communication can be utilized?

II. COMMUNICATIONS NET—WHO NEEDS TO TALK TO WHOM?

A. FORWARD OR ON-SCENE COMMUNICATION

1. Report of Event. Usually, the primary report of a disaster event comes to the authorities via two agents. The first agent on the scene, generally a law enforcement officer, communicates a report of the event to his/her headquarters including all the particulars of what, where, when, estimated damage and casualties, etc. This report activates various other agencies who must respond to the event. The second agent of primary report communication is a lay observer or ambulatory victim who leaves the area and communicates directly with a public agency such as the fire department, hospital, or police, thus activating the disaster chain response.

2. Disaster Command Post Communication. Once disaster response personnel begin arriving on the scene, an on-scene command post (CP), which includes a communications center,

should be established. The on-scene communications center
must maintain communication with

a) Fire and other hazard control personnel
b) Law enforcement personnel
c) Rescue teams
d) Medical command post
e) Rearward command post
f) Evacuation staging area
g) Military
h) Other agencies functioning at the scene (e. g. , Red Cross,
   Civil Defense, etc.)

3. Medical Command Post Communication. The medical command post maintains communication with

a) Rescue teams
b) Triage collecting point(s)
c) Evacuation staging area
d) Field (on-scene) command post
e) Rearward medical command post
f) Rearward disaster command post

B. REARWARD COMMUNICATION

1. Alert Phase. Many potential disasters, such as tornadoes
and floods, have a warning period. When an event has occurred
or is occurring but the extent of damage/injury is not known,
there is also a warning phase.
    There are two aspects of communications during the alert
phase:

a) Securing and opening a communications net by whatever
   means necessary
b) Mobilizing essential personnel

    Key personnel, such as fire and police chiefs, hospital ad-
ministrators, triage officers, and nursing supervisors, are
usually mobilized via a recall system. A recall system may
utilize telephone communication, two-way radios, paging devices, or any combination of these modalities. This system is
also used to recall off-duty personnel required to augment the
usual staff. A recall system must be planned and tested in advance. One must also anticipate other means to reach personnel
if telephone communications should be disrupted, such as the
following:

a) Media announcements (radio, television)
b) Loudspeakers or sound trucks
c) Messengers, such as law enforcement personnel
d) A buddy system, with each key person in the recall net responsible for alerting or confirming the alert of a given number of persons.

2. Hospital Communications

a) Control Hospital-Medical Command Post

One hospital should be designated as the control hospital. All communications from forward areas and rearward disaster agencies come through this control center to coordinate rearward medical operations. The control hospital must be in communication with:

(1) Other Hospitals. To receive reports of bed capacity, medical and surgical capabilities, staffing, blood supplies, the number of casualties received and what each facility needs.

(2) Rearward Command Post. To obtain traffic control, law enforcement support, vehicle coordination, Red Cross assistance, and additional supplies.

(3) Forward Medical Command Post. To obtain information regarding the number of and types of casualties.

(4) Forward Disaster Command Post. To learn of any special hazards such as chemicals or radioactive materials contaminating victims.

(5) Evacuation Staging Areas. To receive reports of which patients are being moved, when, and by what mode of transport, and their destination.

(6) Medical Facilities Outside Disaster Area. To ascertain their ability to provide additional assistance and special care facilities, such as a burn unit.

b) Interhospital Net

Communication between all medical facilities involved in the disaster response is necessary. However, operations are best coordinated through the central control hospital to make optimal use of resources.

c) Intrahospital Net

Each responding hospital must maintain communication with its various patient care and supply areas, especially the emergency treatment area, central supply, operating rooms, laboratory and blood banks, and intensive care units.

Anticipate the disruption of telephone communications and plan for alternate modes within the hospital (e.g., intercom systems and messengers).

C. COMMUNICATION OUTSIDE OF DISASTER NET

A consistent observation made in most disaster studies is that there is a tremendous movement of people, supplies, and messages toward the disaster area. This convergence behavior significantly hampers rescue and relief efforts, especially transportation and communication. One way to control convergence behavior is by managing communication outside of the disaster net.

1. Inquiries about Victims

Numerous people will seek out the hospital to learn if friends or relatives are victims. Multiple inquiries will rapidly jam any hospital switchboard. An information center, using a separate switchboard or telephone trunk line and volunteer personnel, can be established outside the hospital to process the flood of calls.

2. Media

Accurate information from the forward and rearward command posts must be supplied to the radio and television networks. Arranging a brief delay (e.g., 30 mins) in the media announcements of a disaster event would assist disaster personnel in channeling the expected convergence behavior. Law enforcement officers, for example, would have some time to establish roadblocks and checkpoints to control access to the disaster site.

III. NECESSARY COMMUNICATION —
WHAT INFORMATION IS NEEDED?

A. THE EVENT

The initial report of a disaster event must include the following

information: What happened, where, when, estimated number
and type of casualties, a damage report, and description of any
special hazards.

Information regarding the event is continually updated as
the situation changes (worsens, improves, or is resolved).

B. WHAT IS NEEDED?

Initial communication of a disaster event to the rearward agencies may give an indication of what will be needed to cope with
the situation. Once a forward command post is established,
these needs can be further defined and communicated to appropriate rear agencies. Special needs may include:

1. Rescue, clearing, and repair equipment and per-
    sonnel (e.g., firefighters, power companies,
    cranes, earthmovers, etc.)
2. Medical assistance
3. Special hazard control (e. g. , radioactive materials and
    chemical leakage)

C. WHAT RESOURCES ARE AVAILABLE?

A list of resources available to assist in disaster relief must
be communicated to the rear command post and then to the forward command post. The status of the following should be ascertained:

1. Fire and law enforcement agencies
2. Civil Defense groups
3. Red Cross agencies
4. Military units
5. Heavy rescue equipment; utilities repair personnel and
    equipment.
6. Medical resources (personnel, space, and supplies—in-
    cluding blood)
7. Evacuation resources (ground, air, and assets to handle
    special needs such as water or snow)
8. Special agencies (e. g. , to handle radioactive material,
    chemicals, or other contamination)

IV. MODES OF COMMUNICATION

One very important consideration during a disaster is that the
most frequently used mode of communication, the telephone, is
usually disrupted or very easily overloaded. Prepare to

communicate without this valuable link or to utilize it efficiently.

A. EFFICIENT USE OF CONVENTIONAL TELEPHONE LINKS

Convergence behavior will rapidly overload hospital and law enforcement agency trunk lines. This interference with essential communication can be overcome by several methods.

One method is to establish a disaster hotline with unlisted phone numbers between various agencies such as hospitals, ambulance units, and law enforcement headquarters. Hospital pay phones are an important asset; they only require the personnel to commandeer the telephone(s) and a supply of coins (which can be kept in the hospital safe or obtained from the cafeteria, snack bar, or gift shop). Conference lines, teletype, or computer links are other forms of telephone communication that can be used.

B. ALTERNATE FORMS OF COMMUNICATION

1. Two-way Radios with Base Station

This system must be established prior to the event and be in accordance with Federal Communications Commission regulations. * Portable radios must have at least a 2 mile range. Attention must be given to installing equipment with maximum permissible output wattage.

2. Military Resources

If a two-way radio system has not been established prior to the disaster event, the military is a valuable resource. Many active and reserve units are accustomed to field communication and have an available supply of radios, antennas, batteries, and field telephones, as well as trained personnel to establish and operate the equipment.

3. Law Enforcement Agencies

These departments routinely use some form of radio or two-way radio/base station communications.

4. Citizen's Band Radio Operators

---

*FCC: Special Emergency Radio Service. FCC Rules and Regulations. Part 89, Subpart O.

5. Amateur Radio Operators (HAM)

These individuals are extremely valuable resources. They have the required equipment, technical knowledge, and repair ability to maintain communication under adverse conditions.

6. Messengers

Since messengers can use various means of transportation, they should be utilized; however, they must receive careful instructions as to where they are going and to whom the message should be delivered, as well as information and instructions for their return.

7. Megaphones and Sound Trucks

V. SUMMARY

Communication is an extremely important aspect of any contingency medical operation. Success demands innovation and anticipation that conventional means will be unavailable, at least for a portion of the time. Disaster communications are dynamic with a continuous need for update and the relaying of information. A key aspect of disaster planning is the coordination of area-wide disaster communication.

BIBLIOGRAPHY

American Hospital Association: Readings in Disaster Planning for Hospitals. Chicago, 1966.

Garb, S., and Eng, E.: Disaster Handbook. 2d ed. New York, Springer Publishing Co., Inc., 1969.

Gierson, Eugene D., and Richman, Leon S.: Valley triage: An approach to mass casualty care. Trauma 15, 3:193-196, 1975.

National Academy of Sciences: Convergence Behavior in Disasters: A Problem in Social Control. Publication 476. Washington, D.C., National Research Council, 1957.

Storer, Daniel L.: Disaster planning: communications. Ohio State Med J 75:401-402, 1979.

Texas Department of Public Safety: Disaster Emergency Planning: A Manual for Local Governments. Austin, Texas, Department of Public Safety. 1974.

U. S. Department of Health, Education, and Welfare: Hospital Planning for National Disaster. Washington, D. C. , H. E. W. , Public Health Service Division of Health Mobilization, 1968.

Chapter 8

PREEVACUATION AND EVACUATION PLANNING

Part I: Aeromedical Evacuation
Randall B. Case, M.D.

I. INTRODUCTION

The decision to evacuate casualties by aircraft from the site of
a disaster to receiving medical facilities is the final step in the
triage process. It constitutes both a prescription for an individual patient and a transport strategy for a given disaster. It is a
complex, multifactorial decision, involving judgments of an
aeronautical, aeromedical, and emergency medical nature.
This section deals with the aeronautical, aeromedical, and
planning considerations in aeromedical evacuation.

II. AERONAUTICAL FACTORS

A basic understanding of aeronautical factors will help the
physician know what aeromedical evacuation can and cannot do,
and why. These factors are weather, geography, and aircraft.

A. WEATHER

Weather may represent either a contraindication or indication
for aeromedical evacuation.

    1. Poor Visibility. Fog, low cloud cover, haze, precipita-
tion, and dust storms may restrict areas available for safe
takeoff and landing, or necessitate circumnavigation enroute.

    2. Turbulence. Especially prevalent near thunderstorms
and in areas of high winds, turbulence may either exceed the
safe operational limits of the aircraft or require a slower enroute cruise; or in clinical circumstances such as a fractured
cervical spine, it may do the patient definite harm.

    3. Wind. Apart from its potential for inducing turbulence,
strong wind may either prolong or shorten transport time, or
it may exceed the safe operational limits of a given aircraft.

4. <u>Aircraft Icing.</u> Aircraft icing may occur whenever visible moisture (e. g. , fog, clouds) or precipitation exist, in air which is at or within 10°F below freezing, and may prevent safe flight.

5. <u>Precipitation.</u> Snow, sleet, hail, and rain may be associated with poor visibility, turbulence, wind, or aircraft icing. It may also, as in the case of hail, damage the aircraft structure.

6. <u>Situations of Relative Advantage.</u> Conversely, there are certain weather conditions in which aeromedical evacuation is especially advantageous, e. g. , when weather inhibits ground access as with deep mud or flooding following heavy rains, or when roads are impassable following heavy snows or natural disasters. Helicopters are of particular value in such circumstances. Another such situation exists when imminent or existing weather conditions require immediate action, e. g. , in the case of predisaster evacuation or when the rescue involves a problem caused by exposure to extremes of temperature.

B. GEOGRAPHY

Geography may also represent either a contraindication or an indication for aeromedical evacuation.

1. <u>High Altitude.</u> Areas at high altitude may be beyond the performance capability of the available aircraft. The limits of the specific aircraft need to be weighed against the geographical area in question.

2. <u>Landing Site.</u> The geography of a specific landing site may also preclude safe operations. While helicopters are much more flexible than airplanes in this respect, they still require a cleared and reasonably level landing site, free of obstructions such as wires, antennas, and tall buildings in the approach/ departure corridor.

3. <u>Situations of Relative Advantage.</u> There are two geographical situations in which aeromedical evacuation is especially advantageous:

a) Where there is limited or no access via roads, such as in wilderness or mountainous areas, over water, or on islands; in metropolitan areas with congested traffic; or where roads have been destroyed by an enemy or are in enemy hands.
b) Where surface transport covers a significantly

greater distance than direct air transport, such as across a bay or in hilly terrain.

C. AIRCRAFT

The aircraft represents the most variable aeronautical factor. The most significant variables are cabin size, useful load, range, cruising speed, service ceiling, landing site requirements, navigation and communication equipment, and medical equipment. No aircraft is ideal with respect to each of these, and the specific requirements will depend upon the mission at hand. Predisaster familiarization with each type of aircraft potentially available for aeromedical evacuation will enable the physician to obtain best usage when the need arises.

1. Cabin Space. Cabin space often places an undesirable restriction on the amount of equipment and the number of patients, as well as the placement of, and access to, both.

2. Useful Load. The term, useful load, defines limits on the amounts and placement of fuel, equipment, crew members, and casualties. Since cabin space often represents the greater limitation on the number of litter casualties that can be carried, more patients can generally be carried when ambulatory. Furthermore, if the transport distance is relatively short, fuel loads may be limited to enhance carrying capacity.

3. Range. Apart from its relationship to useful load, the range required for a mission may render one aircraft more suitable than another by necessitating a stop enroute for fuel. An aircraft with greater speed, but lesser range may thus effect a slower transport to the destination.

4. Cruising Speed. Cruising speed must be assessed against both transport distance and wind. The longer the distance and the stronger the headwind, the more important cruising speed becomes.

5. Service Ceiling. Service ceiling defines the maximum altitude the aircraft can safely maintain; it must obviously be weighed against origin, enroute, and destination geography.

6. Landing Site Requirements. Landing site requirements impose obvious limitations, both at the scene of the disaster and at the receiving medical facility.

7. <u>Navigation and Communication Equipment</u>. The amount and type of this equipment on board the aircraft influences the degree of adverse weather that can be safely handled, as well as the area of airspace within which the aircraft may be legally operated. A serious operational handicap is imposed if the aircraft is not equipped with the necessary medical frequencies which permit communication with emergency medical personnel both on site, and at the receiving medical facility.

8. <u>Medical Equipment</u>. Medical equipment on board the aircraft may vary from nothing but a litter, to a "mini-ICU," and must be compatible with the aircraft systems.

III. AEROMEDICAL FACTORS

Aeromedical factors encompass altered human physiology under conditions of flight, and the impact of flight upon a wide range of clinical states.

A. AEROMEDICAL PHYSIOLOGY

Aeromedical physiology involves the phenomena of hypoxia, changing gas volumes, accelerative forces, temperature extremes, low humidity, noise, and vibration.

1. <u>Hypoxia</u>. Hypoxia, with its well-known clinical effects, is often encountered in flight as a consequence of altitude. In accord with Dalton's law, in a mixture of inert gases, the total pressure exerted is equal to the sum of the partial pressures of each gas alone ($P_T = P_1 + P_2 + \cdots + P_n$). At sea level on a standard day, atmospheric pressure is 760 mmHg and oxygen concentration is 21%; the oxygen partial pressure is 160 mmHg. Because the body temperature and humidity are nonstandard, and because alveolar CO_2 is also nonstandard, the actual alveolar oxygen partial pressure (PaO_2) is closer to 103 mmHg. But the principle of Dalton's law still applies; as the total atmospheric pressure diminishes with increasing altitude, the PaO_2 diminishes proportionately. These effects are usually experienced less in helicopters than in airplanes, because of generally lower cruising altitudes. Consider two examples at altitudes typical of those to which patients would routinely be exposed during an airplane flight. At 5000 feet MSL (mean sea level), standard atmospheric pressure is 632 mmHg, and PaO_2 is 80 mmHg. At 10,000 feet MSL, standard atmospheric pressure is 523 mmHg, and PaO_2 is 61 mmHg. Given a normal alveolar-arterial oxygen gradient ($AaDO_2$) of 10 mmHg,

possibly more if the patient is ill or injured, the hypoxia expected in flight can be appreciated. In fact, if the patient's baseline arterial oxygen partial pressure (PaO_2) is known (e. g. , from an arterial blood gas), his in-flight PaO_2 may be approximated by the equation:

$$PaO_2 \text{ in-flight} = 20 + (2/3 \times PaO_2 \text{ baseline}) - (3 \times \text{cabin altitude [in thousands of feet]})$$

General approaches to minimizing hypoxia include administration of supplemental oxygen, pressurization of the cabin, and/or cruising at low altitude. Administration of 100% oxygen at 34,000 feet MSL yields a PaO_2 equivalent to breathing air at sea level.

2. <u>Changing Gas Volume</u>. The changes in ambient pressure encountered upon ascent and descent have additional significant consequences, i. e. , changing gas volume and changing solubility of gases in the fluids and tissues of the body. In accord with Boyle's law, the volume of a gas is proportional to temperature and inversely proportional to pressure. ($V = \dfrac{KT}{P}$ where V is the volume of gas, K is a constant, T is temperature, and P is pressure). Given a constant cabin temperature, the volume of a gas expands as the aircraft ascends, and vice versa. In a standard atmosphere, the volume of a gas doubles at 18,000 feet MSL. Since conditions within the body are nonstandard, gas expands 100% above sea level volume at somewhat less than 18,000 feet MSL and expands 50% above sea level volume at approximately 10,000 feet MSL. As with hypoxia, this phenomenon is usually encountered in both pressurized and unpressurized airplanes, but less in helicopters.

General approaches to minimizing changing gas volume and its consequences include: preflight insertion of an NG or chest tube, preflight or in-flight use of decongestants, use of plastic IV fluid bags, filling of ET tube and Foley catheter balloons with saline rather than air, pressurization of the cabin, and/or cruising at low altitude. The remaining aeromedical phenomena apply equally to airplanes and helicopters.

3. <u>Accelerative Forces</u>. Accelerative forces, inherent to transportation of any kind, exert a clinical effect primarily upon the cardiovascular and labyrinthine systems. There are also mechanical effects which alter gravity-driven IV flow rates and render weight-and-pulley traction devices unusable in flight. Accelerative forces in flight derive from several sources.

Turns, take-offs, and landings are associated with predictable accelerative forces. Turbulence induces unpredictable G-forces.

General approaches which may be used to minimize these accelerative forces include gentle pilot technique, avoidance of known or potentially turbulent areas, loading patients transverse to the long axis of the aircraft, and utilizing aircraft with favorable turbulent-ride characteristics.

4. Temperature Extremes. Temperature extremes, which exert well-known effects on metabolism, hydration, and cardiovascular physiology, depend mostly on the individual aircraft and its environmental control systems. While temperature usually decreases with altitude, almost all aircraft have heating systems capable of maintaining cabin warmth. Conversely, many aircraft experience a greenhouse effect in warm, sunny climates, and not all have air conditioning. This can result in heat stress to patients and crew alike. General approaches to minimize temperature extremes include selecting aircraft appropriately equipped for the environment, using sun-reflective liners in aircraft parked out-of-doors, and flying with the cabin doors open.

5. Humidity. The customary lack of humidity in aircraft cabins enhances evaporative loss and predisposes to inspiration of airway secretions and to dehydration, especially in neonates and burned patients. General approaches used to minimize this are anticipation of the problem with appropriate regulation of fluid intake and irrigation/suction of airways.

6. Noise. Noise is quite loud (over 90 db) even in the quietest cabin, and is associated with both clinical and operational effects. Clinically, it represents a potentially permanent hearing loss hazard to neonates and enhances patient anxiety. Operationally, it impedes communication between patient and crew and among crew, as well as rendering certain medical equipment, such as the stethoscope and cardiac monitor or respirator alarms, useless.

General approaches to minimize noise include the use of individual earplugs, of intercom headsets among crew members, and of special medical equipment, such as Doppler blood pressure measuring devices.

7. Vibration. Vibration is variable, depending upon the individual aircraft. Vibration may intensify patient anxiety, impair fracture immobilization, and interfere with medical

procedures, such as starting an IV, performing a cutdown, or intubating a patient. It also may interfere with medical equipment such as EKG monitors.

General approaches to minimize vibration include selection of appropriate aircraft, shockmounting medical equipment, and preflight performance of potentially necessary medical procedures.

B. CLINICAL STATES

Numerous clinical states are altered by the phenomena of aeromedical physiology. Such alteration of both the physiology of acute and preexisting conditions must be taken into account in making a series of related decisions: (1) Should aeromedical evacuation be done at all? (2) If yes, what preflight diagnostic or therapeutic preparations are necessary? (3) What should the inflight circumstances be?

These decisions involve few absolutes; rather, like the decision to perform surgery, they involve judgments regarding relative risks. Contraindications to aeromedical evacuation are only relative, and must be carefully considered in context.

1. <u>Relative Contraindications</u>. The relative contraindications to aeromedical evacuation include decompression sickness, severe respiratory insufficiency, untreated pneumothorax, severe congestive heart failure, recent myocardial infarction, severe anemia, sickle-cell disease, seizure disorder, and impulsive or unruly behavior.

2. <u>Hematologic States</u>. The hematologic states of significance are the anemias and the sickle-cell variants. Obviously, hemorrhage and anemia diminish the body's ability to deliver oxygen to the tissues. Considering that the oxygen requirements of injured tissue exceed those of healthy, resting tissue, the combination of anemia, tissue injury, and hypoxia may result in cellular anaerobic metabolism, with all its sequelae. The sickle-cell variants compound the problems of anemia, with the potential for vasoocclusive crisis, even at altitudes as low as 4000 feet MSL, and even in sickle-cell trait.

3. <u>Cardiovascular Disorders</u>. The cardiovascular disorders of significance are primarily ischemic heart disease and congestive heart failure. Ischemic heart disease is adversely affected by both the hypoxia as well as the hemodynamic effects of accelerative forces encountered in flight. Congestive heart failure of whatever etiology may also be exacerbated by the accelerative forces encountered in flight.

4. <u>Pulmonary Disorders</u>. Most pulmonary disorders are of significance, since they diminish arterial oxygenation. Infections, such as pneumonia or bronchitis; infiltrations, such as sarcoidosis or pulmonary edema; obstructions, such as asthma or emphysema; and mechanical disruptions, such as pneumothorax or flail-chest; are all adversely affected by hypoxia. Some conditions, such as pneumothorax or emphysema, are adversely affected by changing gas volume. Patients with a pneumothorax should have a chest tube with a one-way valve in place prior to aeromedical evacuation.

5. <u>Neurosurgical Conditions</u>. The neurosurgical entities of significance are increased intracranial pressure (ICP), intracranial air, and cervical-spine fracture. The clinical importance of increased ICP is well appreciated. Hypoxia increases ICP, and thus exacerbates ICP-mediated pathology. Intracranial air, whether introduced intentionally during ventriculography, incidentally during recent neurosurgery, or accidentally during trauma, represents a real risk in aeromedical evacuation. Expansion of the trapped intracranial air during ascent may compress neural tissue and/or raise ICP. Cervical spine fractures present practical difficulty with immobilization. In all cases, traction should be maintained by spring devices, rather than weights.

6. <u>Orthopedic Conditions</u>. The above caveats regarding cervical spine fractures apply with respect to other fractures as well. If casts are applied, they should be bivalved (or not be encircling) to accommodate fluid shifts and swelling induced by accelerative forces and changing gas volumes, as well as to enhance emergency egress from the aircraft if needed. Ideally, but this is often impractical in the disaster medicine setting, casts should be dry before flight.

7. <u>Burns</u>. Serious burns present several special considerations for aeromedical evacuation:

a) The low cabin humidity at altitude, or when air-conditioned, and the greenhouse effect in warm, sunny climates, increases evaporative fluid loss. More fluid replacement should be anticipated in flight than in the hospital. If the flight will be of significant duration, a Foley catheter to monitor urine output and a central line to monitor CVP are both desirable in gauging fluid replacement needs.
b) Circumferential eschars, like encircling casts, present a risk of compromising distal circulation or diminishing

respiration in flight. Appropriate escarotomies should be performed before flight.

c) One should consider the possibilities of inhalation injury and carbon monoxide poisoning.

8. ENT Problems. ENT problems are relatively frequent and usually involve changing gas volumes in the middle ear or sinuses. The ear is most commonly affected on descent, the sinuses on either ascent or descent. Preflight prophylaxis with nasal vasoconstrictor spray and/or oral decongestants is often helpful.

9. GI Problems. The GI tract also normally contains some air, which may expand on ascent and cause either pain or rupture of a viscus. The risk of rupture is increased in conditions which weaken the viscus wall, such as in peptic ulcer disease, strangulated hernia, bowel obstruction, acute appendicitis, diverticulitis, typhoid, amoebiasis, and recent GI surgery.

10. Ophthalmologic Conditions. Several ophthalmologic conditions are of significance. Any air in the globe—from penetrating trauma or from surgery—presents the risk of expansion on ascent, with consequent ocular hypertension or rupture of the globe. Hypoxia causes a dilation of retinal and choroidal vessels with increasing introcular pressure. Patients with pre-existing retinal or choroidal hemorrhage are at risk for a re-bleed. Hypoxia also induces miosis which may complicate clinical assessment of head-injured patients. Such miosis is usually bilaterally equal, however. Finally, low cabin humidity enhances corneal drying and ulceration in eyes exposed by ectropion, traumatic flap, or coma. These eyes should have lubricating drops or ointment instilled and be taped shut.

11. Decompression Sickness. Decompression sickness is probably as close to an absolute contraindication for aeromedical evacuation as one can find. Yet, the potential time saved in transport to the nearest hyperbaric chamber might justify aeromedical evacuation if pressurization or low level flight is feasible. When aeromedically evacuated, these patients should be carried with their left side and head down, and breath 100% oxygen.

12. Dermatologic Conditions. The dermatologic conditions of significance are those which enhance evaporative fluid loss and those which produce gas. Such gas-producing infections may be mechanically spread by the expansion of gas in tissues upon ascent.

13. <u>Obstetrical Patients</u>. Apart from the space and equipment limitations of the cabin in the event of delivery, obstetrical patients present no special problems for either mother or fetus, nor does there appear to be any demonstrable risk of premature labor. Patients advanced in pregnancy should be accompanied by appropriate obstetrical equipment.

14. <u>Neonatal Patients</u>. Neonates are actually well-adapted for aeromedical transport. Their left-shifted, hemoglobin-oxygen dissociation curves, higher hemoglobin levels, and tissue adaptation to lower oxygen tensions give them a greater tolerance for hypoxia as compared to adults. Conversely, their less well-developed thermoregulatory mechanisms and greater body surface area/mass ratios require close attention to the maintenance of temperature and hydration enroute.

15. <u>Dental Conditions</u>. The only dental condition of significance is intermaxillary fixation, which requires either a quick-release device or accompanying wire cutters to protect the patient from possible aspiration of vomitus. Some patients will complain of fillings hurting with changes in altitude, but this problem is benign and self-limited.

IV. PLANNING

A. BEFOREHAND

A number of important factors should be considered in the process of planning for aeromedical responses to disasters:

1. What are the terrain features and predominant weather patterns in the region of interest?
2. Where are medical facilities located?
3. What are the expected strengths and weaknesses of aeromedical evacuation in such an environment?
4. What aeromedical resources, both equipment and people, exist in this region and what advance arrangements have been made for their use?
5. What landing sites exist, and in what proximity to medical facilities; under what weather conditions might they be usable?
6. What procedures, if any, might be needed for on-site or medical facility air traffic control, in both favorable and adverse weather?
7. What ground transport, if any, might be required to link landing sites with medical facilities?

8. what communications equipment exists in the aircraft, in the medical facilities, and for disaster control; and how do they interface?

9. What types of training (including aeromedical training) have been, or should be, carried out with which personnel to ensure safe and effective aeromedical operations?

B. DURING A DISASTER

Shifting our perspective to a given disaster, the following factors should be considered to optimize aeromedical operations:

1. What are the aeromedical factors, i. e. , what are the present and forecasted weather and the geography on-site, en-route, and at the receiving medical facilities?

2. What are the number, types, and capabilities of the aircraft now available?

3. Are the weather and geography in any way likely to limit aeromedical operations and, if so, for which types of patients or aircraft?

4. What are the alternate modes of transport available, and how do they compare in these circumstances?

5. What are the number and types of casualties and their location?

6. Who would benefit most from aeromedical evacuation?

7. What preflight preparations are required and for which casualties, to evacuate them safely (see below)?

8. What time and resources will such preparations take?

9. Given the probability that evacuation resources of all varieties will be inadequate, reassess the relative speed of aeromedical evacuation versus other modes of evacuation for a given patient. (It may be faster to send the patient on the first ground ambulance than on the third trip via helicopter.)

10. Establish and continually update the priorities for out-bound transport of each casualty, as well as inbound transport of supplies and personnel required.

V. PATIENT AEROMEDICAL PREPARATION CHECKLIST

A. SUPPLEMENTAL O_2

Supplemental O_2 should be provided to patients with cardiac or pulmonary disease, thoracic injury, anemia, sickle-cell hemoglobinopathy, increased ICP, significant burns, glaucoma, recent retinal or choroidal hemorrhage, decompression illness, seizure disorder, or carbon monoxide poisoning.

B. NG TUBE

NG tubes should be passed on patients with a potential for
ileus (e. g. , major trauma, burns, coma, acute abdomen, etc.),
respiratory embarrassment (e. g. , COPD, pregnant, Pickwick-
ian, thoracic injury, etc.), GI rupture (e. g. , PUD, hernia, obstruction, acute abdomen, amoebiasis, recent GI surgery), or
those who are being mechanically ventilated.

C. CHEST TUBE

Chest tubes should be placed on patients with known or strongly suspected hemo/pneumothorax.

D. DECONGESTANTS

Preflight decongestants should be administered to patients with
sinus or middle ear infections or swelling.

E. OCULAR LUBRICANTS

Ocular lubricants should be instilled in the tyes of comatose
patients or those with ectropion.

F. MOTION SICKNESS PROPHYLAXIS

Motion sickness prophylaxis should be administered to patients
known to be prone to this disorder, especially if turbulent
conditions are anticipated, or if vomiting should be suppressed
(e. g. , intermaxillary fixation, cerebrovascular accident, severe cardiac disease, burns, GI bleeds, or postoperative from
abdominal/thoracic/ophthalmic surgery or from neurosurgery).

G. SEIZURE PROPHYLAXIS

Seizure prophylaxis should be administered to patients with
known, but untreated, seizure disorders, or with significant
head injury.

H. SEDATION/RESTRAINT

Sedation and restraint should be considered for unruly patients.

I. EQUIPMENT

Catheter balloons should be filled with saline rather than air.
IV bags should be plastic (if they are glass, they should be
wrapped with tape and vented). Traction devices should be of
the spring type and casts should be bivalved. Survival equipment should be aboard for each occupant.

J. HEARING PROTECTION

Noise dampening headset/microphone devices should be available for each crew member, and earplugs or earmuffs be provided for patients, when practical.

K. PATIENT POSITIONING

Patients generally should be carried transverse to the longitudinal axis of the aircraft. If this is not possible, cardiac
patients should be carried with head to the rear, and patients
with increased ICP or intraocular pressure with head to the
front. Patients with decompression sickness should be carried
with left side and head down.

L. PRESSURIZATION OR LOW LEVEL FLIGHT

The aircraft should be pressurized to ground level or the flight
conducted at low level (at or below 1000 feet above ground
level) for patients with pneumothorax, intracranial air, intraocular air, gas gangrene, ileus or the potential for ruptured
viscus, a cavitary or cystic lesion, or decompression illness.

BIBLIOGRAPHY

Aeromedical Evacuation. U. S. Army Health Services Command.
28-2038-4, 1980.

Air Ambulance Guidelines. U. S. Dept. of Transportation/
American Medical Assoc. DOT HS 805-703, 1981.

Army Flight Surgeons Manual. U. S. Army Aeromedical Center.
ST 1-105-8, 1976.

Aviation Weather. U. S. Dept. of Transportation, Federal Aviation Administration. AC 00-6, 1965.

Basic Helicopter Handbook. U. S. Dept. of Transportation,
Federal Aviation Administration. AC 61-13A, 1973.

Flight Surgeon's Guide. U. S. Department of Air Force. AFP
161-18, 1973.

Instrument Flying Handbook. U. S. Department of Transportation, Federal Aviation Administration. AC 61-27B, 1971.

Pilot's Handbook of Aeronautical Knowledge. U. S. Dept. of
Transportation, Federal Aviation Administration. AC 61-23A,
1971.

Part II: Ground Evacuation
Patricia H. Sanner, M.D.

I. INTRODUCTION

Medical evacuation in a disaster can have two distinct aspects:
(1) Movement of casualties from the impact area to a safe zone
or medical facility for treatment. (2) Movement of a fixed medical facility to a safe area. Medical contingency planning must
include both of these situations.

II. CONSIDERATIONS IN GROUND EVACUATION PLANNING

A. NATURAL LINES OF EGRESS

Victims of any natural or manmade disaster usually leave an
impact area by predictable routes, such as highways. Inter-
cepting ambulatory casualties along the natural lines of egress
should be anticipated.

B. CONVERGENCE BEHAVIOR

Convergence behavior is a consistent observation made in
most disaster events studied. The tremendous movement of
people, vehicles, and supplies, both authorized and unauthor-
ized, toward the disaster site, may significantly hamper any
movement of casualties from an impact area. Convergence behavior probably cannot be aborted. However, it can be channeled so as not to interfere with rescue and evacuation efforts.
Some ways to channel convergence are as follows:

1. Media Lag Time. With the cooperation of local radio
and TV stations, bulletin announcements of a disaster event can
be delayed for a short period of time. This permits law enforcement agents to establish road blocks and controlled access in
advance of the expected convergence.

2. Controlled Entry and Diversion Routes. Initially, only
authorized personnel should enter an impact area so that effective rescue and relief can occur. This can be accomplished
with controlled entry points and an identification system using
uniforms, reflective vests or caps, a disaster ID card, etc.

Establishing a direct, controlled evacuation route and a
diversion route to control sightseers is another way to channel
convergence behavior. Limit the number of private automobiles
in the area to those required by essential personnel.

III. CASUALTY EVACUATION

A. DIRECT EVACUATION

Certain victims who are minimally injured and ambulatory
leave the impact site on their own along the natural lines of
egress. Other victims are immediately transported by law and
professional rescue personnel. Two problems are inherent in
direct evacuation:

1. It overloads the nearest medical facility without regard
for staffing or capability.
2. Less seriously injured victims are frequently transported first as these casualties are able to ambulate to rescue
vehicles or personnel. No triage occurs with direct evacuation.

B. STAGED EVACUATION

Utilized by the military, staged evacuation is a better method
for casualty movement. The self-selected victims who
have already left the impact area cannot be controlled. However, those along the natural lines of egress and at the impact
site can be handled in an orderly fashion. Staged evacuation has
three aspects:

1. Triage of victims.
2. Establishment of collecting points either by triage or by
sector of the impact area.
3. Movement of triaged patients from collecting points to
facilities most capable of treating the injuries and numbers of
casualties. The appropriate facility for each casualty may not
be the most proximate. Minimally injured patients can be transported to the more distant treatment facilities.

IV. MEDICAL FACILITY EVACUATION

Situations develop in which a medical facility is damaged or in
an endangered area. The term medical facility includes acute
care hospitals and chronic care facilities such as nursing homes,
psychiatric facilities, and rehabilitation centers. Evacuation of
a medical facility involves:

A. SELECTION OF AN EVACUATION SITE

A safe location outside the impact area must be secured.
This may be a single site, such as a school, gymnasium, or
other adaptable structure. Evacuation of a medical facility can
involve movement of patients to several, separate locations,
such as other hospitals, outside the impact area.

B. PREPOSITIONING SUPPLIES AND PERSONNEL

If there is sufficient warning, evacuation can be anticipated.
Specified personnel can proceed to the selected evacuation site
in advance with the equipment and supplies required for initial
operation. Advance personnel could include a nursing supervis-
or to coordinate patient placement; maintenance personnel to
adapt electrical sources, lighting, ventilation, etc. , to patient
care needs; and patient care personnel. Equipment and supplies
needed to begin operation include cots, basic medications and
IV solutions, dressing material, equipment for airway control
and manual ventilation, and food and water. A hospital disaster
plan should incorporate this advance party into its planning.
This can be done by designating specific personnel and tagging
certain equipment and supplies from each hospital area as the
advance group. Another way is to prepare and store an evacuation kit or chest in each unit.

C. ORDERLY EGRESS

Evacuation of a medical facility must proceed in an orderly
manner to avoid further injury and delay. Several methods can
be implemented such as egress by floors, patient care unit
areas, hospital wings, etc. One must determine how patients
are to be moved if elevators are not functioning. It is also very
important to decide what to use in moving nonambulatory patients (gurneys, litters, and wheelchairs are more practical
and mobile than conventional hospital beds).

D. VEHICLES

As patients and personnel are removed from the building, vehicles are required to transport them to the evacuation site(s).
Standard medical vehicles can be utilized to transport the most
critical patients who require ongoing care. Most other patients
may be safely and efficiently transported using other large vehicles, such as buses, trucks, or moving vans. Law enforcement
escort or volunteer traffic control facilitates movement.

V. EVACUATION TRANSPORTATION

A. STANDARD MEDICAL VEHICLES

Standard ambulances can be used, but they are usually limited in number and also in the amount of patients who can be transported per vehicle. Conventional ambulances are best used to transport the most critically injured or the highest priority casualties.

B. OTHER VEHICLES

In mass casualty evacuation, success depends on innovation and adaptation. Many vehicles have been used to move multiple casualties. Private automobiles and taxicabs are one solution. Other ideas follow:

1. Buses. Buses are excellent for transporting large numbers of ambulatory patients. If necessary, litters can be placed across seats. Several attendants can be transported with the patients.

2. Moving Vans. A large number of ambulatory, seated, and litter patients can be transported in a moving van. Lighting and ventilation are improved by opening the side doors.

3. Trucks and Vans. These vehicles are useful to move a variable number and class of patients. Inclement weather restricts the use of open bed trucks.

4. Railroad Cars. Usefulness of rail transportation depends on location and proximity of rail lines to disaster and evacuation sites.

C. SPECIAL CIRCUMSTANCES

Certain disaster situations require special vehicles to evacuate casualties. For example, during a flood, needed boats and rafts can be obtained from private citizens, the U.S. Coast Guard, etc. Snow usually requires special equipment on rescue vehicles such as tire chains or a mounted snowplow. Some snow conditions require more specialized equipment like snowmobiles or sleds. Landslides or volcanic ash may require earthmoving equipment to secure access.

VI. SUMMARY

Successful evacuation of casualties or medical facilities requires planning and creativity. An important aspect is to channel the expected convergence behavior to allow evacuation of
casualties. A staged evacuation with casualty triage, collection,
and movement to appropriate facilities is the most efficient and
effective system.

Standard emergency medical vehicles may be in short supply. Adapting other vehicles expedites orderly movement of
many casualties from the impact area and to treatment facilities.

BIBLIOGRAPHY

Garb, S. and Eng, E. : Disaster Handbook. 2d ed. New York,
Springer Publishing Co. , Inc. , 1969.

McGrath, R. : Use trucks to transport the injured. Mod Hosp
86:70, 1956.

Schwartz, George R. , et al. : Principles and Practice of Emergency Medicine. Vol. II. Philadelphia, W. B. Saunders Company, 1978.

Texas Department of Public Safety: Disaster Emergency Planning: A Manual for Local Governments. Austin, Texas, Department of Public Safety, 1974.

U. S. Department of Health, Education, and Welfare:
Washington, D. C. , H. E. W. , Public Health Service Division of
Health Mobilization, 1968.

Chapter 9

PUBLIC HEALTH AND SANITATION DURING DISASTERS
Craig H. Llewellyn, M.D.

INTRODUCTION

Preceding chapters have emphasized the principles of emergency care of mass casualties using triage. In this chapter the concept of triage is extended to the affected population or community and its health care and environmental health services.

Rapid and accurate initial assessment and prioritization are equally important in both emergency care and in public health activities. Emergency care is essential to the casualties but contributes little to the subsequent relief effort. Triage of community public health problems is fundamental to all subsequent relief efforts. It offers the only real hope of damage limitation and prevention of later secondary health problems which may dwarf the initial emergency care requirements.

There are direct parallels between the physician's approach to the individual casualty in triage and the epidemiologist's approach to the community in assessment and evaluation. The past history for the emergency physician is the baseline of disease and environmental sanitation for the epidemiologist. The emergency physician elicits a chief complaint and performs a physical examination. The epidemiologist carries out rapid assessments, surveys and ongoing surveillance to identify and prioritize problems requiring intervention. Each then monitors the identified problem and the response to intervention. Each is totally dependent upon current and accurate information as a basis for decision. In the public health activities, haste in beginning relief efforts should be traded off for acquisition of good information as the basis for relief actions.

Thus, the message of this chapter is to obtain accurate information, identify, define, and prioritize problems using simple assessment and survey methods. The epidemiologic approach to disaster relief management is indispensible if waste and compounding of the disaster are to be avoided.

DISASTER MYTHS AND REALITIES

During the past decade, the application of epidemiologic and public health techniques to disaster assessment, management, and research has called into question the following assumptions:

1. Disasters cause significant mortality and an associated high number of casualties which require emergency hospitalization.
2. Disasters cause massive social disruption with widespread panic and paralysis of action throughout the community.
3. Epidemic disease is associated with disasters.
4. Disasters leave survivors utterly dependent on outside assistance.

Table 9-1 shows relationships between health effects and types of disasters; particularly in the case of care requirements for severe injuries and the potential for increases in communicable diseases. In the Iranian earthquake of 1968, only 368 (3.3%) of the 11,000 persons treated by emergency services required hospitalization. Experience with recent earthquakes in Peru, Nicaragua, and Guatemala has shown that the requirements for emergency care peaks in the first 24 hrs and returns to normal levels in 72-96 hrs, before any major outside assistance arrives. Floods kill many but injure few. Windstorms cause few deaths or injuries.

Epidemics of infectious disease have rarely been associated with disasters since World War II. However, the risk of increased transmission usually exists, particularly if the disaster causes population relocation; increase in population density; or disruption of normal health care or of environmental health and lifeline services, such as food, transportation, and power. Immunization programs are rarely required as part of disaster relief, but epidemiologic surveillance, disease control, and environmental health surveillance are essential. It is mandatory that normal services, which include vector control, be reinstituted as soon as possible.

Disasters do not produce widespread panic in survivors, nor is the community paralyzed into inactivity. In minutes to hours, spontaneous rescue activities begin; and purposeful, though often inefficient, activity is underway. Thus, the affected population can and will accomplish much of its own rescue and relief, but it will require direction. This direction will only be credible if based upon a sound appreciation of the current situation. Accurate information from repeated assessments is essential to keep the survivors informed, to direct

Table 9-1. Short-Term Effects of Major Natural Disasters*

Effect	Earthquakes	High Winds (Without floodings)	Tidal Waves/ Flash Flood	Floods
Deaths	Many	Few	Many	Few
Severe injuries requiring extensive care	Overwhelming	Moderate	Few	Few
Increased risk of communicable diseases	Potential risk following all major disasters (Probability rising with overcrowding and deteriorating sanitation)			
Food scarcity	Rare	Rare (May occur due to factors other than food shortage)	Common	Common
Major population movements	Rare	Rare (May occur in heavily damaged urban areas)	Common	Common

*Public Document: Emergency Health Management After Natural Disaster—Scientific Publication No. 407, Pan American Health Organization. World Health Organization, Washington, D. C., 1981.

their efforts, and to quell the rumors which abound following disasters. The timely dissemination of accurate information will maintain and enhance cohesion in the affected population.

Many effects of disasters are potential rather than actual health risks. Disruption of normal community behavior, sanitation and health services, combined with crowding and population displacement to areas with inadequate services, are all potential health risks. Unlike the casualties caused at impact, these effects and potential risks can be greatly ameliorated if identified and monitored early in the rescue and relief phase.

Both the actual and potential health risks and attendant relief needs fluctuate at various times during the disaster period; they also vary in their intensity and degree of importance in the disaster area (Figures 9-1 and 9-2). For this reason, repeated assessments and surveillance must be instituted rapidly following impact and must be continued throughout the relief and recovery period.

Rarely are the needs for health care, food, and shelter total in the wake of disaster. Assessments and surveys are indispensable aids to authorities in organizing rescue and relief operations, redistributing resources in the stricken area, setting priorities for outside assistance, and dealing with rumors, both in the affected population and among media representatives. Field hospitals are not required when there are many dead people, but only a few injured survivors. Reallocation of patients to less damaged or better staffed and supplied health care facilities may, however, be indicated.

While each disaster is unique, significant similarities exist. Recognizing these will optimize health relief management and resource allocation. Disaster myths can be dispelled only by the acquisition of appropriate and accurate information. Public health and epidemiologic methods for assessment and surveillance are required for systematic identification and prioritization of problems.

THE ROLE OF THE PHYSICIAN

The nonspecialist in public health or epidemiology has a significant role to play in these actions. Beginning with his/her role in the planning and organizing process, and proceeding through the activities and responsibilities of supervisor, evaluator, and consultant, the physician must continually be prepared to deal with affected community and population problems in the same manner as emergency care requirements. In many instances, he/she will be a participant in a health care team, while in others he/she may be the only available health professional.

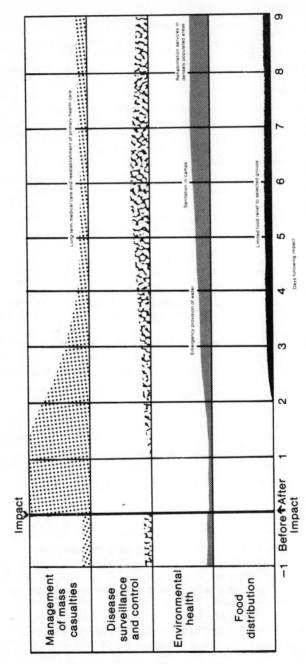

*PUBLIC DOCUMENT: *Emergency Health Management After Natural Disaster* – Scientific Publication No. 407, Pan American Health Organization. World Health Organization, Washington DC, 1981

Figure 9-1. Changing needs and priorities following earthquakes. *

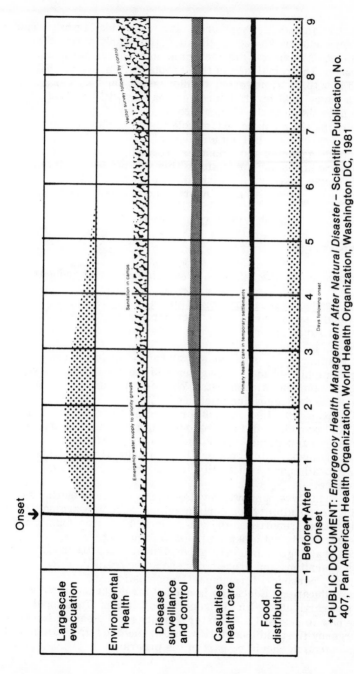

Figure 9-2. Changing needs and priorities following floods/sea surges. *

*PUBLIC DOCUMENT: *Emergency Health Management After Natural Disaster* – Scientific Publication No. 407, Pan American Health Organization. World Health Organization, Washington DC, 1981

The physician should, therefore, have some idea of what needs to be done and how to accomplish it, particularly during the first three days after a disaster—the emergency rescue and relief phase. The remainder of this chapter will address what to do and how to do it; however, the discussion must necessarily be at a superficial level. Interested readers will find basic references listed in the bibliography.

Perhaps the most important role the physician can play is that of reassuring relief authorities, affected population, media, and outside agencies and volunteers regarding rumors of unmet health care needs and epidemics. This will not be possible if the physician restricts his activities to the care of the sick and injured and ignores the remainder of the affected population.

WHAT TO DO AND HOW TO DO IT

PREDISASTER

The emphasis here must be on prevention and preparedness.

1. <u>Conduct a Disaster Threat Assessment</u>. Determine to what disasters the community/region/population is at risk. Review past experiences in the area and similar experience elsewhere.

2. <u>Vulnerability Assessment</u>. What facilities, services, and geographic subunits or segments of the population are vulnerable to the potential threats? What is a conservative estimate of the damage which might occur?

3. <u>Inventory</u>. List available resources to prevent, ameliorate, and provide relief and recovery if a disaster occurs. This includes organizations, agencies, reporting systems, communication, transportation, power, lists of critical individuals, items, location and availability, and sources of possible outside assistance.

4. <u>Plan Development</u>. Develop a broad flexible outline assigning responsibility for certain actions such as warning, alert, mobilization, reporting, and other functions during and after a disaster; this is not a detailed how to document.

5. <u>Training</u>. Managers, supervisors, and workers in emergency operations and procedures should be trained. Develop auxilliary personnel throughout the population.

6. <u>Education</u>. Education is needed for government authorities and particularly for the general population. This should include how to respond to disaster warnings and disaster impact. Emergency first aid, sanitation, water and food protection, and communication should be part of the program.

During predisaster planning maps should be obtained. Background data on water systems; sewage systems; food stocks and distribution modes; chronic and communicable disease data in the community; health care facilities, supplies, and equipment; as well as personnel location and availability should be gathered. Health considerations must be integrated into disaster planning at all levels. Disaster relief authorities must be educated concerning the requirements for rapid initial assessment, specific surveys, and ongoing surveillance to obtain accurate data as a basis for relief operations. Many will be unfamiliar with public health and epidemiologic techniques and think of them only in relation to health activities and not to the overall relief effort. Many will want to do something fast rather than make an organized effort to find out what is needed.

DISASTER AND EMERGENCY RELIEF PHASE

From the time of impact through the next three days, rescue and emergency relief occurs. A major hazard at this point is that rescue and emergency relief activities will be continued longer than necessary. This has often occurred when assessment and surveillance activities have not been organized and initiated in the early phase of emergency relief. The unnecessary continuation of rescue and relief activities is wasteful of resources and postpones restoration of required services, thus increasing health hazards to the survivors; it also invites inappropriate outside assistance.

1. Initial Assessment. Rapid evaluation of all aspects of the disaster, including health, is essential for effective rescue and emergency relief. Accurate information takes precedence over speed. Past relief operations have been plagued by exaggerated and conflicting reports. Inappropriate aid has been rushed to the wrong place to deal with a nonexistent problem while serious problems go unidentified.

The initial assessment should:

Define the affected area and its population.
Identify actual categories of needs based upon damage assessment.
Document potential secondary health risks.

Table 9-2 outlines basic information requirements and relative priorities.
The initial assessment should be carried out by the most

Table 9-2. Information Required for
            Emergency Disaster Relief

---

1. The affected population, its composition and
   geographic location

2. The availability of communication and
   transportation

3. The availability of water, food, shelter, and
   basic sanitation

4. The number of casualties

5. The condition and capability of the health
   care system in the area—personnel, supplies,
   facilities

6. The number and location of displaced
   population

7. The number of dead and missing

---

rapid transportation available (helicopters are excellent for
this purpose) and does not require technical experts. Regular
reporting through preexisting systems should be utilized to the
maximum. Reports from community leaders are often exaggerated in order to get priority attention and disguise ignorance of
the true extent of damage. Based upon information obtained
about the affected area, its population, and the damage to lifeline services (e. g. , health, power, water, food, transportation, communication), significant immediate problem areas
should be identified and resources allocated for intervention.
    Within the first 3 days, based upon the findings of the initial
assessment, a specific multidisciplinary survey of the entire
affected area should be made using technical experts familiar
with local predisaster conditions. Emphasis in the health portion should be given to documenting emergency care needs,
long-term hospitalization requirements, environmental health
system damage, and other potential health risks, such as population displacement with inadequate services and increased
population density. The results of this systematic survey
should indicate any unmet emergency relief needs and will provide the basis for a definitive relief plan.

Concurrent with this survey, epidemiologic surveillance for communicable disease and environmental health surveillance should begin. Preexisting systems, procedures and personnel should be used to the maximum. Both types of surveillance are of the utmost importance in evacuation centers or refugee camps due to the explosive potential for increased disease transmission if basic sanitation is not maintained.

Table 9-3 provides a summary after Nieburg's model of various assessment methodologies. The important point is that assessments must be initiated and then continued by a method chosen for its suitability to the available manpower.

Epidemiologic surveillance should concentrate on reporting by syndrome on a daily basis. An example of a reporting form is shown in Figure 9-3. Further information about communicable disease problems associated with disasters is presented in Table 9-4.

Useful models for environmental health assessment surveillance and operations are provided in the addendum at the end of this chapter. The provision of adequate and accessible amounts of safe drinking water takes precedence. Second in importance is the provision of adequate amounts of water for other requirements. Sanitary food handling and preparation assumes great importance in the prevention of enteric disease transmission, not only in the affected population, but also in the relief workers.

Emphasis must be given to the rapid restoration of environmental health and lifeline services and to the detection of any new environmental hazards caused by the disaster, such as spread of and exposure to toxic industrial substances.

The importance of rapid assessment, survey, and continued surveillance cannot be overemphasized. They must begin concurrently with emergency care of casualties and continue throughout the relief and rehabilitation period. The system established and the data obtained will be useful to both health and other relief activities. While the physician need not be expert in conducting these activities, he/she must be aware of their importance, understand the methods available, and be a vigorous proponent for their inclusion in predisaster plans and postdisaster emergency relief.

Table 9-3.   Nieburg's Model for Data Collection Methods in Disaster Situations*

ASSESSMENT METHOD	REQUIREMENTS		DATA GATHERING TECHNIQUES	ADVANTAGES	DISADVANTAGES
	TIME	RESOURCES	INDICATORS		
1. Predisaster "background" data	ongoing surveillance	trained staff	reporting from health facilities and practitioners; disease patterns and seasonability	provides data base to detect problems/ changes	None
2. Remote: airplane, helicopter, satellite	minutes/hours	hardware	eyes; cameras; destroyed buildings, roads, dams, flooding	quick; useful when ground transport out; useful to identify area affected	expensive; large objective error – minimal specific data
3. On-site "walk-through" (ride through)	hours/days	transport, maps	eyes; talks with local leaders and health workers; deaths, homeless persons, numbers and types of disease problems	quick; visible; does not require technical (health) background	soft, (non-specific) data; potential bias; high error rate; "Most-affected" areas may be unreachable
4. "Quick and dirty" surveys	2-3 days	few trained staff	rapid survey(s); deaths, hospitalized, nutritional status, (see also 3)	quick; hard data; can prevent mismanagement; can form basis of surveillance	not always random; labor intensive; risk of overinterpretation
5. Rapid health screening system	ongoing (as needed)	health workers; equipment depends on needed data	collect data from any fraction of persons passing through screen; nutritional status demography, hematocrit parasitemia, etc.	quickly sets up and functions; collects data and provides services (vaccines, vit. A, triage, etc) in migrating populations	minimal resource needs, useful for "closed populations only;" does not reflect "outside" situation
6. Surveillance system	ongoing	some trained staff; standard diagnoses; method of communicating data	routine data collection in standardized manner; mortality/morbidity by diagnosis and age	timely; expandable; trends visible	takes resources to set up and constant vigilance to run; feedback to workers required
7. Survey	variable hours/days	experienced field epidemiologist/ statistician; reliable field staff	random or representative sample selection specific to problem	much specific data in short time	labor intensive (needs epidemiologist and statistician for data interpretation)

*PUBLIC DOCUMENT: Health Aspects and Relief Management After Natural Disasters. Center for Research on the Epidemiology of Disasters, Bruxelles, Belgium, 1980.

Daily Report by_____ For_____
                        Name of Reporter   Date

From | Locating Address | Phone No. |
☐ Evacuation | | |
  Centre | | |
                    | | |
☐ Hospital OPD | | |
☐ Health Centre | | |
☐ Clinic | | |
☐ Other | | |
  Specify........ | | |

NUMBER OF CASES WITH		TOTAL
(1) Fever (100°F + 38°C +)		
(2) Fever and Cough		
(3) Fever and Diarrhea		
(4) Vomiting and/ or Diarrhea		
(5) Fever and Rash		
(6) Other new Medical Problems Specify.....		

COMMENTS:

Complete. For Evacuation Centres only.
No of persons accommodated today_____
Report significant changes in Sanitation/Food Supply Situation.

NOTE: COMPLETE BACK PORTION OF THE FORM FOR THE FIRST
      REPORT ONLY. PLEASE COMPLETE AND SEND REPORT EACH
      DAY.

Figure 9-3.   Postdisaster surveillance (sample reporting form).

Table 9-4. Communicable Disease Problems Associated With
            Disaster Relief Efforts*

Relief Factor	Disease Mechanism	Specific Disease Example(s)
Shelter	Crowding	Meningococcal* meningitis
Water	Contamination*	"Fecal" diseases
Food	Infant formula, tinned or powdered milk	Diarrhea*
Antibiotics	Excessive use*	Resistant bacteria
Injectible iron	Promotes micro-organism growth	Malaria*
Immunizations	Unsterile needles*	Hepatitis
Arriving susceptibles	Absent immunity	Polio, hepatitis*
Arriving "carriers"	Local vectors, imported organisms*	Malaria, Schistosomiasis
Pseudoepidemics	Heightened surveillance	Any*

*Mechanism or example known to have occurred in disaster
 relief effort.

ADDENDUM

I. SPECIMEN TEXT FOR A PAMPHLET ON EMERGENCY SANITATION AT HOME*

Many public services could be put out of action by
natural disasters. If the water utility serving your community were damaged, your household water supply
would be cut off until repairs could be made. If sewers

*From Guide to Sanitation in Natural Disasters, Assar, M.
WHO, 1974, pp. 93-94.

were broken, it would not be possible to dispose of human wastes by the usual methods. The lack of garbage collection and disposal service would encourage the increase of rats, flies, and other disease-carrying agents. It would be hard to maintain the usual flow of food supplies.

Impure water and unsafe food produce disease. Garbage and human wastes can help to spread disease; a dirty home and an unclean body have the same effect. It is therefore important that families take care of themselves until the situation becomes normal or help is received. To do so, simple sanitation rules should be followed at home. A few simple steps that can protect families are described below.

1. Drink only water or other liquids that you know are safe. Store enough water for the family during the warning period.

2. Know where to find the valve that controls the water supply to your home so that you can shut off the supply, if necessary. Try the valve to make sure it works freely. If a tool such as a wrench is needed to operate the valve, be sure you know where to lay your hands on one quickly in an emergency. Learn where to get water for emergency drinking, cooking, and washing if your outside supply fails.

3. Be prepared to purify water for drinking purposes in your own home. There are various methods that can be used:

Boiling: Water can be made suitable for drinking purposes by boiling for 5-10 min. This will destroy the germs.

Chlorination: Bleach solutions of 5% strength may be available. Add 1 drop of the bleach solution for each liter of clear water (3 drops for turbid water). After adding the appropriate amount of bleach, stir, and allow the water to stand for 30 min. A distinct taste or smell of chlorine, which is the sign of safety, should be detected; if not, add a few more drops, wait for 15 min and taste again.

Purification tablets: Tablets that release iodine may be used safely to purify water. Usually one tablet is enough for 1 liter of clear water; for turbid water two tablets should be used.

Tincture of iodine: Ordinary household iodine can be used to purify water. Add 2-3 drops for each liter of clear water (8-10 drops for turbid water); mix and allow to stand for 30 min.

4. Eat only safe foods prepared under safe conditions. Keep a 2-week supply on hand, and replace the
things you use.
5. Avoid using foods or liquids that might be contaminated.
6. Provide for the disposal of human wastes in
covered containers in case flush toilets are inaccessible
or not working; learn how to make soil bags.
7. Bury excreta and your garbage under at least 30
cm of compacted earth.
8. Listen to and observe the instructions of the
health authorities.

II. GUIDELINES FOR THE USE OF TABLET, POWDER, AND LIQUID DISINFECTANTS IN EMERGENCY SITUATIONS*

Providing tablet, powder, or liquid disinfectants to individual
users should be considered only when distribution can be
coupled with the following:

1. A strong health education campaign in which people are
   instructed about how to use them
2. The distribution of containers for water storage
3. The assistance of public health or auxiliary personnel in
   providing the follow-up needed to ensure proper and continued use of the tablets
4. A network for distribution of additional supplies needed
   throughout the emergency phase and into the rehabilitation phase

   In general, these disinfectants should be considered
during an emergency for disinfecting small quantities of
drinking water in limited and controlled populations, on
an individual basis, and only for the limited time period
of 1-2 weeks. Every effort should be made to restore
normal chlorination facilities and to guarantee that water
sources are protected.
   Whenever disinfection is considered during an emergency, careful attention must be given to the initial

---

*From Environmental Health Management After Natural Disas-
ter, Pan American Health Organization. PAHO. Scientific
Publication No. 430, 1982, pp. 47-50.

condition of the water. Turbidity and color should be reduced as much as possible by allowing the water to settle or by straining it through layers of cloth. Once disinfected, the water should be stored in clear, covered, and noncorrodible containers. Before any form of disinfectant is provided to individual users for emergency treatment, public health personnel must be sure the available sources of water to be used are not, and have not been, chlorinated. The chlorine residual should be determined before any disinfectant is distributed to individual users.

The most common agents that can be used to disinfect small quantities of drinking water under emergency conditions are chlorine, iodine, and potassium permanganate. Detailed discussions of each follows.

CHLORINE COMPOUNDS

Tablets

The most common chlorine compound in use is known as Halazone tablets. Instructions for use of Halazone tablets are usually printed on the bottle. If not, one tablespoon (4 mg) should be used in each liter (approximately 1 quart) of water. If the water is turbid or highly colored, the dosage should be doubled. The water should be stirred and left to stand 10 min before it is consumed.

Halazone tablets lose strength quickly once the wax seal on the bottle is broken. They should, therefore, be used as soon as possible, and the bottle should be capped between uses.

Higher strength tablets (160 mg) are available in larger tablet size. Halazone (160 mg) can be used to disinfect 40 liters of clear water or 20 liters of turbid or highly colored water. Care must be taken not to utilize Halazone (160 mg) in the same tablet-to-water ratio as that prescribed for Halazone (4 mg) tablets. Personnel involved in distribution should be aware of this precaution and should educate users.

Granular Calcium Hypochlorite

This dry powder, called HTH or Perchloron, contains 60-70% available chlorine. It remains quite stable when stored in tightly sealed containers in dark, dry,

cool places. Once the container has been opened, it
loses 5% of its initial available chlorine in 40 days.

Care must be taken not to contaminate the powder
with oil or combustible organic materials when it is
mixed, because to do so may cause a fire. To use HTH,
add and dissolve 1 heaping teaspoon (approximately 1/4
oz or 7 g) per 2 gallons (8 liters) of water, thus producing a stock solution of 500 mg/liter. Add the stock solution to the water to be disinfected in the proportion of 1
part solution to 100 parts water. Let this stand 30 min.
If the taste of chlorine is too strong, allow it to aerate
by standing another few hours or by pouring it from one
clean container to another several times. The stock
solution should be used within 2 weeks after it is prepared.

Sodium Hypochlorite Bleach or "Javel Water"

Common household bleach contains a compound that
can, in emergencies, be used to disinfect water. The
content of available chlorine (usually 3-10%) should be
determined. It should be added to the water according to
the following table:

Available Chlorine	Drops/Liter of Clear Water	Drops/Liter of Turbid or Colored Water
1%	10	20
4-6%	2	4
7-10%	1	2

If the strength of available chlorine in the bleach is
unknown, ten drops of bleach should be added. After
mixing the treated water, allow it to stand for 30 min.
There should be a slight odor of chlorine. If not, repeat
the dosage and allow the water to stand for 15 min.

Iodine

Tablets. The most convenient and reliable iodine
tablet forms are those that contain approximately 20 mg
of tetraglycine hyproperiodine, 90 mg of disodium dihy-
drogen phrophosphate, and 5 mg of talc. These tablets
will dissolve in less than 1 min at about 20°C, liberating
8 mg of elemental iodine per tablet. This amount will

be adequate to treat 1 liter of most natural waters within 10 min.

Solutions. Common household tincture of iodine from a medicine chest or first aid kit (2% tincture of iodine) can be used to disinfect water. Five drops of tincture of iodine will be sufficient to disinfect 1 liter of clear water. For turbid water, however, add 10 drops. Let the water stand for at least 30 min.

Potassium Permanganate (KMnO$_4$)

Potassium permanganate is seldom used because of its long contact time. It is usually considered as a disinfectant for large quantities of water in wells, springs, or storage tanks. Potassium permanganate is of doubtful efficacy against pathogenic organisms, with the possible exception of Vibrio cholerae.

To use the chemical, prepare a solution by dissolving 40 mg of KMnO$_4$ in 1 liter of warm water. The solution will disinfect approximately 1 cubic meter of water after 24 hrs of contact time.

TECHNICAL GUIDE TO ENVIRONMENTAL HEALTH MEASURES TAKEN IN RESPONSE TO NATURAL DISASTER*

This addendum consists of a summary of recommendations which are to be carried out during evacuation and relief operations.

EVACUATION

During evacuation, water from suspicious sources must be boiled for 1 min before it is cooled, or it must be disinfected with chlorine, iodine, or potassium permanganate in either tablet, crystal, powder, or liquid form. The minimum amounts of water to be provided are as follows:

3 liters/person/day in cold and temperate climates
6 liters/person/day in hot climates.

*From Environmental Health Management after Natural Disaster. Pan American Health Organization (PAHO). Scientific Publication No. 430, 1982, pp. 51-55.

Food must be nonperishable and should not require cooking.

Waste disposal should be in a shallow, all purpose trench of the following dimensions:

10 cm deep x 45 cm wide x 3 m long/1000 persons

RELIEF OPERATIONS: TENT CAMPS

During relief operations, sites for tent camps should be chosen where the slope of the land and the nature of the soil favor easy drainage and where there is protection from adverse weather. Sites must be away from mosquito breeding places, refuse dumps, and commercial and industrial zones. The layout of the site should meet the following specifications:

1. Three to four hectares of land/1000 persons
2. Roads of 10 m width
3. Minimum distance between edge of roads and tents of 2 m
4. Minimum distance between tents of 8 m
5. Minimum floor area/tent of 3 m^2

Water distribution in campsites should consist of the following:

1. Minimum capacity of tanks of 200 liters
2. Minimum capacity/capita of 15 liters/day
3. Maximum distance of tanks from farthest tent of 100 m

Solid waste disposal containers in tent camps should be waterproof, insectproof and rodentproof; the waste should be covered tightly with a plastic or metallic lid. Final disposal should be by incineration or burial. The capacities of solid waste units should be 1 liter/4-8 tents; or 50-100 liters/25-50 persons.

Excreta and liquid waste should be disposed in boreholed or deep trench latrines in tent camps. The following are specifications for these:

30-50 m from tents
1 seat/10 persons

Modified soakage pits should be used for waste water

by replacing layers of earth and small pebbles with layers of straw, grass, or small twigs. The straw needs to be removed on a daily basis and burned.

Washing should take place with an ablution bench that is 3 m in length, and double-sided. There should be two benches/100 persons.

RELIEF OPERATIONS: BUILDINGS

Buildings used to accommodate victims during relief should provide the following:

Minimum floor area of 3.5 m^2/person
Minimum air space of 10 m^2/person
Minimum air circulation of 30 m^3/person/hr

There should be separate washing blocks for men and women.

Washing facilities to be provided are as follows:

1 hand basin/10 persons or
1 wash bench of 4-5 meters/100 persons and 1 shower head/50 persons in temperate climates
1 shower head/30 persons in hot climates.

Toilet accommodations in buildings housing displaced persons should meet these requirements:

1 seat/25 women and
1 seat plus 1 urinal/35 men
maximum distance from building of 50 m.

Refuse containers are to be plastic or metallic and have closed lids. There should be one container of 50-100 liters capacity/25-50 persons.

RELIEF OPERATIONS: WATER SUPPLY

Daily consumption of water should be:

40-60 liters/person in field hospitals
20-30 liters/person in mass feeding centers
15-20 liters/person in temporary shelters and camps
35 liters/person in washing installations

Prescriptions for disinfecting water are as follows:

For routine chlorine residual, 0. 7-1. 0 mg/liter
For disinfection of pipes, 50 mg/liter available
chlorine for 24 hrs contact or 100 mg/liter for 1 hr
contact
For disinfection of wells and springs, 50-100 mg/
liter for 12 hrs.

For elimination of high chlorine concentration in
disinfected water, use 0. 88 g sodium thiosulfate/1000
mg chlorine. To protect water, the distance between the
water source and sources of pollution must be at least
30 m. Wells can be protected by keeping the bottoms of
cesspools and latrines 1. 5-3 m above the water table
and with the following:

Impervious casing 30 cm above and 3 m below
ground surface
Concrete platform around well of 1 m radius
Fenced area of 50 m radius.

RELIEF OPERATIONS: LATRINES

Shallow trenches should be:

90-150 cm deep x 30 cm wide (or as narrow
as can be dug) x 3-3. 5 m/100 persons

Deep trenches should be:

1. 8-2. 4 m deep x 75-90 cm wide x 3-3. 5 m/100 persons

Bore-holed trenches should be:

5-6 m deep
40 cm in diameter
1/20 persons

RELIEF OPERATIONS: REFUSE DISPOSAL

Trenches used for disposing refuse should be:

2 m deep x 1. 5 m wide x 1 m long/200 persons

Covered with compact earth 40 cm deep.

With these dimensions, trenches can be filled in one
week. The time to allow for decomposition of the refuse
is 4-6 months.

RELIEF OPERATIONS: FOOD SANITATION

Eating utensils are to be disinfected with the following:

Boiling water for 5 min or
Chlorine solution 100 mg/liter for 30 sec
Quarternary ammonium compounds: 200 mg/liter
for 2 min

RELIEF OPERATIONS: STOCKS

The following are important items of equipment and supply which should be stockpiled for emergency environmental health:

1. Millipore sanitarian kits
2. Comparators for chlorine residual or pH test kits
3. Hach DR/EL field test kits
4. Pocket-type flashlights and spare batteries
5. Water pressure gauges with positive and negative pressure
6. Rapid phosphatase determination kits
7. Mobile chlorinators and/or hypochlorinators
8. Mobile water purification units with a capacity of 200-250 liters/min
9. Tank trucks for water with a capacity of 7 m^3
10. Easy-to-assemble, portable, storage tanks

III. ENVIRONMENTAL HEALTH ASSESSMENT FOLLOWING A NATURAL DISASTER*

INTRODUCTION

All environmental health measures (e.g. , improvement of water quantity/quality, restoration of basic sanitation measures, providing shelter, etc.) following a natural disaster must be assessed in relation to the following factors:

---

*From WHO Course on Health Aspects and Relief Management in Natural Disasters. Brussels, 1980, pp. 148-150.

Changes in population density
Changes in population location
Changes in resources/materials availability

As the above-mentioned factors will vary with time, the intensity of the efforts assigned to each measure must take into account when the action is to take place:

First Priority: 0-3 days (Restore lifeline services, i. e. , food, transportation, and power)

Minimal amounts of safe drinking water
Basic sanitation measures
Minimal shelter

Second Priority: 3-7 days (Restore essential services)

Water for personal hygiene
Institute food protection measures
Institute basic action control measures
Start debris changes
Start solid waste measures

Third Priority: From 7 days on (Restore normal surveillance)

Water quality
Sanitation
Food control

In assigning resources (human material and equipment) the following points must be kept in mind:

What is needed as designed quality standard?
What resources are available in the area NOW?
What additional shifts can be expected in densities, locations, and resources?
When do we expect to reach the service levels existing prior to the disaster?

In preparing its report, a Disaster Assistance Team should develop answers to the following questions for each site they visit.

A. Drinking Water (0-7 days)

 1. From what source will water be obtained?
    a) Wells (Are they protected? What is their
       capacity? How will water be extracted?)
    b) River (What is capacity of intake? What are
       quality variations? Pollution levels?)
 2. How will the water be treated?
    a) Is water bacteriologically safe? ($\pm$ 50 E. coli/
       100 ml?)
    b) What is needed to make it safe? (Protect the
       source?)
 3. Will additional sources be needed?
    a) What materials will be needed?
    b) If it is not safe, what needs to be done to make
       it safe?
 4. How will water be moved from source to user?
    a) Pipe (What size? Where located?)
    b) Truck (Fuel? Maintenance?)
    c) Pumping (Electricity?)
 5. How will water be stored?
    a) Individual basis (In what? How will it be kept
       clear?)
    b) On communal/mass basis (Who will control it?
       How will it be dispensed? What containers?)
 6. What will water be used for?
    a) Individual (Drinking? Hygiene?)
    b) Communal (Bathing? Clothes washing?)

B. Excreta Disposal (0-7 days)

 1. What are the customs of users?
    a) Individual latrines?
    b) Open field defecation?
    c) Communal latrines?
 2. What is the status of existing facilities?
    a) Individual
    b) Community facilities?
    c) Sewerage systems?
 3. How will climate affect excreta disposal?
    a) Hot/dry?
    b) Hot/humid?
    c) Cold?

C. <u>Basic Shelter</u> (0-7 days)

    1. What materials are needed for on-site construction?
      a) How large are families?
      b) What materials are available locally?
      c) How far do they need to be transported?
    2. What are the needs for camp shelters?
      a) Camp site (Food drainage? Siting related to wind? Siting related to water?)
      b) Water supply? (Proposal vs. equipment needed?)
      c) Basic sanitation? (Space available? Can one dig in the soil? Drainage?)

D. <u>Food Protection</u> (0-7 days)
    1. Where/how will food be prepared?
      a) Individual (Fuel? Stoves?)
      b) Camp (Sanitation practices vs. quantities to be prepared?)
    2. Survey food in surrounding area?
      a) Damaged?
      b) Selective use?
      c) Usable quantities?
    3. Establish food handling/storage practices?
      a) Individual education?
      b) Camp instructions?
      c) Food storage? Place?
      d) Mass relief supplies?

E. <u>Personal Hygiene Measures</u>

What is the level of personal hygiene?

IV. ENVIRONMENTAL SANITATION IN REFUGEE CAMPS*

We must recognize the fact that what we are essentially doing is building a new city, therefore, we need to organize an infrastructure for all of the following:

---

*From WHO Course on Health Aspects and Relief Management in Natural Disasters. Brussels, 1980, pp. 131-135.

Drinking water
Excreta disposal
Shelter
Solid waste disposal
Vector control

Building a refugee camp to shelter 30,000 people is a huge task.

A. WATER

1. One public tap per 300 people
2. Need 300 taps
   a) Pipe?
   b) Wells?
   c) At 5 l. p. c. d. (liters per contact day) need 150,000 Lpd (liters per day)

B. LATRINES

1. One latrine per 50 people
2. Must move $\pm$ 16,000 m^3 of earth
   a) Picks, shovels?
   b) Materials for slabs?
   c) Materials for privacy?
3. Must build 600 units

C. SOLID WASTE

1. At 1/2-1 kg/person/day, one must remove 15,000 kg/day
2. Waste must be disposed of in a landfill
   a) How should it be moved?
   b) Where should it be buried?

D. EVALUATION

E. LOCATION

1. Natural drainage
2. Ground space (10-20 m^2 per person)

F. LIVING CONDITIONS

1. 8 m between tents
2. Floor space/person (3 m^2)
3. Drainage canals around houses and roads

G. SANITATION CONDITIONS

1. Adequate water (15/20 l. p. c. d.)
2. Washing facilities (battery of 2 sinks of 1. 5 m per 30 persons)
3. Latrines (1 seat/25 persons)
4. Food hygiene
5. Solid waste collection on sanitary landfill

H. GENERAL

1. Rainwater entered living quarters
2. Problems using showers
3. Problems using laundry facilities
4. Problems using latrines
5. Personal hygiene problems
6. Increased distance from work

I. PROBLEM AREAS

1. Flooding following rains
2. Inadequate quantities of water
3. Contamination of water because of extensive handling and holding
4. Latrine source of infection because of poor design and maintenance
5. Solid waste problems because no collection system; therefore, individual disposal is unsanitary
6. Increase in fly, cockroach, etc. , population

J. GENERAL COMMENTS

1. Boiling water. Where does one obtain a container and fuel?
2. Disinfection.
   a) Where does one obtain a disinfecting agent?
   b) Where does one store the disinfected water?

K. CAMPSITE

1. For good drainage, avoid clay soils.
2. Face south
3. Locate on high ground
4. Subdivide into 1000 person units for administrative purposes

L. GENERAL

1. Health education is very important.

M. WHAT WAS LEARNED

1. Requirements of Campsite
    a) Adequate roads and streets
    b) Adequate drainage over grassy slopes without
       dense vegetation
    c) Space per person of $10/20$ m^2 should be raised
       to $30/90$ m^2 for long-range camps.

2. Water and Basic Sanitation
    a) Water should have adequate treatment and
       piped distribution.
    b) Sanitation facilities should be based on time of
       camp and machine/tools/material/labor avail-
       able at site.
       (1) One latrine/40 people (for short-term)
       (2) One latrine/25 people (for long-term)

3. Solid Waste
    a) Should be based on municipality services of
       collection and disposal. (If this is not possible,
       one must organize a system using sanitary
       landfill.)
    b) Distribute storage containers using communal
       ones if necessary.

4. Other Services

    a) Provide mobile health facility.
    b) Organize camp committee.
       (1) Health
       (2) Security
       (3) Order
       (4) Health education
    c) Food hygiene during distribution and sale
    d) Communal washing and laundry facilities
    e) Vector control facilities
       (1) Control vectors
       (2) Control loose animals

N. DESIGN CRITERIA

    1. <u>Space</u>
       a) 30/40 m^3 per person
       b) 3 m^2 floor space per person
       c) 10 m wide road/streets
       d) 2 m wide sidewalks (tent lones)
       e) 8 m between tents
         (1) Fire protection
         (2) Ventilation

    2. <u>Sanitation</u>
       a) Latrine design
         (1) 1 kg fecal/day/person
         (2) 1 liter urine/day/person
       b) Watertanks of 100 liters within 100 m (use few large rather than many small)
       c) Provide one garbage can (50/100 liters per 25/50 people).
       d) Provide one double-edged wash facility (3 m long) per 50 persons.

O. OTHER REQUIRED SUPPLIES

    1. Pots and pans
    2. Picks and shovels
    3. Quick coupling pipe
    4. Cement
    5. Cement "Y" 4 inch cement mesh rolls
    6. Storage containers (55 gallons)
    7. Handpumps

P. POTENTIAL AREAS FOR CONCERN

    1. MAINTENANCE, MAINTENANCE, MAINTE-NANCE!
    2. Sanitation workers <u>must</u> be protected (they are a basic element).
    3. Take care of the following:
       a) Water storage containers
       b) Excreta disposal

BIBLIOGRAPHY

Assar, M.: <u>Guide to Sanitation in Natural Disasters</u>. Geneva. World Health Organization, 1971.

Bevenson, A.S., ed.: Control of Communicable Diseases in Man, 13th ed. Washington, D.C., American Public Health Association, 1981.

Center for Research in the Epidemiology of Disasters: Health Aspects and Relief Management after Natural Disasters. Bruxelles, Belgium, 1980.

World Health Organization: Emergency Health Management after Natural Disaster. Scientific Publication No. 407. Washington, D.C., Pan American Health Organization, World Health Organization, 1981.

World Health Organization: Epidemiologic Surveillance after Natural Disaster. Scientific Publication No. 420. Washington, D.C., Pan American Health Organization, 1982.

World Health Organization: Environmental Health Management after Natural Disasters. Scientific Publication No. 430. Washington, D.C., Pan American Health Organization, 1982.

Chapter 10

PREPARING AND TRAINING FOR CASUALTY CARE

Frederick M. Burkle, Jr. , M. D. , M. P. H.
Patricia H. Sanner, M. D.
Barry W. Wolcott, M. D.

In 1966, in a special communication to the Journal of the American Medical Association, Roswell Brown aptly asked, "Disaster medicine—What is it? Can it be taught?"[1] Although advances in trauma surgery and the development of the Emergency Medical Services System grew primarily out of our experiences in war, in peacetime our system of military and civilian medical practices remain quite separate. Brown suggested this was due to the fact that "we are so accustomed to fighting our wars elsewhere. "

Our world is presently wracked with conventional war, and with the threat of conflicts in previously peaceful hemispheres. There has been a disturbing increase in the number of refugees around the world as well as an increase in natural and man-made disasters. Along with these problems is the mounting fear of a nuclear war and the hopelessness such a war entails. Yet, despite this, there is still a confused complacency towards disaster medicine among Western medical practitioners.

Most community hospitals have established disaster plans. Physicians responding to recent limited disasters have commented on the ever improving prehospital emergency care systems, a system the primary care provider frequently knows little about. Individual physicians have also become aware of their own deficiencies in the principles and management of mass casualty care, an area in which military physicians are well trained. These principles are obviously needed for the civilian physician population as well. In disasters, all physicians are called upon to care for casualties. Disaster medicine has proven time and time again that there can be no distinction between civilian and military medicine.

Initially, the primary care provider needs to become more familiar with existing, community disaster plans, especially the prehospital EMS system. Physicians involved in the organization and teaching of paramedic personnel have benefited greatly by increasing their knowledge of the functional complexities of this critical area of health care.

162

Secondly, the physician must take advantage of training programs in Advanced Cardiac Life Support[2] and Advanced Trauma Life Support,[3] which exist on both a provider and an instructor level. Every medical provider, no matter what his/her specialty may be, should have a working knowledge of the principles set forth in these programs. These have become the standard procedures of disaster medicine. By right, all physicians should hold provider level certification in both programs if they are to participate knowledgeably in any disaster situation, large or small.

Thirdly, there are those who state that disaster medicine cannot be taught by means of simulated scenarios and drills. These critics suggest that a disaster situation is impossible to predict or simulate well enough to be an efficient teaching tool, and that such simulation will not lead to improved functioning of individuals in actual disasters. Although it is true that an actual disaster is unpredictable by its very nature and each event is therefore unique, certain problems and processes do occur in all. These can be reproduced in simulated disaster scenarios. For example, most disaster operations involving multiple casualties require the following processes: triage, stabilization and evacuation of casualties from the site, and triage and definitive care at receiving facilities. Some problems which are consistently evident in actual and simulated mass casualty situations are: communications, transportation, documentation, coordination of resources, and the difficulty of triage. Physicians accustomed to handling a single, seriously injured patient in a well-equipped hospital facility must learn new triage skills to provide the greatest benefit to the greatest number of patients, rather than focusing on the most severely injured. Knowledge of communication and evacuation systems may be rudimentary. Exposure to these processes and problems in a disaster simulation can provide the potential disaster worker with knowledge of personal deficiencies and also provide the basis for a training program. After-action analysis of the response to a simulated scenario can highlight problem areas and emphasize the need for a systematic approach, planning, prior identification of resources and means of access, innovation, and testing of plans.

A department chief from a hospital in New Brunswick described the benefits of planning after her small Canadian hospital had to evacuate 65 patients due to rising flood waters: "One thing we learned from our experience is that no disaster can be planned to the last detail. Difficulties will always arise that cannot be predicted. But it was a direct result of having an organized plan and of exercising it, that our difficulties were met and so quickly dealt with."[4]

Military medical experience has demonstrated the efficacy of planning, organization, and training by using simulation. Experiences over a 3-year period with senior medical students at the Uniformed Services University of the Health Sciences School of Medicine (USUHS-SOM) have demonstrated the disaster medicine learning process through simulations (Figures 10-1 and 10-2). All senior students are required to participate in a 72-hr field training exercise during which they organize and operate an emergency medical facility which supports a combat unit. They experience all phases of mass casualty care including location of casualties, on-site care, transport to and treatment in the emergency medical facility, and evacuation to more rearward facilities. They face problems of communications, vehicles, climate, evacuation coordination, triage, supplies, personnel and technical limitations. Their response to the initial phase of the exercise is chaotic. By the later phases of the exercise, the students function in a cohesive, creative, and efficient manner despite the increasing complexity of the simulated situations. They develop a solid working knowledge of triage, mass casualty care, communications, evacuation systems, and innovativeness. Whether these students will function better in an actual situation because of this training remains to be tested.

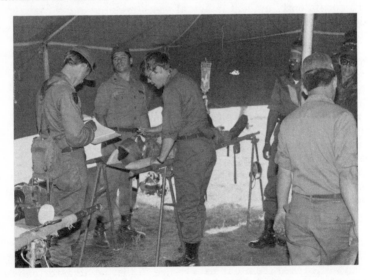

Figure 10-1. A physician-in-training being evaluated by faculty staff. Triage scenario. Combat Casualty Care Course. Fort Sam Houston, Texas. (U. S. Army photograph).

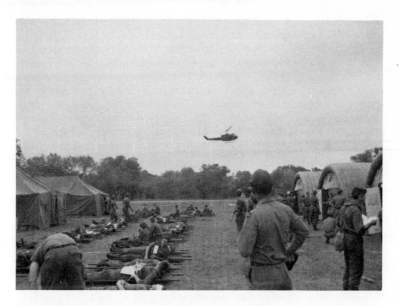

Figure 10-2. Triage scenario organized outside mock mobile hospitals. Combat Casualty Course. Fort Sam Houston, Texas. Principles of military casualty care are easily translated and applied to civilian disaster medicine. (U. S. Army photograph.)

A disaster can be defined as a "situation of massive collective stress ... the consequence of the combined individual stress reactions ...."[5] These stress reactions occur both in victims and in disaster workers. This aspect of disaster operations also appears to be reproducible in simulation. Sanner and Wolcott observed stress reactions occurring in disaster simulation participants which were similar to those occurring in health care workers during actual disasters.

The observations were made during the USUHS-SOM field training exercises described above and another military medical training exercise, the Combat Casualty Care Course. This is an 8-day field training program for physicians and other health care providers from the three military services. During recurrent sessions of both training exercises, several stress reactions were consistently observed: feelings of frustration and futility, loss of confidence, grief reactions to death and dying, physical reactions to unruly patients, "burn-out," and triage stress. These reactions paralleled documented reactions in actual situations. Integration of these observations into the after-action analysis of a mass casualty exercise can provide the participant with some very important psychological preparation for disaster care.

In summary, the editors feel that it is possible to prepare and train for mass casualty care. One can acquire the needed medical skills through participation in emergency care courses such as Basic Life Support, Advanced Cardiac Life Support and Advanced Trauma Life Support. Knowledge of prehospital care systems is mandatory. Military and civilian experiences demonstrate the efficacy of prior planning. Testing disaster response plans using simulated scenarios can highlight problem areas and provide the basis for changes and for improved training programs. Finally, simulations by reproducing disaster stress reactions can provide the potential disaster care provider with some needed psychological preparation for a most demanding and chaotic event.

REFERENCES

1. Brown, R. K. : Special communication: Disaster medicine. What is it? Can it be taught? JAMA 197, 13:133-136, 1966.
2. Advanced Cardiac Life Support Program. American Heart Association, 1981.
3. American College of Surgeons, Committee on Trauma: Advanced Trauma Life Support. 1980.
4. O'Brien, Patricia E. : The hospital isn't closed—we've just relocated—a New Brunswick disaster plan. Can Med Assoc J 120:1138, 1979.
5. Kinston, W. , and Rosser, R. : Disaster: Effects on mental and physical state. J Psychosom Res 18:438, 1974.

SPECIAL PROBLEM AREAS IN DISASTER MEDICINE

Chapter 11

EARLY CARE OF REFUGEES
Frederick M. Burkle, Jr., M.D., M.P.H.

I. GENERAL

The worldwide total of refugees consists of almost 20 million helpless victims of war, famine, natural disasters, and political repression. Eight million of these are Asian refugees.

Priorities in the care of refugees have been singularly responsible for the increased interest and evolution of disaster medicine as a specialty area.

Large scale international relief activities are now commonplace. Agencies maintain a worldwide communications network that allows rapid response potential. Despite this, relief workers rarely become operational in foreign lands before 7-10 days, at best. Indigenous health care providers are overly stressed until outside assistance arrives. Refugee mortality rates are alarmingly high in the first few days postdisaster. Beyond this time, medical personnel may find themselves largely involved in health screening, general ambulatory medical care, and health exams for immigration; not the acute surgical or medical care they anticipated. There is a need to overcome the complexities of providing a more rapid response potential, especially within the first 36 hrs.

In wartime, because of rapidly shifting fronts, refugees may overburden mobile, military medical teams. As a military necessity, military personnel receive priority care. In addition, medical supplies and equipment allocated to military units are rarely used for the refugee population, especially the pediatric segment.

Health care providers from national and international organizations have responded to the challenge of recent natural and military disasters with extensive and unique deployments of short- and long-term services. Lessons learned from these fragmented experiences provide guidelines appropriate to the rapid mobilization of refugee care under any circumstances.

II. RAPID OPERATIONAL REQUIREMENTS

A. Defining the scope of the problem[1]

1. Identify the number of refugees because reliable figures are central to effective planning.
    a) Determine whether these numbers exceed the capacity of existing services.
    b) Update this information constantly.
2. Determine the time available to plan for a response.
    a) Natural disasters rarely allow time for sophisticated planning.
    b) Existing disaster plans must have an immediate response capability.
    c) When time allows, planning should address the uniqueness of the disaster: Special age groups involved; potential for certain injuries predominating, i. e. , an abundance of crush injuries after an earthquake; potential for infectious diseases from migratory refugees.
3. Establish a disaster planning group to oversee the requirements for the disaster response.
    a) Shaw developed a problem and solution priority matrix applicable to the rapid and practical planning of refugee relief care (Figure 11-1). [2] Priority I activities demand urgent solution; priority II is accorded to conditions which require prompt resolution; priority III needs timely correction. Under communications, Shaw assigns priority I to effective communications between refugee shelters and among relief teams; priority II to broader communications between various relief workers and the refugees; and priority III to the development of communications systems among the refugees themselves.
    b) Early attention must be given to preventing misuse of material and personnel resources, as well as to avoiding duplication of services supplied by various relief projects in the disaster area.

B. Communications (see Chapter 7)

1. Lack of effective field communications results in confusion among medical teams and delays in correcting health and sanitation problems. [2,3]
2. Simple portable communications systems should accompany any immediate disaster response (e. g. , medicom, walkie-talkies, CB radios).

Need for Solution to Specific Situation

General Problem Categories	PRIORITY I (Urgent Action)	PRIORITY II (Prompt Action)	PRIORITY III (Timely Action)
1. Communications			
2. Communicable Disease Control			
3. Camp Location and Layout			
4. Civilian and Military Emergencies			
5. Self Sufficient Support			
6. Nutrition			
7. Health Education			
8. Refugee Work and Recreation			
9. Mass Immunization			

Figure 11-1. Problem and solution priority matrix. (Reproduced with permission from Shaw, R.: Health services in disaster: Lessons from the 1975 Vietnam evacuation. Mil Med 142:307-311, 1979.)

      a) Disaster teams should acquire the use of any existing, local communications system.

      b) Portable communications systems must be easily maintained and simple to use.

      c) Maintenance personnel for communications equipment should be identified and easily accessible.

3. A public address system should be installed rapidly wherever large groups of refugees are collected.

      a) Only a few recognizable voices should be utilized to transmit vital information over the PA system.

      b) Early recognition and conscription of a translator or refugee leader to transmit vital information is essential.

C. Rapid assessment of health status and preventive medicine needs of refugees

1. Experience has shown that epidemiological surveillance, specifically the collection, analysis, and dissemination of data is as necessary as acute emergency care in the initial phase of response.[4,6]

    Without this approach both the immediate and delayed mortality and morbidity among refugees will remain high, and recognition of the prime causes of death will be delayed.

2. Specific Measures

      a) Triage all severely ill refugees upon arrival.

      b) Physicians and nurses staffing individual hospital ward tents must triage again and also log the age, sex, and diagnosis of all patients admitted.

      c) Data from all tents must be reviewed at a central location. Logbooks should be surveyed to identify diagnoses of increased prevalence, morbidity, and mortality.

      d) Burial data (age, sex, and diagnosis) will help identify those at greatest risk of death and the responsible diagnosis. Infectious disease precautions must be taken when examining autopsy material.

      e) Laboratory data surveillance will identify early patterns which lead to high morbidity and mortality. Numerous positive malaria smears, anemia, requests for type and crossmatch, positive CSF smears may rapidly identify patterns of disease from widely scattered wards. Such early surveillance should lead to the rapid deployment of personnel, supplies, and therapies to deal with these problems (e.g., establish

a walking blood-bank, provide antimalarial and antibiotic supplies, contact infectious disease consultants,
and provide proper isolation techniques).

f) A close working relationship between acute care providers and surveillance personnel should provide the
following:

(1) Rapid decline in mortality
(2) Rapid decline in morbidity
(3) Improved triage potential
(4) Reduction in inappropriate admissions
(5) Rapid evaluation of therapy effectiveness
(6) Modification of therapies and priorities

D. Communicable disease control

1. Refugee camp conditions are both rudimentary and
crowded. Early identification and control of communicable diseases are critical.

2. Skilled public health personnel maintain early priorities
in assisting in the planning, construction, and layout of
the refugee camps. [2,3,7] These are essential for sewage, sanitation, and the control and reduction of communicable disease. Military, mobile, preventive medicine units are expert in rapidly deploying such services.

E. Water

Guidelines recommend that permanent refugee installations
provide 150 gallons of water per person per day. In the
first 36 hrs and possibly more, water usage will be restricted to human consumption, hygiene, and cooking, thus
requiring only 75-100 gallons per person per day. [7]

F. Nutrition

1. Relief foods may accompany the initial influx of health
workers. Preliminary triage should include recognition
of dehydration, emaciation, edema, anemia, or vitamin
deficiencies among refugees.

2. A separate triage category may be established whereby
individuals or groups of refugees receive rapid fluid
and/or nutritional attention in separate quarters.

3. Attention must be given to the potential misuse of
relief foods. Powdered milk, often in abundant supply
and easily distributed, may cause serious harm in the

gastrointestinal tracts of children and adult refugees who are unaccustomed to milk. Asian, African, Indian, and tropical populations have experienced violent diarrhea, dehydration, electrolyte imbalance, vomiting, aspiration, and allergic reactions as a consequence of ingesting it. Similar problems will also result when formulas are mixed with contaminated water. [8]

4. Simplified oral hydrating solutions include the following:
    a) A general, mildly hypotonic solution may be prepared by adding[9]
        2 level tbsp glucose
        1 level tsp salt
        1/2 tsp soda bicarbonate (baking soda)
        1/4 tsp potassium citrate
        1/8 tsp magnesium sulfate may be added to each liter (1000 cc) of previously boiled water.
    b) A simple sugar-salt solution for children is prepared by adding[10]
        2 level tbsp sugar
        1 salt tablet (2. 6 g)
        2 potassium chloride tablets (1 g) to 1 liter (1000 cc) of previously boiled water
            May be given as is or with sweetened condensed milk diluted 1 in 8.
            Fed to child as 1 oz (30 cc) for every kg, every 3 hrs, with a maximum of 8 oz (240 cc).
    c) Parents are taught to measure 1. 5 g of salt by using one "three-finger pinch" (thumb and two finger pinch) into a pint of previously boiled water. This simplified rehydration formula is easily taught to refugee parents in underdeveloped countries. [10]
    d) Oral solution for mass casualty care
        1 level tsp salt
        1/2 tsp soda bicarbonate (baking soda)
        1 gallon of previously boiled water
            Provide individuals with 1-2 glasses of this solution.

G. Immunizations

1. Attention to mass immunization for refugee populations is rarely necessary in the first 36 hrs of disaster or refugee relief care. Mass immunizations do not prevent disease epidemics. [2]
2. Careful analysis of the refugee population needs must be carried out before mass immunization is decided upon.

3. Mass immunizations require an abundance of medical personnel, recordkeeping chores, and supplies. None are priorities in the first 36 hrs, nor possibly at any time, unless preventive medicine analysis dictates otherwise. Medical personnel must never be diverted to such tasks during the acute phase.

4. It is more practical for health care teams and disaster relief workers to have updated immunization records as part of prior ongoing disaster planning. Catching up on immunizations at the time of worker deployment is neither practical nor necessary.

H. Mental health priorities

1. The psychological stresses experienced by refugees are greater and more intrusive to the personality than that seen in disaster victims who remain in their own locale, or country, or in their original social status (see Chapter 15). Reasons given for this include the following:[11,15]

   a) Stress of witnessing the disaster or military conflict first hand
   b) Stress of the experience of fleeing
   c) Loss of ability to attain basic survival needs: food, water, shelter, security
   d) Loss of social status, self-identity, and individuality within a cohesive community
   e) Stress of exposure to a new language, new race, and new cultural demands
   f) Sense of frustration and isolation in expressing their needs in the context of a foreign land and language. (This may lead to paranoia, a common symptom seen in refugee populations.)
   g) Separation from or loss of family members
   h) Inability to communicate with separated relatives or friends
   i) Stress of prolonged crowded conditions and lack of privacy
   j) Physical fatigue, sleep deprivation, and poor nutritional status all contribute to a lack of psychological well being
   k) Stress of being a burden to, or unwanted by, the host country
   l) Competitiveness, hoarding, selfishness, violence, and guilt experienced by the threat to survival
   m) Ego disruption from fear of, or actual, illness or injury

2. Psychological well being may determine the refugee's response to medical aid. Health workers should recognize that refugees, many of whom experience a sense of helplessness and hopelessness, may not survive their physical illness or injury despite adequate medical attention. Early recognition of this possibility is critical.

   a) Pay attention to communication to be sure that it includes reassurance and the recognition that you, as a health worker, recognize the refugee's isolation and helplessness.

   b) Provide suspect patients with the company of a nurse's aide, volunteer, or refugee translator. If it is culturally acceptable, develop a buddy system among isolated refugees; this is a helpful technique.

   c) Orient refugees to their surroundings. Inquire as to their family members; inquire and show interest in their prerefugee lives and occupations. Openly discuss the immediate plans for their care and disposition.

   d) Be an active listener; encourage verbalization and the expression of emotions. Do not walk away from emotional expression or grief. Respect the refugee's overwhelming sense of loss.

   e) Become knowledgeable on the accepted cultural expressions of emotional reactions.

   f) Provide refugees with access to religious worship and counselors.

   g) Involve refugees in duties related to their occupations.

   h) Be aware that despite heroic attempts to reach a place of refuge, helplessness, and hopelessness may occur when refugee center conditions fail to meet their expectations. Also, remember that refugees may first learn of the loss of a relative upon arrival at the refugee center.

III. PERSONAL CARE

A. Health workers are susceptible to physical and emotional exhaustion (see Chapter 15).

B. Heat exhaustion and dehydration in new climates require attention to the use of salt tablets or oral electrolyte solution.[9] Workers must be reminded to use safe water supplies. Surprisingly, they frequently pay less attention to these basic guidelines than the patients they are instructing and caring for.

C. The author's recommendations are as follows:
  1. Develop a survival language of medical and social phrases that will assist you in your work. Without it, you will remain isolated.
  2. Become informed in a credible way about the cultural demands of the country and the people you are treating.
  3. Be an active listener and practice humility. Frequently, relief workers, possibly because of a feeling of power, treat refugees as foreigners even in their own country.
  4. Learn the skills of triage, both for your patient care, and for the overwhelming demands placed upon you.
  5. Improve your physical diagnosis. It will be your greatest tool. Laboratory and x-ray facilities will be lacking or nonexistent.
  6. Dare to be creative in overcoming barriers to supply and equipment needs.
  7. Learn some psychiatric skills, not only to understand the victims, but as a better observer to your own reactions.
  8. Remember that alcohol and drugs are devastating to personality integration, especially when combined with fatigue, yet they may both be used by some workers to buffer anxiety and feelings of incompetence in a new and overwhelming environment.
  9. Establish personal friendships. There is no time when you will need a friend more. Use this friend to verbalize your anger. The more you verbalize your anger, the less harm you will bring to your patients.
  10. Provide leadership, if you can.
  11. Know how and when to delegate tasks to others.
  12. Provide frequent rest periods for those who are constantly working with acute trauma.
  13. Develop adaptive defense mechanisms:
      a) Suppression: Develop the ability to avoid repressing the surrounding emotional and physical threats to your ego.
      b) Accept absurdities: Don't ruminate about what you have absolutely no control over or about what you cannot change.
      c) Sense of humor: Find humor in your own vulnerability; this will help to solidify confidence from other team members and to relieve tension.

IV. PROTECTION OF REFUGEES IN ARMED CONFLICTS[17]

A.   Both the United Nations High Commissioner for Refugees, under provisions of the United Nations Covenants on Human Rights, and the International Committee of the Red Cross, under provisions of the Geneva Convention, recognize the basic human rights instruments for individuals. Therefore, they provide that refugees and stateless persons shall be protected persons; and they otherwise provide for their welfare.

B.   International Refugee Law, along with the Law of Human Rights and the International Humanitarian Law, provides that refugee law, with all its guarantees is authoritarian and embodies customary law, or the general principles of law recognized by civilized nations.

      Such law, however, has no enforcement mechanisms.

REFERENCES

1. Stalcup, S. A., et al. : Planning for a pediatric disaster—experience gained from caring for 1600 Vietnamese orphans. N Engl J Med 293, 14:691-695, 1975.
2. Shaw, R. : Health Services in a disaster: Lessons from the 1975 Vietnamese evacuation. Milit Med 142:307-311, 1979.
3. Shaw, R. : Preventive medicine in the Vietnamese refugee camps on Guam. Milit Med 141:19-29, 1977.
4. Glass, R. I., et al. : Rapid assessment of health status and preventive-medicine needs of newly arrived Kampuchean refugees, Sa Kaeo, Thailand. Lancet 24, 1:868-872, 1980.
5. Goodman, R. A., and Speckhard, M. E.: Health needs of refugees. Letters to the Editor. Lancet 24, 1: 1139, 1980.
6. Ebrahim, S. : Health needs of refugees. Letters to the Editor. Lancet 24, 1:1139-1140, 1980.
7. Gaydos, J. C., et al. : A preventive medicine team in a refugee operation—Fort Chaffee Indochina refugee camp. Milit Med 143, 5:318-321, 1978.
8. Heyneman, D. : Mis-Aid to the third world: Disease repercussions caused by ecological ignorance. Can J Public Health 62:303-313, 1971.
9. Dahlberg, K. : Medical care of Cambodian refugees. JAMA 243, 10:1062-1065, 1980.
10. Morley, D. : Pediatric Priorities in the Developing World. London, Butterworths, 1973.

11. Harding, R. K. , and Looney, J. G. : Problems of Southeast Asian children in a refugee camp. Am J Psychiatry 134, 4:407-411, 1977.
12. Edwards, A. T. : Paranoid reactions. Med J Aust 1:778-779, 1956.
13. Meszaros, A. F. : Types of displacement reactions among the postrevolution Hungarian immigrants. Can Psychiatric Assoc J 6:9-19, 1961.
14. Rahe, R. H. , et al. : Psychiatric consultation in a Vietnamese refugee camp. Am J Psychiatry 135, 2:185-190, 1978.
15. Pederson, S. : Psychopathological reactions to extreme social displacements. Psychoanal Rev 36:344-354, 1949.
16. Chamberlain, B. C. : The psychological aftermath of disaster. J Clin Psychiatry 41, 7:238-244, 1980.
17. Patrnogic, J. : International protection of refugees in armed conflicts. Ann Droit Int Med 29:95-105, 1980.

Chapter 12

ENVIRONMENTAL CASUALTIES
Patricia H. Sanner, M.D.

I. HEAT ILLNESS

Heat illness is not a single entity but rather a spectrum of disturbances in the homeostatic mechanism of heat exchange in the body. Environmental heat illness can be prevented by educating the individual; by assessing the heat stress potential of the environment and planning work, sports, or military operations accordingly; and by allowing time for acclimatization.

A. ACCLIMATIZATION

An individual develops improved heat tolerance through a process called acclimatization. This is a result of four physiologic responses which begin with the first heat exposure and are well developed in one week. Full acclimatization, i.e., the ability to perform the maximum amount of strenuous work in a hot environment, requires 2-4 weeks to achieve, depending on the heat sensitivity of the individual. Full acclimatization can be achieved in this time with as little as two 50-min periods of aerobic work per day. The four physiologic processes are as follows:

1. Increased skeletal muscle efficiency results in increased aerobic metabolism.
2. Maximal sweat production increases in the acclimatized or heat-adapted person from approximately 1.5 liters/hr in the unadapted state to approximately 3.0 liters/hr.
3. Increased aldosterone secretion causes plasma volume expansion through decreased renal Na+ excretion and decreased Na+ concentration in sweat.
4. Plasma volume expansion improves myocardial efficiency and results in increased cardiac output with decreased peak heart rate when an individual works in a hot environment.
The net effects of the physiologic responses of acclimatization are increased aerobic metabolism, increased sweat volume, and increased cutaneous circulation. Thus, acclimatization

improves heat tolerance by increased heat dissipation and decreased heat production.

B. CLINICAL SYNDROMES

There are basically three heat syndromes which represent a spectrum of disturbances in homeostasis: heat cramps, heat exhaustion, and heat stroke.

1. Heat Cramps

   a) <u>Signs and Symptoms</u>. The patient complains of brief, intermittent, very severe muscle cramps after work in a hot environment. The cramps usually occur in the muscle groups involved in the work. The patient's core temperature remains normal and there are no associated systemic symptoms.

   b) <u>Etiology</u>. Heat cramps are a result of Na+ depletion. An individual working in a hot environment has been replacing salt and water losses (sweat losses) with H_2O alone. Heat cramps, for this reason, are more frequent in acclimatized persons because of the markedly increased volumes of sweat.

   c) <u>Treatment</u>. The patient should be placed at rest in a cool environment and receive oral or IV electrolyte solution. Oral replacement is usually adequate. Possible oral fluids are lemonade, tomato juice, and commercial athletic drinks. A saline solution of 0.1% may be prepared by dissolving 2 $\overline{X}$ grain salt tablets in 1 quart of water or 1 1/3 mess kit spoonfuls of salt in 5 gallons of water.

   d) <u>Prevention</u>. Instruct the person working in a hot environment to drink <u>both</u> water and electrolyte solution. Preparing many of the proprietary electrolyte replacement solutions at one-half strength is adequate. Salt tablets are <u>not</u> recommended.

2. Heat Exhaustion

   a) <u>Signs and Symptoms</u>. The patient with heat exhaustion presents with a variety of systemic manifestations with or without muscle cramps. The systemic signs and symptoms may be as follows:

   (1) <u>CNS.</u> Headache, faintness, dizziness, vertigo, irritability

(2) <u>Volume depletion</u>. Thirst, hypotension, tachycardia, syncope

(3) <u>GI</u>. Nausea, vomiting, anorexia

(4) <u>Constitutional</u>. Weakness, malaise

Body temperature may be normal to slightly elevated and sweating is present.

b) <u>Etiology</u>. There are two types of heat exhaustion.

(1) <u>Water depletion type</u>. This course is a situation of limited H_2O availability (e. g. , desert) or when an individual cannot obtain or make the need for water known (e. g. , an infant or an elderly, confused patient). These patients have hypernatremic dehydration. Their body temperature is slightly elevated (100-101°F) (37. 7-38. 3 C). This type of heat exhaustion may rapidly progress to heat stroke.

(2) <u>Sodium depletion type</u>. This is a continuum of the heat cramps process of sweat losses replaced by H_2O alone. The patients demonstrate signs of volume depletion and hyponatremia. Their body temperature is normal. This type of heat exhaustion is not likely to progress to heat stroke.

c) <u>Treatment</u>. The patient should be placed at rest in a cool environment. IV fluid and electrolyte replacement is preferred although oral solutions may be given to alert patients in the field if IV fluid is unavailable. Normal saline is the usual IV fluid used although 3% saline may be required to correct severe hyponatremia. Oral fluids are as discussed above in the treatment of heat cramps.

d) <u>Prevention.</u> Assure adequate water and electrolyte replacement as in prevention of heat cramps. Caretakers of infants and elderly or disabled people must be very attentive to their fluid need.

3. <u>Heat Stroke</u>

Heat stroke is an acute medical emergency with a mortality rate of 17-70% depending on the series reviewed. A patient presenting with <u>any</u> loss of consciousness associated with heat stress should be regarded as a heat stroke victim until proven otherwise.

a) <u>Signs and Symptoms</u>. There are two clinical presentations of heat stroke.

(1) <u>Classical Heat Stroke</u>. The patient is usually at the extremes of age, often with some underlying systemic disease. Classical heat stroke occurs in an epidemic pattern during heat waves. The patient has a rectal temperature greater than 105°F (40. 6°C) and the skin is hot and dry without sweating. CNS signs are prominent (e. g. , confusion, coma, grand mal seizures, dilated or poorly-reactive pupils).

(2) <u>Exertional Heat Stroke</u>. The patient is usually a normal, healthy, young individual performing intense muscular exertion in a hot environment (e. g. , a marathon runner). Exertional heat stroke occurs sporadically. The patient presents with a rectal temperature greater than 105°F (40. 6°C); hot, <u>moist</u> skin; and CNS signs, such as confusion, coma, and grand mal seizures. In addition, these patients often develop severe rhabdomyolysis, acute tubular necrosis (ATN), disseminated intravascular coagulation, and severe electrolyte and acid-base disturbance. There is a 30% incidence of ATN in exertional heat stroke, probably secondary to myoglobinuria. Initially, this patient may have hypo- or hypernatremia and hypokalemia. Later hyperkalemia supervenes due to massive tissue destruction and renal failure. Usually, a mixed respiratory alkalosis and metabolic acidosis occurs due to combined heat-induced hyperventilation and lactic acidosis. Lactic acidosis may be marked in exertional heat stroke with mean levels of 14. 7.

Both types of heat stroke may be associated with cardiac arrhythmias, including conduction defects, ventricular ectopy, and tachyarrhythmias.

b) <u>Management</u>

(1) <u>Prehospital</u>

(a) Rapid cooling is the most important procedure and must be started immediately. Place the patient in a cool environment such as a tent with fans or a recreation vehicle with air conditioning that operates off engine source. Use any cool water source available, such as hoses or field water tanks, and ice if this can be obtained. <u>Methods</u>:

i) Ice water bath immersion with assistants vigorously massaging the patient's extremities.
ii) Ice water massage and exposure to circulating air (e. g. , a fan) to increase evaporation.

(b) Assure airway and ventilation; administer O_2 if available.

(c) IV with Ringer's lactate (RL) or normal saline (NS) to deliver approximately 1000-1200 cc in the first 4 hrs.

(d) Rapid transfer to hospital-type facility.

(2) Hospital

(a) Continue cooling with goal of decreasing core temperature to 102°F (38.9°C).

(b) Ventilatory support as needed.

(c) Conservative fluid replacement: Usually the hypotension seen in these patients is due to marked cutaneous vasodilation and will respond to cooling alone. The usual fluid replacement in the first 4 hrs is 1000-1200 cc of Ringer's lactate or normal saline. If blood pressure does not increase with cooling, administer a careful fluid challenge of 250-500 cc normal saline. If there is still no blood pressure improvement with fluid challenge, administer isoproterenol at 1 mg/min IV drip with careful monitoring. Patients with exertional heat stroke often have greater fluid requirement than those with classical heat stroke.

(d) Measure temperature with high rectal thermistor probe.

(e) Continuous cardiac monitoring.

(f) Lab: CBC with platelets, serum electrolytes, BUN, creatinine, ABGs, and urine specific gravity as baseline studies.

(g) Osmotic agents: In cases of exertional heat stroke, ATN is likely. Administer 25 g of 20% mannitol solution IV and furosemide 40-120 mg IV.

(h) Give $NaHCO_3$ if pH is less than 7.20.

c) Prevention

(1) Classical heat stroke. Some ways to prevent classical heat stroke are:

(a) Identify the population(s) at risk when heat waves are anticipated. Usually, elderly people living in low income, high density areas are most susceptible. Provisions for alternate living facilities, fans, etc., could significantly decrease the incidence of heat stroke in this population.

(b) Instruct emergency medical personnel in recognition and field treatment of heat stroke. Emergency vehicles should carry ice at all times during heat waves.

(c) Emergency rooms should prepare to manage heat stroke with ice, tubs, fans, etc., set up or easily accessible in the area.

(d) Careful monitoring of chronic care facilities to assure adequate environmental cooling is indicated. Attendants should receive specific instructions to give fluids at designated intervals.

(2) <u>Exertional heat stroke</u>. Some methods to prevent this type of heat stroke are:

(a) Allow time for acclimatization to a hot climate by designing a gradual training program for the first 2-4 weeks.
(b) Prohibit the use of restrictive clothing (e. g. , football pads) during the period of acclimatization.
(c) Prohibit the use of sweat suits in athletic training.
(d) Recognize adverse environmental conditions and plan athletic or other training programs accordingly.
(e) Since exertional heat stroke has occurred with marathon running, the guidelines of the American College of Sports Medicine should be carefully followed by race sponsors and participants. These guidelines are abstracted as follows:

i) Distance races (greater than 10 miles or 16 km) should not be held when the WBGT Index* is greater than 82. 4°F (28°C).
ii) Distance races should be held before 9:00 a. m. or after 4:00 p. m. if daytime dry bulb temperature** is greater than 80°F (27°C).
iii) Runners should be instructed to drink fluids at completion and at least 400-500 ml (13-17 oz) of fluid 10-15 min before the event.

WBGT Index = 0. 7 WB + 0. 2 BG + 0. 1 DB

WB (wet bulb) = Reading from a conventional thermometer bulb covered with a moist wick and exposed to ambient air. Accounts for air movement effects.
BG (black globe) = Reading from a conventional thermometer at the center of a 6 inch copper sphere painted flat black. Accounts for radiant heat effects.
DB (dry bulb) = Reading from a conventional thermometer. Measures air temperature.

---

*<u>WBGT Index</u>. Wet bulb globe temperature index is the best indicator of environmental heat stress potential.

**Dry bulb temperature is the air temperature reading from a conventional thermometer.

iv) Water stations with water and electrolyte solution should be set up at 2-2. 5 mile (3-4 km) intervals.

v) Race sponsors should make advance arrangements for treatment of heat illness.

C. GENERAL PREVENTIVE MEASURES FOR HEAT ILLNESS

1. Educate individuals (e. g. , athletes, hikers, soldiers) and supervisors (e. g. , coaches, drill instructors) regarding the signs and symptoms of heat stress and first aid measures.

2. Assess the environmental heat stress potential using WBGT index.

3. Adjust duration of exposure and activity level according to the estimated heat stress level.

4. Allow 2-4 weeks for acclimatization with gradual increase in duration and level of exertion in a hot climate.

5. Institute a specific oral fluid discipline program during athletic events, work details, etc.

SUMMARY: FIELD AND CONTINGENCY MANAGEMENT OF HEAT ILLNESS

The diagnosis and prehospital treatment of heat illness have been discussed above. This section will summarize some specific aspects of contingency care relative to personal protection, field resources, and triage of heat casualties.

A. PERSONAL PROTECTION

Avoid having medical or rescue personnel become heat casualties. All the preventive measures discussed previously are applicable. Personnel should be especially careful to do the following:

1. Maintain adequate hydration with fluid and electrolyte solutions.
2. Avoid excessive direct sun exposure.
3. Utilize sunscreen and shading head gear.
4. Rotate medical and rescue personnel to decrease prolonged exposure to the high heat stress environment.

B. FIELD RESOURCES NEEDED

1. Cool Environment

This can be a tent with fans powered from portable generators or recreational vehicles or buildings with independent power sources.

2. Cooling Supplies

    A. Cool water source (e. g. , hose or portable water tank)
    B. Ice if possible. (This can be obtained from hospitals, convenience stores, restaurants, mess halls, etc. , and transported to the scene in portable ice chests.)
    C. Fans (electrical or manual)

3. Replacement Fluids

    A. IV solutions: Ringer's lactate/normal saline
    B. Oral solutions: Lemonade, tomato juice, commercial athletic solutions prepared at one-half strength in large containers.
    C. Salt tablets or table salt so that a 0. 1% salt solution can be prepared at the scene.
    D. Cool water

C. TRIAGE

1. Heat Stroke

Immediate treatment and urgent evacuation to hospital facility.

2. Heat Exhaustion

Immediate treatment but can be adequately treated in contingency facility if necessary. Patient can be returned to duties with proper protective measures and instructions.

3. Heat Cramps

Minimal treatment needed which can be completed in short period of time (hours) in a contingency facility; the individuals can also be returned to duties as above.

II. LOCAL COLD INJURY

Local cold injuries, like heat illness, are preventable forms of environmental trauma. Injury involves peripheral parts (e. g. , hands, feet, ear lobes) and core temperature remains normal. Several environmental factors contribute to local cold injury, including degree and duration of cold applied to tissues; wind chill factor; skin contact with metal, water, or cold petroleum products; immobilization and dependency of extremities. Host factors that may predispose to local cold injury are previous local cold injury; lack of acclimatization and cold weather education; other physical factors such as peripheral vascular disease, alcohol ingestion, and cigarette smoking.

A. NONFREEZING INJURIES

The combination of cold temperatures (above freezing), wetness, dependency and constriction from boots or other clothing produces tissue damage by vasoconstriction and thrombosis. There are three main types of nonfreezing local injuries: chilblains, trench foot, and immersion foot.

1. Chilblains

a) Signs and Symptoms. This is the mildest form of local cold injury. The patient complains of painful, pruritic, reddened skin in exposed areas. These skin areas are tender, swollen, erythematous, and blanche with pressure. Vesicles, bullae, and ulceration may also be present.

b) Treatment. The affected areas should be massaged and have local heat applied. The skin should be protected from repeated cold exposure.

2. Trench Foot

a) Signs and Symptoms. Trench foot is observed among individuals immobilized for long periods in a cold, wet environment. The patient complains of cold, numb feet and leg cramps. On examination, the extremities are swollen and erythematous with vesicles and possible gangrenous changes noted. Arterial pulses are absent.

b) Treatment. Wet garments must be removed and the patient placed at rest in a warm environment. The affected extremities should be elevated. No surgical debridement or amputation should be performed as it may take one month or more for nonviable areas to demarcate.

3. Immersion Foot

Individuals who have had their extremities immersed in water,
dependent and stationary, for long periods may develop immersion foot. Signs, symptoms, and treatment are the same as for
trench foot.

B. FREEZING INJURIES

Tissue damage in freezing local cold injuries is a result of both
vasoconstriction and thrombosis as well as extracellular ice
crystal formation. Three types of injuries are distinguished,
but they actually represent a spectrum of freezing damage
rather than distinct processes. These are frostnip, superficial
frostbite, and deep frostbite.

1. Frostnip

    a) Signs and Symptoms. This is the mildest form of frost-
bite, usually affecting the fingertips, toes, earlobes, nose, and
cheeks. A sensation of severe cold progresses to numbness followed by pain. The skin is erythematous and tender without
edema or vesicles.
    b) Treatment. This is the only form of frostbite that can be
completely and adequately treated in the field. Remove wet
clothing. Warm the affected area by placing it against the warm
skin of the trunk or axillae.

2. Superficial Frostbite

    a) Signs and Symptoms. Superficial frostbite involves the
skin and subcutaneous tissues. The patient describes a cold
sensation followed by numbness which progresses to a warm
sensation in the affected body part. This is the most specific
symptom that distinguishes frostbite from frostnip. On examination, the skin is blanched and waxy-hard in texture. Generalized edema and vesicle or bullae formation occur 24-36 hrs after injury.

3. Deep Frostbite

    a) Signs and Symptoms. Injury extends below the subcutan-
eous tissue layer. Symptoms are the same as for superficial
frostbite. The skin is blanched, anesthetic and rock-hard with
delayed edema and blistering.
    b) Treatment. (Includes superficial frostbite)

(1) Remove all constricting and wet garments. Wrap affected body part(s) in dry clothing or blanket.

(2) Do not rub affected part with snow, apply dry heat, or expose part to open flame or vehicle exhaust.

(3) Prohibit alcohol and cigarettes. Encourage hot liquids if available.

(4) Rewarm rapidly, but this rapid rewarming must only be done once. It should not be initiated in the field if there is any risk of refreezing. An individual can walk a long distance on frozen feet without further injury; however, once the feet are thawed, the person becomes a litter case. The affected extremity or extremities are immersed in a water bath at 105-110°F (40. 6-43. 3°C) for 20-40 min in a container large enough to permit immersion without the part's touching the sides or the bottom. Immersion is continued until color returns to the affected part or it has been immersed for 40 min. If no warm water bath and thermometer are available, use the warm parts of the body to rewarm (e. g. , axilla).

(5) Handle thawed tissues in a careful, sterile manner as follows:

(a) Separate digits with sterile cotton padding and elevate the extremity.

(b) Use a loose, padded dressing if needed, but only for patient movement. It is preferable to leave the affected area exposed to air.

(c) Leave blisters intact unless the contents become turbid.

(d) Do not apply any ointments to affected tissues.

(e) Administer tetanus prophylaxis as indicated.

(f) Delay any surgical debridement/amputation until demarcation is complete (this may take more than 1 month).

III. HYPOTHERMIA

Hypothermia is a condition of core temperature decrease to less than 95°F (35°C) as a result of cold exposure. Detection of hypothermia often demands a high index of suspicion because a conventional thermometer may only register down to 94°F (34. 4°C) and some electronic models only as low as 90°F (32. 2°C). Hypothermia is a true medical emergency with a mortality rate of 21-87% depending on severity. Mild hypothermia (temperature of 90-95°F [32. 2°C-35°C]) is associated with decreased mortality and morbidity, but severely hypothermic patients (core temperature less than 90°F [32. 2°C]) are at extremely high risk.

A. PREDISPOSING FACTORS

1. <u>Hosts</u> are at extremes of age or are outdoor sportsmen, seamen, or divers.
2. <u>Toxic states</u> (e. g. , drug and alcohol intoxication) may predispose to prolonged exposure.
3. <u>Chronic illnesses</u> (e. g. , hypothyroidism, hypopituitarism)
4. <u>CNS</u> disease may alter central temperature regulation.
5. <u>Drugs</u>, especially phenothiazines and barbiturates, which interfere with central temperature regulation.
6. <u>Trauma</u> may predispose to prolonged exposure.

B. CLINICAL FEATURES

1. Very cold, cyanotic skin and mucous membranes
2. Respiratory rate markedly decreased; apnea occurs at 75°F (24°C)
3. Hypotension
4. Heart rate markedly decreased; at 86°F (30°C) or less, there is increased myocardial irritability with arrhythmias; asystole occurs at 59°F (15°C)
5. CNS: Altered mental status (difficulty in concentrating, apathy, etc.); coma; DTRs decreased or absent; pupils poorly reactive.
6. Shivering ceases at 86-91°F (30-33°C) and is replaced by muscle rigidity.

The hypothermic patient should not be pronounced dead unless there is no response to resuscitation after rewarming to 86°F (30°C).

C. COMPLICATIONS

There are multiple complications of hypothermia which adversely affect prognosis. Some of these are the following:

1. <u>Cardiac</u>: Arrhythmias, arrest, myocardial infarction
2. <u>Pulmonary</u>: Arrest, aspiration, bronchopneumonia, pulmonary edema
3. <u>Renal</u>: Acute tubular necrosis
4. <u>GI</u>: Bleeding, pancreatitis
5. <u>Local cold injuries</u>

D. TREATMENT

1. Prehospital

Place the patient in a warm environment or shelter from the wind as much as possible. Remove any wet clothing and wrap the patient in dry blankets or extra warm, dry clothing. One can also place the victim and a rescuer skin-to-skin in blankets or a sleeping bag, or between two rescuers. Building a fire with a reflector placed behind the victim is another method of warming. Apply basic manual skills of cardiopulmonary resuscitation if needed. Establish an adequate airway and give supplemental O_2. Administer IV solutions cautiously and warm the fluids if possible (e. g. , using a blood warmer, the surface of a warm vehicle, etc.). This patient requires urgent evacuation to a hospital facility.

2. Hospital

Rewarming is the most important and urgent aspect of treatment. There are three basic rewarming methods:

   a) Passive external. Application of blankets at room temperature to conserve endogenous heat; this can be utilized in a prehospital situation.
   b) Active external. Application of heating blankets or immersion in warm water bath.
   c) Active core. There are multiple procedures to rewarm the heart and brain first. Active core rewarming may be carried out by administering heated, humidified O_2 at $40^{\circ}C$ by local mask or ETT; by administering heated IV fluids at $40-46^{\circ}C$; or by performing gastric lavage, peritoneal dialysis, or hemodialysis with heated fluids. Two more advanced techniques are extracorporeal circulation and thoracotomy with heated lavage of the mediastinum.

   Multiple studies have shown that mildly hypothermic patients (temperature $90^{\circ}F$ [$32. 2^{\circ}C$] or above) may be safely rewarmed with the passive, external method. Patients who have core temperatures less than $90^{\circ}F$ but with stable cardiovascular function may be rewarmed by a combination of passive external rewarming and simple active core methods such as heated O_2 or IV fluids. Patients with core temperatures of less than $90^{\circ}F$ and cardiovascular instability require active core rewarming, usually with a combination of techniques, including heated peritoneal dialysis or hemodialysis.

Two problems occur with rewarming:

(1) <u>Afterdrop</u>. This refers to a 0.5-3.0°F (16.1-17.9°C) decrease in core temperature after rewarming due to peripheral vasodilation and release of cold blood to the body core.

(2) <u>Rewarming shock</u>. This is a sudden decrease in blood pressure, asystole, or arrhythmias occurring shortly after rewarming is initiated. Again, this is probably a result of release of cold blood back to the body core. As would be expected, the afterdrop and rewarming shock are most frequent with active external rewarming and are minimal with active core techniques.

3. Careful Monitoring

VS, CVP, urine output, ECG monitoring, and ABGs should be corrected for the patient's temperature or a falsely increased PO_2 and decreased pH will be reported.

4. Vigorous Supportive Measures

CPR, mechanical ventilation, and IV fluid should be used as supportive measures. It has been observed that arrhythmias can be induced during procedures such as intubation, nasogastric tube placement, etc. The incidence of these induced arrhythmias is decreased if the patient is well oxygenated before any procedure. Atrial fibrillation is the most common arrhythmia and usually does not require treatment. Defibrillation is usually not affected until the patient's core temperature is 82°F (27.7°C) or greater. Antiarrhythmic drugs and vasopressors are usually not indicated.

5. Treatment of Complications and Underlying Diseases

Sepsis and pneumonia need to be treated if they occur.

SUMMARY:
FIELD AND CONTINGENCY MANAGEMENT
OF COLD TRAUMA

The diagnosis and prehospital treatment of local cold trauma and hypothermia have been discussed above. Some specifics of contingency care are outlined in this section including personal protection, field resources, and triage.

A. PERSONAL PROTECTION

Medical and rescue personnel must avoid becoming cold trauma casualties. Preventive measures include:

A. Having adequate cold weather clothing and equipment and understanding their use.
B. Wearing nonconstricting, dry clothing applied in layers. This increases heat conservation via air trapping. Layering also facilitates gradual removal of clothing to prevent sweating.
C. Covering head, ears, and hands to decrease radiant loss.
D. Using a protective ointment on the nose, lips, and cheeks to decrease convective heat loss.

B. FIELD RESOURCES AND SUPPLIES

A. Warm environment or shelter (e. g. , heated tent, heated recreational vehicle, etc.)
B. Blankets
C. Sterile, nonocclusive dressing material
D. Analgesics, tetanus prophylaxis
E. IV solutions and administration sets
F. Airways and O_2 source
G. Warm water rewarming unit (not necessary as warm body may be used to rewarm frostbite areas)

C. TRIAGE

A. Hypothermia requires immediate treatment and urgent evacuation to a hospital facility.
B. Frostbite, trench, and immersion foot should receive delayed treatment especially if the patient has other more urgent injuries or if there is a chance of the extremity's refreezing after thawing.
C. Frostnip and chilblains need minimal treatment. These patients may be adequately treated in a contingency facility and then released to return to their duties with adequate, dry, protective clothes/equipment.

BIBLIOGRAPHY

HEAT ILLNESS

American College of Sports Medicine: Position Statement. Prevention of heat illness during distance running. J Sports Med 16:345, 1976.

Clowes, G. , and O'Donnell, T. : Heat stroke. N Eng J Med
291, 11:564-566, 1974.

Knochel, J. : Environmental heat illness: An eclectic review.
Arch Intern Med 133:841-864, 1974.

O'Donnell, T. : Acute heat stroke: Epidemiologic, biochemical,
renal and coagulation studies. JAMA 234, 8:824-828, 1975.

O'Donnell, T. , and Clowes, G. : The circulatory abnormalities
of heat stroke. N Eng J Med 287, 15:734-737, 1972.

Schrier, R. , et al. : Renal, metabolic, and circulatory responses to heat and exercise. Ann Intern Med 73:213-223, 1970.

Stine, R. J. : Heat illness. JACEP 8:154-160, 1979.

LOCAL COLD INJURIES AND HYPOTHERMIA

Abramowicz, M. (ed.): Treatment of frostbite. Med Lett Drugs
Ther 18, 25:105-106, 1976.

Adams, T. : Mechanism of cold acclimatization in the cat. J
Appl Physiol 18:778-780, 1963.

Boswick, J. A. : Cold injuries. Major Probl Clin Surg 19:96-
106, 1976.

DaVee, T. , and Reieberg, E. : Extreme hypothermia and ventricular fibrillation. Ann Emerg Med 9, 2:100-102, 1980.

Departments of the Army, Navy, and Air Force: Technical
Bulletin. Cold Injury (TM MED 81, NAVMED 5052-29, AFP
161-11) Sept. 30, 1976.

Maclean, D. , and Emslie-Smith, D. : Accidental Hypothermia.
London, Blackwell Scientific Publications, 1977.

Miller, J. , et al. : Urban accidental hypothermia: 135 cases.
Ann Emerg Med 9, 9:456-460, 1980.

Skitkata, J. , et al. : Studies in experimental frostbite. Arch
Surg 89:575-584, 1964.

Stine, R. : Accidental Hypothermia. JACEP 6, 9:413-416, 1977.

Ward, M. : Frostbite. Br Med J 1:67-70, 1974.

Welton, D. E. , et al. : Treatment of profound hypothermia. JAMA 240:2291-2292, 1978.

Chapter 13

RADIATION CASUALTIES
William A. Alter III, Ph. D.
James J. Conklin, M. D.

I. INTRODUCTION

Accidental or purposeful exposure of man to ionizing radiation
may cause injury or even death. Instability in world politics
and the marked proliferation in nuclear weapons have increased
the risk that health professionals may have to deal with situations of mass casualties that have radiation injuries alone or in
combination with blast and thermal injuries. In addition, mankind is at risk from many other radiation sources in use today
within the medical and industrial communities. Although the
possibility of radiation injuries from peacetime radiation accidents is much greater than a nuclear explosion, the numbers of
potential casualties should be far fewer for any one incident.

In the event of an accident, the physician's primary task
will be to assess the severity of the radiation injury, as well as
to determine the etiology of a pattern of symptoms that may be
associated with other disease states or injuries. Significant and
even potentially lethal doses have been received by individuals
who were unknowingly exposed to a radiation source. Unfortunately, improper diagnoses have delayed the onset of treatment
or even permitted the exposure to continue.

A far different picture emerges when the problem of nuclear
war is considered as the source of radiation casualties. In this
situation, health care personnel will face the ultimate challenge.
Casualties will be many and resources will undoubtedly be inadequate. Of prime importance will be the salvaging of victims
who require only minimal initial treatment and resources. Further complicating this situation will be the fact that most of the
radiation casualties will have additional injuries resulting from
the blast and thermal effects of the detonation itself.

Information contained within this chapter will be useful to
medical personnel who face the prospect of handling radiation
casualties from any source.

For the physicians who are required to function in a field
setting, some preliminary sorting of casualties is necessary.

197

This is based on symptoms seen within the first few hours after irradiation in which the exposure was whole-body or at least involved a major portion of the chest and abdomen.

For the physician who has the resources of a hospital, initial screening of patients will be similar to that seen in the field setting. However, additional testing can be performed on those individuals suspected of having a radiation injury. Specifically, this involves sampling for analysis of changes in concentrations of blood cells and platelets.

Considering that there isn't any immediate life-threatening hazard for the individual who has the potential to survive a radiation injury, the physician should be initially concerned with primary resuscitation. Only then should time be spent in assessing the possibility of radiation injury. In either setting (field or hospital), health workers should not delay handling victims of a radiation accident or nuclear weapon detonation. By wearing surgical attire and utilizing dosimetry equipment, these patients can be handled in an appropriate manner. The care of irradiated and contaminated patients is described with regard to the procedures applicable during the first two days of exposure.

II. THE ACUTE RADIATION SYNDROME

A. BIOLOGICAL EFFECTS OF IONIZING RADIATION

Radiation sensitivity is generally related to the mitotic rate of the different tissues and the degree of cell differentiation within any cell line. In order of radio-sensitivity, those tissues most critical to survival include:

1. Hematopoietic tissue
2. Mucosal lining of the gastrointestinal tract
3. Endothelial lining of the vasculature
4. Nervous tissue

As a result of damage to these tissues, whole-body irradiated individuals will experience symptoms during the overt clinical phase of the acute radiation syndrome. The onset of this phase will vary from a few hours to several weeks postexposure. These symptoms are rarely useful in the immediate time frame when initial sorting and diagnosis is undertaken. Of significant value will be those prodromal symptoms which appear within the first few hours to days after exposure. The rate of onset and duration of prodromal symptoms will be helpful in making preliminary diagnosis of radiation injury and severity.

B. PRODROMAL SYMPTOMS OF RADIATION INJURY

Due to the difficulty in establishing an early definitive diagnosis,
it is best to function within a simplified tentative classification
system based on three possible patient categories. Table 13-1
contains these radiation injury categories in a dose versus
symptoms matrix. More detailed information on latency, duration, and severity of these symptoms appears in the text.

1. Radiation Injury Unlikely. Due to the absence of any
symptoms associated with significant radiation injury, patients
are judged to be at minimal risk for radiation complications.
These patients should be handled according to the severity of
other medical problems which preexisted or occurred at the
time of the event in question. If free of any other injuries or
disease states that require treatment, they should be released
and asked to return for follow-up testing once the emergency
situation subsides.

2. Radiation Injury Probable. Symptoms associated with
radiation injury are present. Anorexia, nausea, and vomiting
will be the primary prodromal symptoms associated with this
category. These patients are prioritized for further evaluation
after all life-threatening injuries are stabilized. In this group,
a blood analysis provides the best biological indicator of radiation injury. Patients in this category will not require any medical treatment within the first few days for their radiation injury.
Patients may be either released or removed to a holding area.
Evidence to support the diagnosis of significant radiation injury

Table 13-1 Preliminary Triage of Casualties with
Possible Radiation Injuries

Symptoms	Unlikely	Probable	Severe
Nausea	-	++	+++
Vomiting	-	+	+++
Diarrhea	-	$\pm$	$\pm$ to +++
Hyperthermia	-	$\pm$	+ to +++
Hypotension	-	-	+ to ++
Erythema	-	-	- to ++
CNS dysfunction	-	-	- to ++

will be obtained from subsequent blood samples taken over the next two days. Once the evidence indicates that a significant radiation injury was received, these patients need to be monitored for pancytopenic complications.

   3. <u>Radiation Injury Severe</u>. These patients are judged to have received a radiation dose which is potentially fatal. Nausea and vomiting will be almost universal for this group. In addition, the prodromal phase may include prompt explosive diarrhea, significant hypotension, and signs of neurologic injury. These patients should be triaged according to the availability of staff and resources. Patients should receive symptomatic care. Blood analysis is necessary to support this initial classification.

C. SYMPTOMS WHICH FREQUENTLY OCCUR IN WHOLE-
   BODY IRRADIATED PATIENTS WITHIN THE FIRST FEW
   HOURS POSTEXPOSURE

   1. <u>Nausea and Vomiting</u>. These symptoms occur with increasing frequency as the radiation exceeds 100-200 rads. Onset may be as long as 6-12 hrs postexposure, but symptoms usually subside within the first day. Occurrence of vomiting within the first two hours is associated with a severe radiation dose; its occurrence within the first hour, especially if accompanied by explosive diarrhea, is associated with a dose range that frequently proves to be fatal. Due to the transient nature of these symptoms, it is possible that the patient will have already passed through this initial phase of gastrointestinal distress prior to being seen by a physician. It will be necessary to inquire about these symptoms at the initial examination. Emotional stress may also precipitate a similar gastrointestinal response.

   2. <u>Hyperthermia</u>. Casualties who have received a potentially lethal radiation injury show a significant rise in body temperature within the first few hours postexposure. Although the number of cases is few, this appears to be a consistent finding. Occurrence of fever and chills within the first day postexposure is associated with a severe and life-threatening radiation dose. Hyperthermia may occur in patients who receive lower but still serious radiation doses (200 rads or more). Present evidence indicates that hyperthermia is frequently overlooked.

   3. <u>Erythemia</u>. Individuals who received whole-body radiation doses in excess of 1000-2000 rads will experience erythema

within the first day postexposure. This is also true for patients who have received comparable doses to a local body region, where the erythema is restricted to the affected area. In doses lower but still in the potentially fatal range (200 rads or more), erythema is less frequently seen.

4. <u>Hypotension</u>. A noticeable and sometimes clinically significant decline in systemic blood pressure has been recorded in victims receiving a supralethal whole-body radiation dose. A severe hypotensive episode was recorded in one individual receiving several thousand rads. In those receiving several hundred rads, a systemic blood pressure drop of above 10% is noted. Severe hypotension after irradiation is associated with a poor prognosis.

5. <u>Neurologic Dysfunction</u>. Experience indicates that virtually all individuals who demonstrate obvious signs of central nervous system damage within the first hour postexposure have received a supralethal dose. Symptoms include mental confusion, convulsions, and coma. Intractable hypotension will probably accompany these symptoms.

D. HEMATOLOGIC CHANGES

Providing that the physician has the resources of a clinical laboratory, additional information can be obtained that will support the original working diagnosis suspected by the presence of prodromal symptoms. An initial blood sample for concentration of circulating lymphocytes should be obtained as soon as possible from all patients classified as "radiation injury probable" and "radiation injury severe." At the completion of the initial assessment, or at least no later than 24 hrs after the event in question, additional comparative blood samples should be taken.

Circulating lymphocytes are very radiosensitive. Considerable evidence has been accumulated that shows an excellent correlation between changes in the concentration of peripheral lymphocytes and the whole-body radiation dose. Figure 13-1 estimates the lymphocyte changes occurring over 24-48 hrs and relates it to exposure dose.

1. <u>Lymphocyte levels in excess of $1500/mm^3$</u>. Minimal likelihood of significant dose that would require treatment.

2. <u>Lymphocyte levels between 1000 and $1500/mm^3$</u>. May require treatment for moderate depression in granulocytes and platelets within 3 weeks postexposure.

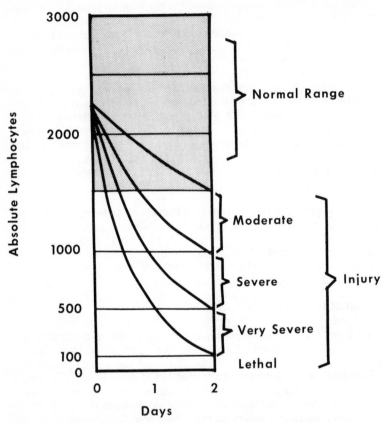

Figure 13-1. Patterns of early lymphocyte response in relation to radiation dose. Data obtained from radiation accident victims. (Reprinted with permission of the publisher from: The Medical Basis for Radiation Accident Preparedness by Hubner, K. F., and Fry, S. A. (eds.), 1st Edition, 1980. Copyright by Elsevier Science Publishing Co., Inc.)

3. Lymphocyte levels between 500 and 1000/mm^3. Will require treatment for severe radiation injury and should be hospitalized to minimize the complications from hemorrhage and infection that will arise within 2-3 weeks postexposure.

4. Lymphocyte levels of less than 500/mm^3. Have received a radiation dose that may prove fatal. All need to be hospitalized for the inevitable pancytopenic complications.

5. Lymphocytes are not detectable. Have received a supralethal radiation dose and survival is very unlikely. Most patients have received severe injuries to their gastrointestinal
and cardiovascular systems and will not survive for more than
2 weeks.

Further analysis of blood samples is performed over the
next 2 weeks to assess the decline in granulocytes and platelets.
Symptoms that accompany pancytopenia include:

1. Fever
2. Oral ulcer formation
3. Widely distributed petechiae
4. General malaise

Use these symptoms as a guideline for further therapy.

E. SUMMARY

In summary, patients who have received a potentially fatal dose
of radiation will most likely experience a pattern of prodromal
symptoms which are associated with the radiation exposure itself. Unfortunately, these are nonspecific and may be seen with
other forms of illness or injury. This may complicate the diagnostic process. Therefore, the physician must determine the
symptoms which have occurred within the first day postexposure, evaluate the possibility that they are indeed related to
radiation exposure, and then assign the individual to one of
three categories: radiation injury unlikely, radiation injury
probable, radiation injury severe. In the latter two categories,
study of changes in circulation lymphocytes will support or rule
out the original working diagnosis. All combined injury patients
should be treated initially as if there were not any significant
radiation injury present. Triage and care for any life-
threatening injuries should be rendered without regard for the
probability of radiation injury. Only in those patients where
radiation is the sole source of the problem should the physician
make a preliminary diagnosis of radiation injury. This is based
on the appearance of nausea, vomiting, diarrhea, hyperthermia,
hypotension, and neurologic dysfunction.

F. INITIAL TREATMENT FOR PATIENTS WITH
    WHOLE-BODY RADIATION INJURY

For those receiving whole-body radiation doses of more than
100-200 rads, gastrointestinal distress will predominate in the

first 2 days. Antiemetics may be effective in reducing symptoms. Unless severe radiation injury has occurred, these symptoms will usually subside within the first day.

For those patients who continue to experience gastrointestinal distress, parenteral fluids should be considered. If explosive diarrhea was present within the first hour postexposure, the use of fluids and electrolytes should be dictated by the availability of these resources. Under the demands of triage, the presence of explosive diarrhea (especially bloody) is likely to be related to a fatal radiation dose.

Cardiovascular support for those patients with clinically significant hypotension accompanied by neurologic dysfunction should be undertaken only when resources and staff allow for it. These patients are not likely to survive their radiation injuries. The effects of injury to the vascular and gastrointestinal linings, combined with marrow aplasia, is rarely survivable.

G. DIAGNOSIS AND TREATMENT OF THE PATIENT WITH COMBINED INJURIES

In the event of a radiation accident or nuclear detonation, there is every likelihood that many patients will suffer additional injuries. Initial triage classification is based on the existence of the conventional injuries and then further reclassification may be warranted on the basis of prodromal symptoms associated with radiation injury. Animal studies indicate that infections are much more difficult to control and that wounds and fractures heal more slowly with sublethal doses if radiation. Potentially survivable burns and trauma will be fatal in a large percentage of subjects who receive significant sublethal radiation injury. Patients requiring surgical intervention should have the procedures performed as soon as possible (i. e. , within 36 hrs) due to the risk of complications arising from pancytopenia. With severe radiation injury, patients are classified expectant despite potentially survivable conventional injuries.

III. THE CONTAMINATED PATIENT

Radiation injury per se does not imply that the patient is a health hazard to the medical staff. Studies indicate that the levels of intrinsic radiation present within the patient (after exposure to neutron and proton sources) are not life-threatening hazards for health workers.

In a disaster where the nature of the radiation source is unknown, patients entering a medical treatment facility should be routinely decontaminated if radiation monitoring is not

available. The simple expedient of removing the patient's clothing will usually reduce most of the contamination. Washing exposed body surfaces will further reduce this problem. Both of
these procedures can be performed in the field or on the way to
the treatment facility. Once the patient has entered the treatment facility, care should be rendered on the basis of obvious
injuries. In no case should care for life-threatening injuries be
delayed until decontamination procedures are completed.

In those situations where radiation safety personnel are
available, decontamination procedures will be established to
assist the physician in rendering care while minimizing the
hazard from radioactive contaminants. More extensive decontamination procedures include scrubbing the areas of persistent
contamination with a mild detergent or diluted solution. Caution
should be taken not to disrupt the integrity of the skin while
scrubbing. This could lead to incorporation of the radioisotopes
into the deeper layers of the skin. Contaminated wounds should
be addressed first; these sites will be the ones in which the
contaminant is rapidly incorporated. Washing, gentle scrubbing,
or even debridement are necessary to reduce the contaminant
level.

Wearing surgical attire will reduce the possible contamination of health personnel. If additional precautions are warranted,
rotation of the attending personnel will further reduce the possibility of contamination or exposure.

Inhalation or ingestion of radioactive particles is a much
more difficult problem. Sufficient information must be available
to indicate the type of substance, route of uptake, time since
exposure, and resources available to remove the contaminant.
Blocking agents can reduce the potential for uptake into target
tissues; chelating agents can form complexes with the trans-
uranics; diuretics and hydration can enhance the clearance of
agents; and purgatives can enhance the clearance of agents
present in the gastrointestinal tract. Specific details on the appropriate management of internal contamination[1] should be a
mandatory reference for any hospital at risk to receive radiation casualties.

IV. POTASSIUM IODIDE FOR PREVENTION
OF THYROID INJURY

The Federal Drug Administration is currently recommending
potassium iodide be considered in radiation emergencies for
individuals likely to receive more than 25 rem to the thyroid
gland from radioiodine released into the environment.

The FDA feels the risks from short-term use of low dose

potassium iodide outweigh the risks of radioiodine-induced
thyroid nodules or cancer.

State and local public health officials should be consulted to
determine feasibility of use. Potassium iodide does not prevent
or reduce the uptake or storage by the body of other radioactive
materials.

Dose: Adults and children over 1 year: 130 mg/day
Children under 1 year: 65 mg/day

V. WHERE TO GET ADDITIONAL HELP IN HANDLING THE IRRADIATED OR CONTAMINATED PATIENT

Radiation accidents can happen on virtually any major roadway
where radioactive materials are transported. Radiation sources
are widely distributed across the country in medical facilities,
university laboratories, and industrial plants. Every hospital
should have an emergency plan which includes radiation casualties. The authors recommend perusal of the article "Emergency Department Radiation Accident Protocol,"[2] as an important
first step in developing a sensible hospital plan.

Department of Energy regional offices are available through
emergency numbers that provide 24-hr assistance for any potential or actual radiation exposure (see Figure 13-2).

Assistance is available on a 24-hr basis with the Radiation
Emergency Assistance Center/Training Site (REAC/TS). This
facility is located at Methodist Hospital, Oak Ridge, Tennessee
(Contact Area Code 615-482-2441, Extension 502, or Beeper
#241 during off hours).

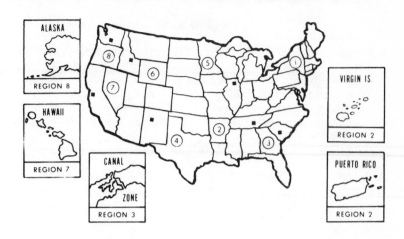

Regional Coordinating Office	Post Office Address	Telephone
1 Brookhaven Area Office	Upton, L.I., New York 11973	(516) 345-2200
2 Oak Ridge Operations Office	P.O. Box E, Oak Ridge, Tennessee 37830	(615) 576-1005 or (615) 525-7885
3 Savannah River Operations Office	P.O. Box A, Aiken, S.C. 29801	(803) 725-3333
4 Albuquerque Operations Office	P.O. Box 5400, Albuquerque, N.M. 87115	(505) 844-4667
5 Chicago Operations Office	9800 S. Cass Ave., Argonna, Ill. 60439	(312) 972-4800 Off Duty Hrs. (312) 972-5731
6 Idaho Operations Office	P.O. Box 2108, Idaho Falls, Idaho 83401	(208) 526-1515
7 San Francisco Operations Office	1333 Broadway, Oakland, California 94612	(415) 273-4237
8 Richland Operations Office	P.O. Box 550, Richland, Washington 99352	(509) 376-7381

Figure 13-2. Department of Energy regional coordinating offices for radiological assistance and geographical areas of responsibility. (U.S. Government publication.)

REFERENCES

1. National Council on Radiation Protection and Measurements: Management of Persons Accidentally Contaminated with Radionuclides. Recommendations of NCRP. NCRP #65. Washington, D.C. , 1980.
2. Leonard, R.B. , and Ricks, R.C. : Emergency department radiation accident protocol. Ann Emerg Med 9:462-470, 1980.

BIBLIOGRAPHY

Andrews, G.A. : Medical Management of Accidental Total-Body Irradiation. In The Medical Basis of Radiation Accident Preparedness. Hubner, K.F. , and Fry, S.A. , eds. New York, Elsevier North Holland Inc. , 1980.

Andrews, G.A. , and Cloutier, R.J. : Accidental acute radiation injury: The need for recognition. Arch Environ Health 10:498-507, 1965.

Conklin, J.J. , Walker, R.I. , and Hirsch, E.F. : Current concepts in management of radiation injuries and associated trauma. Surg Gynecol Obstet. 156:809-829, 1983.

International Atomic Energy Agency: Manual on Early Treatment of Possible Radiation Injury Safety. Series #47. Vienna, International Atomic Energy Agency, 1978.

Mathe, G. , Amiel, J.L. , and Schwarzenberg, L. : Treatment of acute total-body irradiation injury in man. Ann N Y Acad Sci 114:368-389, 1964.

Messerschmidt, O. , and Stahler-Michelis, O. : Effects of ionizing radiation combined with other injuries. Acta Anesthesiol Belg 19:308-314, 1968.

Poda, G.A. : Decontamination and Decorporation: The Clinical Experience. In The Medical Basis for Radiation Accident Preparedness. Hubner, K.F. , and Fry, S.A. ,eds. New York, Elsevier North Holland Inc. , 1980.

Thoma, G.E. , and Wald, N. : The diagnosis and management of accidental radiation injury. J Occup Med 1:421-447, 1959.

Voelz, G. L. : Current Approaches to the Management of Internally Contaminated Persons. In <u>The Medical Basis for Radiation Accident Preparedness</u>. Hubner, K. F. , and Fry, S. A. , eds. New York, Elsevier North Holland, Inc. , 1980.

Chapter 14

CHEMICAL CASUALTIES
Douglas Stutz, Ph.D.
Frederick M. Burkle, Jr. , M.D. , M.P.H.

I. INTRODUCTION

Chemicals are the essence of existence in today's world. New
materials being manufactured to meet the requirements of today's living frequently have dangerous properties. Other chemicals have been and are being produced for use in warfare.
Everyday the media carries stories about incidents which involve hazardous chemicals somewhere within the United States;
it may be a gas leak, an explosion in an industrial or manufac-
turing plant, or a highway tanker accident. The size of the
community doesn't matter, nor does the location. These incidents involving hazardous chemicals play no favorites; all have
potential for disaster, whether they be small or large. Medical
and paramedical personnel must have knowledge about hazardous chemicals—what they are; how they will basically act; and,
how injuries created by those chemicals can be managed—in
order to insure that when an incident occurs, it will not become
a disaster.

Dangerous chemicals are classified as hazardous materials
and can be defined in a number of ways. The Department of
Transportation has defined what hazardous materials are only
in relation to transportation, i.e. , any substance or material
in quantity or form that imposes unreasonable risk to safety,
health, or property when transported in commerce should be
considered as a hazardous material. One must consider, however, that any chemical or combination of chemicals which is
flammable, corrosive, etc. , and which, during handling, storage, or processing, could have detrimental effects on the operations of personnel in the immediate environment, emergency
personnel, the public in general, equipment, or the environment should be considered hazardous. Most official definitions
refer primarily to materials being transported. However, in
reality, a large number of incidents occur in storage facilities
and during use. As a result, these cannot be ignored and one

must consider that all substances which can be potentially dangerous should be considered as hazardous materials, or in the case of this chapter, dangerous chemicals.

For purposes of this discussion, chemicals can be broken down into two general classifications: chemicals used as weapons and other hazardous chemicals. Chemical weapons can further be classified by either their physiological action or their military use.

When classified by their physiological activity, they are considered to be nerve agents, blister agents, choking agents, or blood agents. When classified by military use, they are classified as toxic chemical agents or casualty-producing agents because they produce serious injury or death. These also include nerve agents, blister agents, choking agents, and blood agents. There is a second military use which is that of incapacitation. Incapacitating agents produce temporary physical or mental effects, or both.

There are over 70,000 chemicals commonly found in use in commerce today. No single individual can tell what physiological reaction to expect as a result of an acute exposure to any more than a relative few of those agents. Some of the more harmful chemicals have been identified as a result of various disasters or by the increased rate in incidents of irreversible, delayed carcinogenic effects.

It is only recently that the science of toxicology has expanded to consider the synergistic, additive, or antagonistic effects which various industrial chemicals may have upon the individual being exposed. We can predict the health effects resulting from acute exposure to a few of the chemicals if we know what that chemical is, its concentration at the time of exposure, the duration of exposure, and the route of exposure. Unfortunately, many chemicals have more than one hazard, all of which can be equally dangerous. As an example, hydrogen cyanide is not only highly flammable, and under some conditions explosive, but it is also extremely toxic.

A chemical may frequently be more dangerous in one form than another as is the case of gaseous metal relative to solid metal. Some agents are extremely hazardous when dry, but when wet with water solvent are relatively safe.

Chemicals can be classified in a number of ways, but for the purposes of our discussion we will consider them as follows:

1. Poison
2. Flammable agents
3. Explosives
4. Noxious gases
5. Corrosives

II. SCOPE OF THE PROBLEM

During the first half of the decade of the 70s, over 32,000 hazardous material incidents were reported to the Department of Transportation. These dealt specifically with chemicals being transported and did not include incidents for storage, manufacture, or use. Since that time, the trend in every state has been for a steady increase in the number of incidents. A portion of this increase can obviously be ascribed to better reporting procedures; however, there is a definite trend for increase. It is estimated that in 1980 over 2.7 billion tons of hazardous materials were shipped in the United States; the majority of that was chemicals. Again, consider that this is a figure for shipment and does not include that material maintained in storage, or during its manufacture, or while it was being used.

III. MANAGEMENT OF CHEMICAL HAZARD AREAS

A. CHEMICALS USED AS WEAPONS

Chemical agents can be used tactically or strategically under a nuclear or nonnuclear environment anywhere within the range of weapons and aircraft. Chemical operation scope is broad, aims at groups rather than individuals, and can be directed against civilian populations. Chemical agents can be disbursed by a variety of means, including explosive shells, rockets, missiles, aircraft, bombs, mines, and spray devices. Because of this variety of delivery possibilities, a chemical agent cannot always be assessed and identified. Therefore, in a wartime or combat situation, anytime a spray or cloud even appears to be delivered by aircraft, shells, or bombs, it should be a signal for putting on protective masks immediately. Vapors delivered from aircraft may not be visible, and vapors and sprays may be hidden by various atmospheric conditions.

1. The first priority upon arrival on the scene, whether it be in a military situation involving warfare or whether it be in a civilian incident, is self-protection. The rescuer must provide adequate protection for him/herself prior to entry into the area where the agent has been disbursed.
     Let us deal first with any situation which involves a wartime atmosphere. In this case, you should put your protective mask on if any of the following conditions exist: if you enter a war zone; if your position is such that you are hit by significant concentrations of artillary mortar, rocket fire, or bombs from aircraft; if a spray is laid down over your area or an area

which you are going to enter; if a suspicious odor or liquid is present; if you are entering an area known or suspected to be contaminated with toxic chemicals; or if you have one of the following symptoms: unexplained runny nose, feeling of choking or tightness in the chest or throat, dimming of vision, difficulty in focusing your eyes on close objects, eye irritation, unexplained difficulty in breathing, or increased rate of breathing. Keep in mind also that the casualties who have been contaminated with a chemical agent may endanger unprotected personnel. Anyone handling these patients must wear a protective mask, chemical protective gloves, and chemical protective clothing until the contaminated clothing has been removed and disposed of properly. If possible, any gathering station or aid station should be established upwind from heavily contaminated areas.

2. The second priority is specific identification of the agent which can be done through the proper use of signs and symptoms in the individual as well as by the mechanism of exposure. Signs and symptoms will be discussed in detail later in this chapter.

The primary rescuer should consider the fact that most personnel who are military, in this type of situation, will have, if possible, already administered self-aid and first aid to their buddies. However, it is the rescuer's responsibility to follow up with proper triage and diagnosis of the injuries and to provide medical treatment. At the same time, it is necessary for those providing the rescue, whether it be in a military situation or otherwise, to supply protection for themselves and for other rescuers and to ensure that other persons don't become contaminated and therefore exposed.

B. CIVILIAN CHEMICAL CASUALTIES

When in a nonwartime situation, the rescuer may, upon arrival at the scene of an incident, find major complications in the form of hazardous chemicals; these may be the primary problem or may merely be involved in the overall incident. For example, in the case of the overturned tank truck where the driver has been injured and other automobiles were involved, there may be a danger of the truck's leaking hazardous material. Again, the first step is to provide adequate protection for all personnel involved prior to establishing a rescue attempt. This means everyone must remain far enough away from the scene of the incident to be safe until a decision can be made as to the proper method for handling the problem.

1. <u>Identification of Toxic Chemicals</u>. It is vitally important
that the agent or agents involved be identified. The material,
its properties, and the extent of the hazard to personnel or
property in an existing emergency must be determined. Identification can be accomplished through a number of resources.

a) First, attempt to obtain a shipping manifest; this will
provide the necessary information about the type of chemical
that is being carried. These manifests are usually very accurate; however, on occasion they will be mislabeled to ensure
that a lower tariff be paid. A second resource is the plaques or
signs which are placed on the side and end of the vehicle to announce what is being carried within the vehicle. The new marking system, as explained in the 1980 <u>Emergency Response</u>
<u>Guidebook for Hazardous Materials</u>, published by the Depart-
ment of Transportation, provides a fairly clear way of identifying many chemicals. The rescuer must be familiar with the
proper placarding system to ensure that he or she knows how to
identify the material involved.
If the incident is not a transportation incident but involves a
static location, then personnel who work at that location are an
excellent resource for providing information about the chemicals or agents involved. Quite frequently a trade name or chemical name will be noted on the container. These names can be
then used to determine what the agent is and what its potential
effects are.

b) The second major problem is that of determining the
physical properties and the amount of material involved. You
need to know if it is a gas, solid material, or liquid; the amount
of material, which includes the area covered by the spill or the
incident; the total amount of materials involved; if it is a leak;
the rate of leakage, etc.

c) Thirdly, the chemical properties must be established.
Hazardous materials can be divided into four categories for
identification purposes; however, it is essential to check more
than one category for any chemical. The categories are:

1. Flammability
2. Toxicity for health hazard
3. Reactivity (such as with other chemicals or water)
4. Radioactivity

d) The fourth item that must be determined is the extent of
the hazard involved. After having determined the first three

phases, the rescuer will be able to ascertain which of the following categories apply:

(1) Extremely Dangerous. Can cause death or disabling injury on brief exposure; or are extremely volatile flammable liquids, flammable gases, or materials that would detonate.

(2) Dangerous Materials. Could cause injury from exposure, have detrimental effects, or are highly flammable or highly self-reactive materials.

(3) Hazardous Materials. Can cause temporary disability or injury, which presumably would heal without permanent effects.

(4) Nuisance Hazard. Could cause temporary irritation or discomfort which would clear up when exposure is ended; includes materials which are only slightly combustible.

2. Evaluation Phase. The next process in scene management is to evaluate what you have determined in the identification phase.

a) Determine the degree of involvement.
b) Evaluate the hazard caused by the material.
c) Determine the primary contributing factors which will affect the incident.

Any evaluation must include the following contributing factors which must be analyzed to determine what the effect will be or is upon the incident itself:

(1) Wind factor
(2) Drainage
(3) Amount involved
(4) Humidity
(5) Density of population

3. Decision Phase. Once you have identified the material and evaluated the situation, a decision, based upon this information, must be made about the means for accomplishing a rescue. With major situations, never concern yourself about planning too big; plans may always be scaled down and are sometimes difficult to scale up.

Major problems that must be covered when considering these situations are:

(1) Evacuation of the area. Remembering to start close to the incident, to consider wind direction, and to ensure people are directed away from the immediate area.

(2) Containment, if possible. If not, you must be able to control the total amount of area involved.
(3) Rescue, when immediate removal is necessary.
(4) Additional support if required.

4. Implementation Phase. Implementation of decisions developed in earlier phases must be given careful thought. At this point any wrong move could wipe out all the plans and be dangerous to all personnel involved.

a) Initiate the rescue and ensure that the rescue is performed systematically, utilizing teamwork, a planned search pattern, and orderly removal of the victims.

b) Initiate evacuation orders, if necessary, keeping in mind the necessary environmental conditions to ensure that all personnel are evacuated sufficiently far from the incident so that they will not be exposed.

c) Provide exposure protection for those individuals who must participate in the rescue. This can be done primarily through the use of proper protective clothing and equipment; secondarily by the use of the proper support unit (e. g. , fire departments).
It is important throughout the course of the incident to maintain a proper time record for calculation of exposures, to obtain the names and addresses of all persons exposed, and to try to retain those people at the site, until they have been thoroughly checked out and decontaminated (if possible, in the field). Ensure that support personnel involved in providing medical needs are notified of any incident as early as possible. All medical facilities that will be involved in treatment of patients should be notified in advance so that they may adequately prepare for the influx of patients.

d) Assess the need for EMT and paramedic teams and coordinate the use of these teams. The first team to arrive on the scene should be used as a triage team to ensure the proper evaluation and treatment of patients. Additional support ambulances should be requested to be sure that an adequate amount of transportation is available.

e) A prime part of scene management is ensuring that all personnel involved and equipment to be used are adequately prepared for the type of incident involved. A major part of management is planning for these emergencies. Planning will

provide you with necessary information which would be difficult
to obtain at a moment's notice. If disaster plans and hazardous
material incident management plans are developed ahead of
time, then the medical respondent will be adequately prepared
upon arrival at the scene and when patients arrive in the emergency room for treatment.

IV. TRIAGE AND IMMEDIATE MANAGEMENT

Similarities between military and civilian chemical disasters
can be predicted. The principles of triage and management are
the same for both.

In general, Armed Forces personnel are trained to provide
personal decontamination for themselves. Furthermore, corpsmen are trained in the complexities of resuscitation and the decontamination of physically disabled personnel (Figures 14-1
and 14-2).

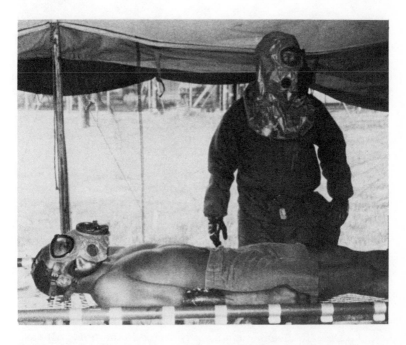

Figure 14-1. Physician-in-training and "actor-casualties" participate in chemical decontamination scenario. Combat Casualty Care Course, Fort Sam Houston, Texas (taken by author: F.
M. Burkle, Jr. , M.D.).

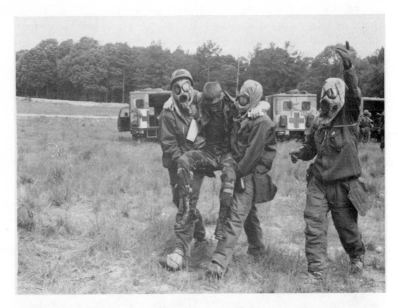

Figure 14-2. Chemical treatment scenario. Combat Casualty Care Course. Fort Sam Houston, Texas. With the increasing use of industrial chemicals and the added threat of chemical warfare, training in chemical disaster management becomes a priority (U.S. Army photograph).

A. RESPONSIBILITIES OF MEDICAL PERSONNEL AT THE FIELD SITE

    1. Attend to the ABCs.
    2. Counteract any toxic reactions with specific antidote.
    3. Decontaminate face, eyes, exposed skin.
    4. Rapidly remove contaminated clothing and place on clean litter.
    5. Outline the areas of contamination with skin marker.
    6. Continue first aid measures and transport following general triage-transport principles (see Chapter 4).

B. PROCEDURES TO BE FOLLOWED

    1. Despite cleaning methods reported in the field, all casualties should be received at one central area. Due to expected confusion in the field, contaminated casualties will arrive at the hospital by ambulance or private vehicle.

2. The receiving area should be designated and clearly marked as contaminated or dirty.
3. Toxic reactions should be counteracted with specific antidotes.
4. Further decontamination, undressing, and showering should be done or repeated before triage to a clean area.
5. The skin should be cleaned with large amounts of soap or detergent with water. Skin abrasion should be avoided. Since many poisons are more soluble in alcohol than in water, the skin should be washed with alcohol. Eyes should be irrigated with normal saline or tap water. Several casualties can be washed together by means of a hose.
6. ABC and triage priorities should decide whether to manage the surgical conditions or chemical hazard first; but in general, if the situation allows, decontamination should be the initial procedure.

C. TRIAGE CATEGORIES

In chemical disasters, the majority of casualties arrive free of associated medical or surgical complications. Unfortunately, this is not the case in military conflicts, vehicular accidents, or explosions. Triage categories in mixed disasters are illustrated in Table 14-1.

D. SPECIFIC ANTIDOTE TREATMENT

Nerve gas and anticholinesterase agent (e. g. , organophosphate pesticides and chemicals) poisoning may require immediate administration of atropine.

1. Atropine inhibits the action of excess acetylcholine. It benefits the critical central nervous system and respiratory depression but will not inhibit the peripheral neuromuscular paralysis.
2. Where respiratory failure occurs, atropinization and artificial respiration will be necessary.
3. Atropine alone is effective only in the mild to moderately severe cases of suffering respiratory failure.
4. In field situations, personnel are trained to administer atropine 2 mg IM (by syrette, automatic injector, or syringe) at the earliest signs of symptoms (tightness and constriction of chest). This is followed by one atropine tablet.
5. Severe cases with cyanosis, respiratory depression, or coma require

Table 14-1. Triage Categories

Mixed Chemical/ Medical-Surgical	Chemical Alone	Medical-Surgical Alone
Contaminated/ minimal	Contaminated	Minimal
Contaminated/ expectant		Expectant
Contaminated/de- layed treatment		Delayed
Contaminated/im- mediate treatment		Immediate

    a) Secretions to be suctioned and airway to be maintained
    b) O_2, intubation if necessary
    c) With improvement of cyanosis, atropine 2-4 mg IV.
       Repeat dose every 5-10 min until there are signs of
       atropinization (dry mouth, throat, flushing, rapid
       pulse, difficulty in swallowing). Maintain slight de-
       gree of atropinization for 48 hrs.
  6. Pralidoxime chloride (2-PAM-Cl, Protopam), a therapeutic oxine, is used as an adjunct to atropine.
    a) Adults: 1 gm in 100 ml of sterile water, normal
       saline or D5W, slowly (15-30 min) IV, or deep IM (1
       gm in 3 ml distilled water) repeated every 30 min if
       respiratory depression, muscle fasciculation, or
       seizures occur.
    b) Children: Dose is 20-40 mg/kg.

E. SELF-CARE FOR MEDICAL PERSONNEL

  1. Medical personnel must take precautions to protect
     themselves. Initially the exact nature of the chemical
     involved may be unknown. There should be no hesitation
     in using protective clothing, masks, and a thick layer of
     skin ointment.
  2. Once the casualties have passed through the triage sys-
     tem, medical personnel and others who have handled the
     casualties should be triaged through the system them-
     selves. Determine and triage first any personnel inad-
     vertently contaminated, no matter how small the contact.
  3. Contaminated clothing and gear must be placed in a
     designated dump area in tightly closed metal cans if
     possible.

SELECTED REFERENCES

Departments of the Army, Navy, and Air Force: Treatment of
Chemical Agent Casualties and Conventional Military Chemical
Injuries. TM 8-285, NAVMED P-5041, AFM 160-12,
Washington, D. C. , Departments of the Army, Navy, and Air
Force, May, 1974.

Doull, J. , Klaassen, C. D. , and Amdur, M. D. : Casarett and
Doull's Toxicology. 2d Ed. New York, MacMillan Publishing
Co. , Inc. , 1980.

Department of Transportation: Emergency Response Guidebook
for Hazardous Materials. Washington, D. C. , Department of
Transportation, 1980.

Ayerst Laboratories: Protopam Chloride. Professional bro-
chure. New York, Ayerst Laboratories, 1973.

Chapter 15

NEUROPSYCHIATRIC CASUALTIES
Frederick M. Burkle, Jr. , M. D. , M. P. H.

I. GENERAL

One of many definitions for a disaster is that it is a "situation of massive collective stress. "[1] There is a disruption in the existing social system. Neuropsychiatric casualties are a predictable consequence of such disruption. Unfortunately, many health care providers are poorly prepared to understand or deal with these victims.

Current knowledge of civilian disaster responses are attributed to research initiatives and concepts derived primarily from military psychiatry. Initial studies from WW II focused on intrapsychic processes that lead to the concepts of stress-related disorder (traumatic war neurosis). [2] Postwar disaster-related experiences incorporated this wartime knowledge. Whether secondary to combat or civilian disaster situations, stress reactions were first regarded as transient states. The tendency to correlate neurosis with a long-term illness and poor prognosis did not justify the earlier designation of these reactions as neurotic. Traumatic emotional responses were subsequently grouped under gross stress reactions. [3] Follow-up studies, however, have indicated that some victims retain and suffer their original symptoms for many years after the initial traumatic event (posttraumatic stress disorder). [4-8] Some researchers have retained the term, traumatic war neurosis. * The author suggests that this is a misleading designation which should be replaced by the terms, reaction or disorder (i. e. , traumatic war reaction), unless future long-term assessment should prove otherwise.

---

*Traumatic Neurosis: Criteria[9] are insomnia, nightmares irritability, startle patterns, anxiety, depressive mood, low self esteem, guilt feelings, loss of interest and motivation, contraction of ego functioning.

The disaster stress may be the one factor necessary to precipitate a chronic mental disorder in an individual otherwise predisposed to such premorbid risks (i. e. , genetic predisposition or personality disorder).

It has become apparent, however, that classic mental disorders are not produced by external danger. Records from WW II indicate the rate of psychosis among military personnel is the same in peace as in war. [10] Transient emotional reactions, some of which manifest severe psychotic behavior, may begin to improve as soon as the assumed or real danger subsides.

During WW II and the Korean War, soldiers with combat-related psychoses were frequently evacuated with the diagnosis of "acute schizophrenia." These soldiers were remarkable (often to the chagrin of military physicians) for their rapid reintegration and the complete resolution of their psychotic behavior. Unfortunately, the diagnostic label of "schizophrenic" frequently remained on their permanent record.

With the increasing awareness of the emotional responses to war and civilian disasters, psychiatric practitioners have changed their thinking. The inclusion of brief reactive psychosis in the current DSMIII[11] terminology provides an alternative to the former limiting and often inaccurate category of acute schizophrenic episode of DSMII.

The reader should understand that reaction to the overwhelming stress of combat or civilian disasters has an effect on everyone. Susceptibility is universal. Bourne believes that the neuropsychiatric casualty in war (and in civilian disasters) can be conceptualized as an "adaptive failure, often of a temporary nature. "[12] There is no such thing as "no response. "

In the acute situation (i. e. , the first 36 hrs), it is better to leave the patient undiagnosed than to use a diagnosis which may label the individual forever. It is recommended that the clinical impression be a brief description of signs and symptoms, and that treatment modalities be focused on those target symptoms which are most urgent or critical.

II. PSYCHOLOGICAL THEORY

A. INTRAPSYCHIC PROCESSES

1. Stimulus Barrier Concept. [13,14] Theories suggest that each individual's mind has a unique stimulus barrier which reflects those cumulative experiences in his/her life that have dealt with the input of emotional stimuli. This stimulus barrier appears to have both conditional and adaptive responses. The responses

are integrated with an individual's sense of self (ego) and personality organization.

2. <u>Phases</u>. [13] There are three stages in personality dysfunction: disorganization, reorganization, and reintegration.

Everyone is vulnerable to trauma, whether emotional or physical or a combination of both, that may challenge the limits of the stimulus barrier. Under severe stress, every individual is subject to some degree of disorganization of his/her ego function. Reactions may be transient, prolonged, delayed, acute, or chronic. They may or may not be recognized by the victim. Reorganization and reintegration may occur rapidly, or the ego may find it difficult to reconstruct adaptive defenses essential for the refunctioning of the stimulus barrier. Once the stimulus barrier has been exceeded,[15] a person may be more vulnerable to a secondary traumatic stress.

III. CIVILIAN DISASTER-RELATED NEUROPSYCHIATRIC CONCEPTS

Shock trauma occurs where there is a single massive experience.[1] Natural disasters, such as earthquakes, floods, or tidal waves, are usually responsible for shock trauma. Despite the widespread devastation, hope is generated from the expectation that the traumatic event is a temporary one. Civilian disasters, as a rule, do not result in widespread neuropsychiatric decompensation. Only a relative minority of individuals are able to grasp the relevant aspects of a disaster situation quickly, and to utilize this understanding for immediate and appropriate constructive action. However, this phase quickly passes and more than 90% of individuals reintegrate and function well in the postimpact phase. [16]

There was no increase in the rate of psychosis or psychiatric admissions during the bombings of England during WW II, as a result of the atomic devastation of Japan, or with major civilian disasters worldwide. [10]

Few civilian hospitals are equipped to handle the mental health aspects of a disaster or to participate in assisting other health care professionals in the evaluation and treatment of physically traumatized casualties with additional acute psychological problems. As a result, responses are both misinterpreted and compounded causing unnecessary admissions, treatments, and logjams in the triage process.

Civilian disaster experience has shown that one-third of the population experiences little emotional stress; two-thirds experience stress and mild depression; and less than 1% suffer any severe impairment. [17] Tyhurst reports that at the time of the disaster, 12-25% of individuals will remain "cool and collected" while a more normal 75% will be temporarily stunned and bewildered. [16]

Civilian disasters result in intense stress from:

1. Sudden loss of loved one(s)
2. Severe disruption in expected routines
3. Sudden loss of basic security needs (e. g. , home, food supply, etc.)
4. Possible sense of loss from bodily injury

People exhibit the following symptoms during civilian disasters:

1. Acute grief
2. Severe anxiety/panic reactions
3. Both #1 and #2 may approach or assume transient psychotic or psychotic-like behavior that would warrant the diagnosis of brief, reactive psychosis.

Tyhurst and Glass describe the disaster syndrome present in up to 75% of victims during the impact phase. [10,16] It includes the following: absence of emotion, inhibition of activity, docility, indecision, lack of responsiveness, automatic behavior, and physiological manifestations of fear. Table 15-1 and 15-2 illustrate these phases and their resultant behavior.

IV. COMBAT-RELATED NEUROPSYCHIATRIC CONCEPTS

Basic military and survival training are designed to expose military personnel to stress they are likely to experience in the event of war. [18] Training processes select out, over time, those individuals who would not function well under wartime stresses. In one study, 1. 8% of recruits were admitted for psychiatric appraisal. [19] The U. S. Military Academy identifies up to 4% of each class as "stress reactors. "[20] Air recruits may develop the classic symptoms of traumatic war disorders while still in training. [21] Soldiers with a history of poor adaptation in society were at greater risk of poor adaptation to combat situations. [10,26] In WW II, Marshall found that only 15-25% of combat infantrymen exhibited "appropriate aggressive action" in battle. [22]

Although it has been suggested that training is the primary factor in protecting an individual from neuropsychiatric disruption, everyone's stimulus barrier can be exceeded.

Table 15-1.   Phases of a Disaster*

Phase	Stress	Psychological Behavior
Preimpact	Worry	Denial or anxiety
Warning	Anticipation of stress	Denial or protective action
Impact	Maximum, unavoidable, direct physical stress	12-25%: Remain calm, collected and busily function 75%: Temporarily stunned and bewildered 12-25%: Inappropriate behavior, confusion, pananxiety, hysteria
Recoil	Stress subsides	90%: Awareness returns; self-conscious of immediate past; express emotions for first time
Postimpact	Residual effects of primary and secondary stress	Grief, depression, posttraumatic stress syndrome, psychosomatic complaints, varied responses

*Modified from the classification of Tyhurst and Glass. [10,16]

A. CONTRIBUTING COMBAT FACTORS[12]

1. Total Days in Combat. After 80-100 days in combat, risk of neuropsychiatric problems increase markedly.

2. Quality of Leadership. [31]

3. Unit Morale

4. Unit Cohesiveness and Support. Literature from the Yom Kippur War shows marked differences were found in the psychological reactions of the members of elite combat group units where there was considerable social support compared to the physiological reactions of members of reserve units where the

Table 15-2. Phases of a Disaster

Phase	Psychological Behavior
Preimpact phase	Awareness of impending stress
Impact phase	Stimulus barrier is over-whelmed
Acute disorganization phase (usually transient)	Disoriented, blunting of aware-ness, memory disturbances, disturbance in judgment, fluctuating affect, and, dis-turbance in perception of events
Regression phase	Ego constriction utilized to re-sist further disorganization
Reconstitution phase	Ego reintegrates

*Modified from the classification of Titchener and Ross.[13]

soldiers were total strangers to each other. The reserve units experienced an increased rate of traumatic neurosis.[9]

5. Static Battle Lines Increase Rate of Neuropsychiatric Casualties. Movement, whether forward or in retreat, decreased this rate. [12]

6. Meanings of Combat for Each Individual. The combat experience and the direct adaptation to it are not in themselves sufficient to explain the soldiers' reactions. The varied reactions became understandable only when the meanings of combat for each individual are recognized.[23]

B. CONTRIBUTING NON-COMBAT FACTORS[24]

1. Isolation, boredom, inadequate diet, chronic physical discomfort, exhaustion, and physical illness contribute to the problem.
2. Personnel with preexisting neuroses have a 7-8 times greater probability of developing overt neuropsychiatric symptoms. [25]

3. The lack of close friendships is another contributing fac-
    tor. In the Vietnam War the buddy system was often
    nonexistent due to the constant staggering of new troops
    to combat units. [12]

In previous wars, combat neuropsychiatric casualties
ranged upwards to 23%. [12,30] Field commanders expected at
least a rate of 10%. [27] The neuropsychiatric casualty rate in the
Vietnam War was an alltime low of 6%. [12,30] The reasons given
are as follows:[27]

1. One year tour of duty
2. Improved psychological awareness of the military com-
    mand
3. Improved training
4. Improved equipment
5. Improved leadership
6. Rapid medical evacuation
7. Improved morale of combat troops
8. Brief battles with emphasis on mobility
9. R & R (rest and recreation) policy
10. Improved psychiatric training of general medical offi-
    cers

C. CATEGORIES

Pettera observed three general categories of emotional reactions from forward combat areas in Vietnam. [28]

1. Combat Fatigue (Exhaustion) with Psychic Distress

a. Secondary to frequent, prolonged contact with enemy
    forces
b. Combined physical and emotional fatigue (primarily
    physical)
c. Symptomatology is uncontrollable crying, hyperventila-
    tion, extreme tremulousness, and acute incapacitating
    anxiety (commonly termed "clutching" or "freezing").

2. Combat Reaction

Pattera recognized the limitation of neurosis in describing this
phenomenon and substituted the term, reaction.

a) Occurs only in combat unit personnel
b) Precipitated by repeated, severe psychic trauma
c) Develops over prolonged period of time
d) Symptom progression is illustrated in Figure 15-1. [28] It
   includes reliving the combat psychic trauma through
   nightmares, depression, guilt, and shame over subjec-
   tive performance in combat; the fact of having broken
   down when others did not; incomplete bereavement over
   loss of a friend in combat—all provide stimulus to progression. Ineffectiveness in combat is recognized by the
   soldier and by unit leaders. Both the thought of combat
   and combat itself provoke deep fear. [28]

3. Transient Anxiety Reactions

a) Acute and moderately incapacitating
b) Little or no recognized etiology

Eiseman emphasized the role of sensory deprivation from
studying the role of isolated night sentry positions in precipitating stress-related anxiety. He found that there is a tendency to
hallucinate under such conditions. [27]

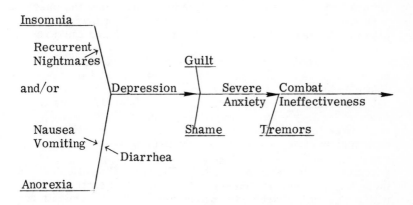

Figure 15-1. Symptom progression

Table 15-3. Diagnostic Categories as Related to
            Hospital Treatment

Diagnosis	%	Duration of Hospitalization
Psychosis	44%	14 days
Nonpsychotic acute situational reaction	17. 5%	6 days
Psychoneurosis	12. 3%	8 days
Character-behavior disorder	11. 2%	8 days
Alcohol and drug problems	6. 8%	2 days
Combat exhaustion	5. 7%	3 days

Bloch further delineated the acute diagnostic categories (see Table 15-3) generally seen in those individuals evacuated from outlying posts and admitted for neuropsychiatric evaluation:[29] 56% of those initially diagnosed as psychotic were returned to duty; 28% with a new diagnosis of acute situational reaction. One hundred percent of those with "combat exhaustion" were returned to duty. Treatment programs "emphasized the inter-personal dimensions of a soldier's illness rather than the intra-psychic components," with the treatment goal being rapid re-turn to duty. [29]

In other studies, character and behavior disorders led other categories (40%),[32] and only 13 were classified as psy-chotic or neurotic. [33] Tischler revealed that approximately one-half of the neuropsychiatric casualties in his study had been in Vietnam for less than 4 months, were young (17-20 years), came from intact nuclear families, had positive relationships with their parents, and were more often single with a high school education. [33] In contrast, Schramel studied 100 neuro-psychiatric patients evacuated from Vietnam. His patients were more likely to be nonvolunteer, married, significantly older with a history of disrupted family and marital life, and with an 80% alcohol abuse rate. Schramel's findings were similar to those found in the Korean War. [34] In Marine and Navy personnel, Strange described three categories of patients seen on the hos-pital ship, Repose:[35]

1. Character and behavior disorders: 69%*
2. Psychoneurotic: 23%
3. Psychotic: 8%

Combat stress was a major precipitating factor in 49% of character and behavior disorders and 47% of psychoneurotic disorders. It was further determined that many of these individuals would have escaped psychiatric hospitalization had it not been for their traumatic combat experience. Combat-related experience was deemed relatively unimportant as a precipitation in those patients with psychosis. [35]

V. TREATMENT MODALITIES

A. NONPHARMACOLOGIC TREATMENT OPTIONS

1. All patients require

a) Encouragement to ventilate their experience and feelings as soon as possible

b) Reassurance that their reaction is normal and understood by the health care providers; that vulnerability to loss of emotional control is universal when the stress exceeds a certain limit

c) Reassurance that their reaction is not shameful

d) Encouragement to return to purposeful activity or active military duty as soon as possible

e) During the process of reassurance assess and rule out whether a more severe emotional response exists (i. e. , intrusive psychotic thinking or behavior that might limit rapid recovery)

f) Pharmacologic management should be avoided until a careful physical examination has been completed to rule out postconcussion syndromes, CNS bleeding, and early hypotension that may present as a change in mental status and anxiety

2. The psychological first aid approach offered by the disaster plan for Montgomery County, Maryland has practical adaptability for the myriad of responses seen in disaster victims[36] (see Table 15-4).

3. Up to 10% of victims may be so disturbed as to require additional rest, removal from the site, physical restraint, sedation, and/or antipsychotic, antianxiety medications.

---

*Character and behavior disorders predominate in the noncombat military psychiatric population as well.

Table 15-4. Psychological First Aid for Disaster Situations*

Reaction	Symptoms	Do	Don't
Normal	Trembling	Give reassurances	Don't show resentment
	Muscular tension	Provide group identification	Don't overdo sympathy
	Perspiration	Motivate	
	Nausea	Talk with him	
	Mild diarrhea	Observe to see that individual is gaining composure, not losing it	
	Urinary frequency		
	Pounding heart		
	Rapid breathing		
	Anxiety		
Individual panic (flight reaction)	Unreasoning attempt to flee	Try kindly firmness at first	Don't use brutal restraint
	Loss of judgment	Give something warm to eat or drink	Don't strike
	Uncontrolled weeping	Get help to isolate if necessary	Don't douse with water
	Wild, running about		Don't give sedatives

Reaction	Signs	What to do	What not to do
Depression (underactive reactions)	Stand or sit without moving or talking	Be empathetic	Don't tell him to "snap out of it"
	Vacant expression	Encourage him to talk	Don't overdo pity
	Lack of emotional display	Be aware of your own limitations	Don't give sedatives
		Get control quickly	Don't act resentful
		Secure rapport	
		Get him to tell you what happened	
		Be empathetic	
		Recognize feelings of resentment in patient and yourself	
		Find simple, routine job. Give warm food and drink	
Overactive	Argumentative	Let him talk about it	Don't suggest he is acting abnormally
	Talks rapidly	Find him jobs which require physical effort	Don't give sedatives
	Jokes inappropriately	Give warm food and drink	Don't argue with him
	Makes endless suggestions		

Table 15-4. Psychological First Aid for Disaster Situations (cont'd)

Reaction	Symptoms	Do	Don't
Overactive (cont'd)	Jumps from one activity to another	Supervision is necessary Be aware of own feelings	
Conversion reaction	Severe nausea and vomiting Can't use some part of the body	Show interest in him Find some small job for him to make him forget Make him comfortable Get medical help if possible Be aware of own feelings	Don't tell him there is nothing wrong Don't blame him Don't ridicule him Don't ignore disability openly

* Modified from: M51-400-603-1: Triage Plan: Montgomery County, Maryland. Dept. of NM — Resident Instruction, Med. Field Man., U.S.A. Med. Cntr., Fort Sam Houston, TX.

B. PHARMACOLOGIC TREATMENT OPTIONS

1. Acute Anxiety Reactions

a) <u>Benzodiazepines</u> are the drugs of choice:
   (1) Chlordiazepoxide (Librium): Well absorbed from GI tract with peak blood levels in 2-4 hrs. IV route is rapid and effective. IM route contraindicated due to slow and erratic absorption.
   <u>Dose</u>: 5-25 mg q. i. d. orally, 50-100 mg IV
   (2) Diazepam (Valium): Similar to the absorption and preparation preference of chlordiazepoxide. Half-life is longer (20-50 hrs). Possible cardiorespiratory depression. Requires extreme care in administering IV.
   <u>Dose</u>: 2-5 mg q. i. d. orally, 5-10 mg IV
   (3) Flurazepam (Dalmane): Sleep adjunct where antianxiety component is desired. Little or no effect on REM sleep.
   <u>Dose</u>: 15-30 mg orally
b) <u>Antihistamines</u>. Less effective as an antianxiety agent. May be useful substitute when benzodiazepines are not available.
   (1) Hydroxyzine (Vistaril and Atarax)
   <u>Dose</u>: 50-100 mg IM initially, then 10-25 mg q. i. d.
   (2) Benadryl
   <u>Dose</u>: 50-100 mg IM or IV initially, then 25-50 mg q. i. d. orally
c) <u>Barbiturates</u>. Prior to discovery of benzodiazepines, barbiturates were considered a first line antianxiety medication. Will produce CNS depression and sedation. Useful substitute when benzodiazepines are not available.
   (1) Phenobarbital
   <u>Dose</u>: 65-135 mg initially IM
d) <u>Narcotics</u>. Meperidine (Demerol) and morphine are powerful antianxiety medication that are understandably not used routinely due to their addictive nature and abuse potential. However, in a disaster situation where routine antianxiety medications may not be readily available, and restrictions for their use are no longer justified, their use may be critical in the control of recalcitrant cases. Due to the risk of respiratory and circulatory depression, use in the critically injured is contraindicated. In such cases, anxiety suggests impending shock.
   (1) Meperidine (Demerol)
   <u>Dose</u>: 50-100 mg IM, SC, or PO

(2) Morphine
Dose: 5-10 mg IM

2. Panic Reactions

Panic reactions are similar to acute anxiety attacks; however, the patient exhibits intense fear that may lead to disorganization with or without paranoia, delusions, hallucinations, and bizarre behavior. These victims may be destructive or self-destructive. The disorganization and altered thinking is a painful state that must be treated without delay.

   a) Antianxiety Medications. If the anxiety component predominates, these medications applicable for acute anxiety attacks should be utilized. If psychotic behavior predominates or limits the victim's acceptance of oral medication, antipsychotic medications must be used.
   b) Antipsychotic Medications. High-potency neuroleptics are used for their antipsychotic effect, not their sedative effect. Seventy-five percent of an IM dose may be absorbed within 30 min. Monitor BP q 30 min.
      (1) Haloperidol (Haldol)
          Dose: IM 5-10 ml initially. May be repeated in 30 min to 1 hr if severe agitation persists. 5-10 mg may be given every hr until symptoms subside or victim falls asleep (up to a total of 60 mg). Monitor BP q 30 min.
      (2) Perphenazine (Trilafon)
          Dose: Same as for haloperidol.
      (3) Other high potency neuroleptics, such as trifluoperazine (Stelazine) and fluphenazine (Prolixin), may also be used.

3. Rapid Intramuscular Neuroleptization Should Produce:[37]

   1. A calming effect
   2. A change in mood
   3. A beginning remission of psychotic symptoms

   When these occur, oral medication is prescribed. With panic states accompanied by psychotic behavior, only antianxiety medications need be given if reintegration was rapid and if agitation and erratic or diminished sleep are not present. If behavior or sleep patterns indicate that the psychosis remains in the acute phase, oral antipsychotics should be prescribed. Oral medication prescribed in the next 24 hrs is double the total

IM dose that was required in the first 24 hrs to achieve symptomatic control.

Side Effects: Drug-induced parkinsonism, common with high-potency neuroleptics, may develop soon after IM injection and is more common in the very young, elderly, or injured victim. Akathisia (i. e. , highly distressing motor restlessness, fidgeting, pacing) may occur along with, or slightly later than, drug-induced parkinsonism. These extrapyramidal reactions should be promptly reversed with the following:

> Diphenhydramine (Benadryl) 50 mg IM or IV
> Cogentin 2 mg IM or IV
> Diazepam (Valium) 5-10 mg IV

4. Brief Reactive Psychosis.

The use of high-potency neuroleptization (see above) is usually humanely required in these victims. Where sleep deprivation is a factor, lower potency phenothiazines (chlorpromazine, thioridazine) are necessary for sedation. * Prolonged sleep (24-48 hrs) may be necessary to reverse this process. Neuroleptics should be discontinued or substituted by flurazepam as soon as possible in order to promote REM sleep.

> a) Chlorpromazine (Thorazine)
>   Dose: 50-75 mg IM, then 100 mg q. i. d. orally
> b) Thioridazine (Mellaril)
>   Dose: 50-75 mg IM, then 100 mg q. i. d. orally

The emergency use of IV haloperidol (Haldol) may be required in victims with life-threatening or seriously disabling medical problems whose treatment is delayed or impeded by a neuropsychiatric condition. [38] The rate of administration is 5 mg/min IV, and it takes effect in 10-40 min. The upper rate of administration is 5 mg/30 sec or 10 mg/min. Although this rate appears to have a benign effect on BP and heart rate, these parameters should be monitored closely, especially in the multiply-injured victim. The use of halperidol concentrates via nasogastric tube in 2-5 mg doses may rapidly and sufficiently sedate the multiply-injured patient when a nonparenteral route is preferred and when sedation is required without fear of respiratory depression (e. g. , chest or abdominal injured victim). [39]

---

*These medications are more sedating and cause more hypotension than the high-potency neuroleptics.

5. Combat Related Disorders

Combat Fatigue (Exhaustion). These victims require prolonged sleep (24-48 hrs). Complete recovery and rapid return to duty is expected.[28] Suggested medications are secobarbital (Seconal) 200 mg, or chlorpromazine (Thorazine) 100 mg, thioridazine (Mellaril) 100 mg, or flurazepam (Dalmane) 30 mg, thioridazine time dose may be all that is required.

It is critical that a natural REM pattern sleep be established without delay.

Combat Reaction (Neurosis)

   a) Judicious use of both antianxiety and sleep medication is recommended
   b) The majority of victims return to duty within three days.
   c) Positive reinforcement is often necessary along with prolonged sleep, regular meals, and diversion through recreation.
   d) Fifteen percent remain combat ineffective.[28]

VI. SPECIFIC POPULATION RESPONSES

A. CHILDREN

As a group, children are usually quite resilient, although short- and long-term neurotic responses have been recorded. Children with prior emotional problems, who are separated from their parents, and who reflect the psychopathology of their parents are at greater risk.[40,41]

B. ELDERLY

Studies tend to confirm suggestions that the elderly victim will experience a greater sense of loss to property and feeling of loss of time itself.[41] The elderly may profit from working with children in the postimpact phases.

C. MENTALLY ILL

Some psychotic patients evidence transient improved functioning during disasters, and can assist relief workers and other patients.[42] Not enough data exists on the neurotic, depressed, or characterological patient to provide accurate predictions. If psychiatric beds must be vacated to make room for the critically injured, psychiatric patients must be screened for potential

out-of-hospital risk by a psychiatrist familiar with their case,
or they must be temporarily transferred to a nursing or group
home.

D. HEALTH CARE PROVIDERS

In the single massive experience, the mind set, anticipation,
and organization for medical care is for the short haul. Acute
care predictions can be correlated with the nature of the event
that caused the disaster. Indigenous medical personnel can be
anticipated to assume care once the situation has stabilized.
Relief workers are able to remain objective observers maintaining adaptive psychological distance from this phenomenon.
Physicians, especially surgeons, may be regarded as insensitive and detached. Some degree of detachment is necessary for
the physician to fulfill the demands during a disaster; however,
no health care provider is immune from the emotional impact.
Edwards reports sources of stress for nurses during short-
term civilian disasters to be:[41]

1. Concern over their own safety
2. Concern over the safety of their own families
3. Concern over deficiencies in the relief organization and
    supplies
4. Increased responsibility
5. Excessive demands
6. Need to avoid role-conflict with other workers
7. Nurse-patients identifying with pediatric victims
8. Need to do something significant
9. Feelings of possessiveness toward victims

In wartime, the objectiveness seen in the distancing behavior of physicians, so necessary in the medical center in which
they trained, is lost when they become an integral part of the
social sequence. If basic biological and social needs are not
met, health care providers will cease to function in that role
and simply look after themselves. This occurred in Hiroshima,
where out of a population of 245,000, 75,000 people were killed
and 100,000 were injured in the atomic blast. Of 150 physicians
in Hiroshima, only 30 were left alive. Of 1,780 nurses, only
126 survived. [43]

VII. PREVENTION

Tyhurst stated that in a disaster situation physicians can prevent more cases of psychiatric disability than psychiatrists can
later treat. [16]

Edwards suggests that neuropsychiatric management should include:

1) adopting a sensitive, sympathetic, and flexible attitude towards the wide variety of reactions that may be encountered.
2) ensuring that injured and frightened survivors are nursed together and are not left alone.
3) provide rest, blankets, and hot drinks as appropriate.
4) encourage timely ventilation of the affective component of the experience.
5) use reassurance and suggestion during the period of heightened suggestibility.
6) adopt the leadership role, issuing confident and easy to follow instructions and encouraging purposive activity.
7) conveying accurate and responsible information to survivors, their loved ones, and the media and squashing rumors as they emerge.
8) transferring disturbed and disturbing patients to a special treatment center.
9) using psychotropic drugs conservatively and only when definitely indicated.
10) referring patients showing emotional sequelae for psychiatric assessment or treatment, or both. [41]

VIII. TRIAGE OF NEUROPSYCHIATRIC CASUALTIES

PRINCIPLES

A. Neuropsychiatric casualties will be relatively few in number.
B. The disruptive or agitated behavior of a small number of these victims has the potential of impeding the progress of triage and the care of the more critically ill.
C. Emotional reactions must be treated expediently since the psychiatric staff may be needed in other more urgent medical and surgical capacities.
D. The psychiatrist or generalist should recognize and treat the most urgent and critical of target symptoms and pass the victim on to nurses, aides, or medical students for further evaluation and treatment under the supervision of a psychiatrist.
E. In a field situation the triage officer should attempt to place victims with emotional reactions into functioning roles where they are expected to care for others, assist in transport, or fetch equipment.
F. Victims triaged as neuropsychiatric are frequently a

distraught spouse, exhausted rescue workers, lost children, or angry and litigious parents.[44]

G. Every disaster plan for a general community hospital should include planning for the triage of neuropsychiatric casualties via essential units:[44]

1. Psychiatric ambulatory assessment unit
2. Crisis information unit
3. Relatives and visitor reception area unit
4. Psychiatric crises support team
5. Psychiatric casualties unit

REFERENCES

1. Kinston, W., Rosser, P.: Disaster: Effects on mental and physical state. J Psychosom Res 18:437-456, 1974.
2. Grinker, R.R., and Spiegel, J.P.: Men Under Stress, New York, McGraw-Hill, 1945.
3. Archibald, H.C.: Gross stress reaction in combat—a 15 year follow-up. Am J Psychiatry 119:317-322, 1962.
4. Cavenar, J.O., and Nash, J.L.: The effects of combat on the normal personaltiy: War neurosis in Vietnam returnees. Compr Psychiatry 17:647-653, 1976.
5. Borus, J.R.: Incidence of maladjustment in Vietnam returnees. Arch Gen Psychiatry 30:554-557, 1974.
6. Solomon, G.F.: Three psychiatric casualties from Vietnam. Arch Gen Psychiatry 25:522-524, 1971.
7. Van Putten, T., and Emory, W.H.: Traumatic neuroses in Vietnam returnees. Arch Gen Psychiatry 29:695-698, 1973.
8. Nash, J.L., and Walker, J.I.: Stress disorders in Vietnam returnees: The problem continues. Milit Med 146:582-583, 1981.
9. Steiner, M., and Newmann, M.: Traumatic neurosis and social support in the Yom Kippur War returnees. Milit Med 143(12):866-868, 1978.
10. Glass, A.J.: Psychological aspects of disaster. JAMA 171:222-225, 1959.
11. American Psychiatric Association: Diagnostic Criteria from DSM-III. Washington, D.C., APA, 1980.
12. Bourne, P.G.: Military psychiatry and the Vietnam experience. Am J Psychiatry 127:481, 1970.
13. Titchener, J.L., and Ross, W.D.: Acute or chronic stress as determinants of behavior, character, and neurosis. In American Handbook of Psychiatry. Vol. 3. Arieti, S., and Brody, E., eds. New York, Basic Books, 1974.

14. Chamberlin, B.C.: The psychological aftermath of disaster. J Clin Psychiatry 41, 7:238-244, 1980.
15. Grauer, H.: Psychodynamics of the survivor syndrome. Can Psychiatric Assoc J 14:617-622, 1969.
16. Tyhurst, J.S.: Individual reactions to community disaster: The natural history of psychiatric phenomena. Am J Psychiatry 107:764-769, 1951.
17. Hartmann, K., and Allison, J.: Expected psychological reactions to disaster in medical rescue teams. Milit Med 146:323-327, 1981.
18. Boydstun, J.A., and Perry, C.J.G.: Military Psychiatry. In Comprehensive Textbook of Psychiatry. 3rd ed. Kaplan, H.I., et al., eds. Baltimore, Williams and Wilkins, 1980.
19. McCabe, M.S., and Board, G.: Stress and mental disorders in basic training. Milit Med 141:686, 1976.
20. Conrad, F.E., et al.: Stress adjustment and attrition at West Point: Clinical aspects. Milit Med 141:864, 1976.
21. Leiken, S.J.: Traumatic War Neurosis Revisited. In Proceedings of the 12th Annual Conference of Air Force Behaviorial Scientists. Perry, and Jennings, eds. Brooks Air Force Base, Texas, United States Air Force School of Aerospace Medicine, 1965.
22. Marshall, S.L.A.: Men Against Fire: Problem of Battle Command in Future War. New York, William Morrow and Co., Inc., 1947.
23. Hendin, H., et al.: Meanings of combat and the development of posttraumatic stress disorder. Am J. Psychiatry 138, 11:1490-1492, 1981.
24. Menninger, W.C.: Psychiatry in a Troubled World, New York, Macmillan Co., 1948.
25. Brill, N.Q., and Beebe, B.W.: A Follow-up Study of War Neuroses. V.A. Medical Monograph. Washington, D.C., U.S. Government Printing Office, 1955.
26. Strange, R.E.: Effects of combat stress on hospital ship psychiatric evacuees. In Psychology and Physiology of Stress. Bourne, P.G., ed. New York, Academic Press, 1969.
27. Eiseman, B.: Combat casualty management in Vietnam. J Trauma 7, 1:53-63, 1967.
28. Pettera, R.L., et al.: Psychiatric management of combat reactions with emphasis on a reaction unique to Vietnam. Milit Med 134:673-678, 1969.
29. Block, S.H.: Army psychiatry in the combat zone—1967-1968. Am J Psychiatry 126, 3:289-298, 1969.
30. Tiffany, W.J.: The mental health of army troops in Vietnam. Am J Psychiatry 123:1585-1586, 1967.

31. Bey, D.R.: Change of command in combat: A locus of stress. Am J Psychiatry 129:698, 1972.
32. Bourne, P.G.: Men, Stress, and Vietnam. Boston, Little, Brown and Co., 1970.
33. Tischler, G.L.: Patterns of psychiatric attrition and behavior in a combat zone. In Psychology and Physiology of Stress. Bourne, P.G., ed. New York, Academic Press, 1969.
34. Schramel, D.J.: U.S. Military Psychiatric Patients: Southeast Asia. In Proceedings of the 13th Annual Conference of Air Force Behavioral Scientists. Jennings, C.L., and Perry, C.J.G., eds. Brooks Air Force Base, Texas, U.S. Air Force School of Aerospace Medicine, 1973.
35. Strange, R.E.: Hospitalship psychiatry in a war zone. Am J Psychiatry 134:281-286, 1967.
36. Montgomery County, Maryland: Triage Plan. Modified from M51-400-603-1. Dept. of Non-Resident Instruction. Medical Field Manual. Fort Sam Houston, Texas, U.S. Army Medical Center.
37. Ayd, F.J., ed.: Guidelines for using shortacting intramuscular neuroleptics for rapid neuroleptization. In International Drug Therapy Newsletter. 12 (2&3), 1977.
38. Dudley, D.L., et al.: Emergency use of intravenous haloperidol. Gen Hosp Psychiatry 3:240-246, 1979.
39. McDanal, C.E., et al.: Near-drowning from ding string surfboarding: A case report. Letter to the Editor. JAMA 238, 5:398, 1977.
40. Newman, C.J.: Children of disaster: Clinical observations at Buffalo Creed. Am J Psychiatry 133:306-312, 1976.
41. Edwards, J.G.: Psychiatric aspects of civilian disasters. Brit Med J 1:944-947, 1976.
42. Koegler, R.R., and Hicks, S.M.: The destruction of a medical center by earthquake: Initial effects on patients and staff. Calif Med 116:63-67, 1972.
43. Lown, B., et al.: Sounding board—The nuclear arms race and the physician. N Engl J Med 304, 12:726-729, 1981.
44. Martin, R.D.: Disaster planning for psychiatric casualties for general hospitals with psychiatric services. Milit Med 145(2):111-113, 1980.

Chapter 16

EMERGENCY TROPICAL MEDICINE
Andre J. Ognibene, M.D.

I. INTRODUCTION

Tropical and subtropical areas harbor an inordinate number of natural disasters such as cyclones and earthquakes, as well as manmade conflicts. In addition to managing multiple traumatic casualties, disaster teams or field medical personnel will face additional problems when operating in a tropical environment. They must recognize, treat, and contain unfamiliar diseases in both disaster victims and relief workers. This same problem supervenes when the disaster is the influx of a large number of refugees from a tropical locale. In order to function effectively in either of these situations, the physician must be familiar with disorders of tropical origin. Some common tropical diseases have been selected for discussion here.

II. MALARIA

A. INTRODUCTION

Malaria is one of the most common, global, febrile disorders; it is capable of presenting anywhere in the world. The failure of American physicians to recall lessons learned from the often dreary tropical medicine lectures in medical school was partially responsible for the malaria-caused deaths of nine American civilians in 1969. This is almost as many deaths as those occurring among U.S. military personnel who were engaged in an endemic area in Vietnam during the same period of time.

B. PRESENTATION AND CLASSIFICATION

While periodic fever and chills are quoted in major texts, presentation may range from low grade fever and backache to a disastrously acute onset with coma or convulsions. The combination of fever and working in or traveling from an endemic area are sufficient to provoke further study of the blood smear.

Plasmodium vivax malaria is generally benign and does not

produce the serious complications and fatality rate associated with Plasmodium falciparum disease. P. vivax malaria may be confused on smear with Plasmodium malariae, but should never be confused with P. falciparum. While P. malariae may produce a nephrotic syndrome, the most complex and malignant disorder remains P. falciparum malaria. If it is undiagnosed and the patient is untreated, the resulting complications can be fatal. The thin, counterstained blood smear is easiest for the physician to examine although the thick smear is more likely to be positive. The thick smear, however, is best left for capable laboratory technicians to review. Since P. falciparum invades cells of all ages, trophozoites are found in all sizes of red cells. In P. vivax infection, large red cells (neocytes) are infected with single trophozoites. P. falciparum infections may place multiple trophozoites in one cell. Applique forms, where the trophozoite is pinned against the red cell wall, are characteristic of P. falciparum infection and should be sought when the slides are reviewed. This universal parasitemia of P. falciparum disease predisposes patients to overwhelming infections in which parasite counts can be exceptionally high.

C. COMPLICATIONS

There are no life-threatening complications to P. vivax infection, and clinical response to Chloroquine is dramatic. Primaquine 15 mg daily for 2 weeks is required to eliminate the exoerythrocytic phase which is harbored in the liver. P. malariae is responsive to similar therapy. P. falciparum is capable of producing severe hemolysis, renal failure, pulmonary involvement, and severe cerebral disease. In general, the parasite count per high power field roughly correlates with severity. With counts over 10/hpf in the presence of complications noted, the case fatality rate is quite high. Since some degree of hemolysis is universally present, anemia is characteristic of P. falciparum disease and is generally absent in patients with P. vivax.

D. ACUTE PRESENTATION

Cerebral malaria constitutes a medical emergency requiring immediate therapy. Most patients, on arrival, are febrile and comatose. Examination of the spinal fluid is negative and opening pressures are only slightly elevated or normal. The comatose state may be unusual in that the patient may appear to be awake, with eyes open but roving and simulating a postictal state or pseudobulbar palsy. In some patients, the presentation may be an acute paranoid state or other organic mental disturbance. Fever is universal and should prompt detailed examination of the patient and the blood smear. In a number of patients, renal failure may complicate the cerebral disease. In any patient with P. falciparum infection, including those on therapy, a pulmonary distress syndrome may supervene in the first 72 hrs, requiring careful monitoring of respiratory rate and PO$_2$ where indicated.

E. THERAPY

For uncomplicated P. falciparum, quinine sulfate 650 mg q8h, plus Primethamine 25 mg bid for 3 days and sulfadiazine 500 mg q6h for 5 days, are recommended. If cerebral manifestations are present, the quinine must be given intravenously until oral therapy can be resumed (600 mg in 300 cc of saline over 1 hr, 3 times daily). Decadron 4 mg IV q6h has been used in the first 24 hrs of therapy for cerebral disease or overwhelming respiratory distress syndrome but probably offers no advantage. Maintenance of PO$_2$ by respirator care, if required, and the use of positive and expiratory pressure are critical in patients with severe pulmonary complications. In the presence of renal failure, reduce quinine dosage to 650 mg daily and consider early peritoneal or hemodialysis. When pyrimethamine is used, small doses of folic acid may forestall a pyrimethamine-induced megaloblastic anemia without affecting the antimalarial action. The anemia of P. falciparum disease rarely requires therapy other than for the primary illness. If disseminated intravascular coagulopathy (DIC) is suspected, heparin therapy may be useful. However, it is well to recall that thrombopenia occurs without relation to DIC in P. falciparum disease.

III. ENCEPHALITIS

A. INTRODUCTION

The presentation of an acute cerebral episode does not always indicate cerebral malaria in a tropical environment or traveler. The worldwide occurrence of encephalitides requires consideration in the differential diagnosis. These include Japanese B, West Nile, St. Louis, Western and Eastern equine, Venezuelan equine, and Murray Valley among others. In general, mosquitoes of the genus Culex are the principal vectors. Those mosquitoes are urban dwellers and, therefore, the patient does not have to have been in the bush to acquire the disease.

B. PRESENTATION AND DIAGNOSIS

The presence of moderate to severe headache, fever, photo-
phobia, eye pain, and neck stiffness should alert the physician
to the possibility of encephalitis. Lumbar puncture is essential
to the diagnosis. In most cases, a lymphocytosis will be present;
however, polymorphonuclear leucocytes may predominate, both
in the spinal fluid and the blood. The cerebrospinal glucose is
generally preserved and the protein elevated. The opening pressure is almost always elevated. The gram stain of the fluid for
bacteria is negative. Depending on when patients present, the
mental status examination can be entirely normal. Usually,
high fever and progressive deterioration are noted in the first
36 hrs.

C. THERAPY

The early care of the patient is critical. It is during this period
that hyperpyrexia occurs, with temperatures as high as
106°F (41.1°C). The febrile course is associated with deterioration of mental faculties and frank coma may supervene. It is
imperative that hypothermic therapy be applied and the body
temperature maintained at 100°F (37.7°C). In the absence of a
mechanical hypothermia apparatus, any ingenious method will
suffice. The early hours are critical and require meticulous
nursing care. Those patients who are maintained in good hydration at controlled body temperature appear to do somewhat better, manifesting less residua than an untreated group. Seizures
during the hyperpyrexic stage herald a good prognosis and
should be controlled acutely with diazepam and chronically with
phenytoin. Focal neurologic signs appear with sufficient frequency so as to require careful and continuing neurologic assessment with attention to vital functions. In most encephalitides
of viral origin, late morbidity, such as personality changes,
persistent memory loss, early dementia, parkinsonism and
dyskinesias occur in 10-20% of patients. Differential diagnosis
depends on the specific area of operation/travel and on later
results of serologic study.

IV. OTHER VIRAL SYNDROMES

A. INTRODUCTION

While viral disorders such as encephalitis can present catas-
trophically, physicians generally do not consider common viral
disorders high on the list of overwhelming infections.

Occasionally, the unusual presentation of a laboratory worker
with monkey B virus disease or Lassa fever will offer a rare
challenge. The initial paresthesias of rabies are usually
coupled with a history of innoculation provided by the excited
and frightened patient. In such cases, despite rapid provision
of antiserum, the prognosis is dim. A patient presenting in
peripheral vascular collapse with fever, especially a child, is
not likely to be considered to have a viral disorder. In the
presence of prolonged travel or residence in Asia or India, the
shock syndrome of Dengue does become a consideration.

B. DENGUE PRESENTATION AND PATHOGENESIS

The prodome includes a headache, cough, and vomiting, usually
with a petechial rash. Meningococcemia is usually suggested.
The presence of abdominal pain and severe lethargy may pre-
cede the peripheral vascular collapse. The shock state results
from massive activation of C3a and C5a anaphlylatoxins by the
virus in the presence of an anamnestic antibody response initiated by a second challenge from the same virus. It is usual for
youngsters with this disorder to have resided long enough in an
endemic area to have suffered a second infection. The vector is
the Aedes mosquito found not only in remote areas of the world,
but also in the United States. Fortunately, those areas of the
U. S. harboring the mosquito are not hyperendemic for the disease since it is hyperendemicity which predisposes to reinfec-
tion and the shock syndrome. The virus can be recovered from
the blood if cell culture systems are available; otherwise diagnosis is delayed until serologic confirmation can be obtained.

C. THERAPY

The shocklike state is dramatic and associated with a severe
intravascular coagulopathy, profound acidosis, hemoconcentra-
tion, and renal failure. Therapy must address each metabolic
abnormality individually. Heparin, steroids, bicarbonate, volume replacement, or transfusion for hemorrhage are the basis
for therapy. The requirement to manage heparinization during
bleeding and volume replacement with renal shutdown are the
key management challenges. The consumptive coagulopathy
must be terminated, volume restored, and renal output re-
gained without provoking pulmonary edema or fatal hemorrhage.
Intensive care monitoring capability are prerequisite.

V. BACTERIAL DISEASE

A. INTRODUCTION

While shocklike presentations of infectious viral disorders are
unusual, the occurrence of shock in overwhelming bacterial infection is commonly a challenging problem in emergency care.
Present training alerts the physician to the pneumococcus or
the Gram-negative pathogens as etiologic agents of such presentations. However, in a tropical environment, the onset of
explosive fever, chills, headache, and subsequent vomiting
should suggest other bacterial organisms.

B. PLAGUE

1. <u>Pathogenesis and Presentation</u>. The severe and utter prost-
ation of the patient, the leucocytosis of 30,000-50,000/mm^3,
and the blood smear's swarming with unphagocytosed organisms
are characteristic of septicemic plague. Although bubonic
plague accounts for 85% of the cases seen in the United States,
it is the septicemic form which is most dramatic. No disease
develops symptoms so rapidly and so overwhelms and prostrates
a patient, bringing him to the verge of death, as quickly as
septicemic plague. Although phagocytosis does occur when the
bubonic plague bacillus initially enters the body, killing in the
phagocyte is later blocked. The plague bacillus elaborates factors which render its progeny immune to further phagocytosis
and, on release from the infected cells, they reproduce rapidly
and unhindered in the human host. Plague in the U.S., although
sporadic, has been associated with infected wild mammals and
their fleas. Plague in wild rodents is found in a wide area of
the southwestern United States, as well as throughout Asia and
Africa.

2. <u>Therapy</u>. To the physician, two immediate challenges are
apparent on receiving an infected patient. The first is to treat
the patient successfully, and the second is to protect himself
and his co-workers from materials such as sputum, blood, or
aspirated materials from bubo sites if they are present. Material from patients is hazardous and must be handled with aseptic
technique. In the bubonic form, presentation is less acute, although overlap occurs. In some critically ill patients, abdominal, chest, and neck pain may well be due to massive buboes
in the abdomen, chest, and neck. The trachea can be compressed to compromise respiration. Involvement of the lungs
may take the form of a transient pneumonia, a congestive form

associated with sepsis, or a primary pneumonic form with large amounts of sanguine-purulent sputum. It is this latter form which is highly contagious and requires rigid respiratory isolation and protection of contacts. Because of the early onset of DIC, shock, digital gangrene, and severe acidosis, therapy must be aggressive. Fluid volume replacement and antibiotic therapy are mandatory. While a number of antibiotics are effective, combined therapy with Tetracycline 4-6 g daily or chloramphenicol 50-75 mg/kg daily, given with streptomycin 0.5 g q4h for the first 36 hrs and then q6h, is recommended. Sulfonamides do not seem as protective against the development of plague meningitis. Therapy should be given for a minimum of 10 days. In the presence of persistently positive sputums or other cultures, continuation of antibiotics is mandatory. Public health authorities must be brought in to investigate the possibility of community spread whenever such assistance is available.

C. TYPHOID FEVER

1. Presentation. Characteristically, the diagnosis can be missed even during an epidemic. The classic onset is insidious, with headache, malaise, and anorexia as prominent symptoms. Many patients (and some physicians) ignore this prodome, only to suffer onset of fever to 104°F (40.0°C), severe cough, meningismus (with normal CSF), mental confusion, apathy, abdominal distension, and a sallow, pasty appearance which is quite striking. The characteristic rose spots are infrequent. Since Salmonella typhosa is spread primarily by human contamination of either water or food, a history of exposure to unsanitary environments is important. Where public water supply and food handlers are well-screened, the disease is rare. With a breakdown of sanitation, clusters of cases appear.

2. Diagnosis and Therapy. The cornerstone of diagnosis is culture of the blood, urine, and stool. Clinically, the relative bradycardia and lack of a rise in blood leucocytes in the face of a severe illness may be helpful. The most urgent and catastrophic presentation includes abdominal pain with signs of perforation and/or massive gastrointestinal hemorrhage. Once formed, small bowel lesions are relatively unaffected by antibiotic therapy. Since perforation and hemorrhage are responsible for over three-quarters of the deaths from typhoid fever, rapid diagnosis and therapy are essential. Perforation should be treated surgically under antibiotic coverage. If susceptibility is known, chloramphenicol can be used; otherwise, ampicillin

is the drug of choice. The patient should be hydrated, trans-
fused if indicated for the provision of oxygen-carrying capacity,
and taken to surgery. This same approach is required in un-
abated hemorrhage of 5 or more units. There is general agree-
ment that delay in definitive surgery increases mortality. For
those patients who cannot be resuscitated to the point that surgery is feasible, prognosis is dismal. Each patient requires an
individual decision; however, every resuscitative effort to allow surgical therapy of significant hemorrhage or perforation
should be made.

D. AMEBIASIS

1. Introduction. Typhoid is not the only bowel disease requiring urgent action to save a patient. Like typhoid fever, amebiasis may present, not as a diarrheal syndrome, but as acute
appendicitis, regional enteritis with right lower quadrant mass,
chest pain with pleural effusion, toxic megacolon, or an acute
meningoencephalitis. The disease is worldwide in distribution
and in tropical areas, replaces Shigella as the primary cause
of dysentery. Because of simple and effective therapy available
in the form of metronidazole, 2. 25 g a day in divided doses,
early diagnosis is critical.

2. Presentation and Diagnosis. The clinical presentation with
amebic dysentery is most common, but diagnosis is difficult if
routine stool collections are relied upon. Any suspect case requires action by the physician in order to obtain direct procto-
scopic material, preferably from an ulcer site. Cotton swabs
should not be used. Scraping or aspiration of material is preferred.
    Since perforations occur primarily in the cecal area, there
may be local tenderness in the right lower quadrant associated
with gastrointestinal upset and a mild leucocytosis. To the un-
inquiring physician and the eager surgeon, this can be construed as appendicitis. Surgery in untreated cases may be
disastrous and result in postoperative fistulae and abscess formation. Individuals with these symptoms should first be studied
for amebiasis.
    Similarly, an ameboma with bowel symptoms may mimic
Crohn's disease while fulminant infections with toxic megacolon
require distinction from ulcerative colitis. When immediate
laboratory support for review of specimens is unavailable, PVA
(polyvinyl alcohol) in equal parts with collected material will
preserve trophozoites for later review.

E. CHOLERA SYNDROMES

1. Introduction. While amebiasis stands as the most common dysenteric disease in the tropical environment, cholera and Vibrio parahaemolyticus are the most dramatic in their presentation to emergency care. There is a tendency for cases to cluster, and a group of patients presenting together can rapidly deplete the capability of any emergency treatment facility to care for additional patients.

2. Pathogenesis and Therapy. Cholera vaccine affords only partial protection and only for a short time; therefore, there is no immunization requirement for travelers from endemic areas reentering the United States. In both classic cholera (El Tor or O') and Vibrio parahaemolyticus (seafood diarrhea), the rapid loss of water and electrolytes may reach 20 liters or more in 24 hours. This massive fluid depletion in a stool that, upon examination, is free of leucocytes, is almost pathognomonic. Because the colon is normal, the small bowel is incriminated as the site of the fluid loss. The enterotoxin of the organism binds rapidly to the small bowel wall and adenyl cyclase activation generates large quantities of cyclic AMP, impeding sodium absorption at the brush border. Fortunately, sodium absorption with glucose carriers is unimpeded, thus allowing repletion of the patients orally with a glucose-electrolyte solution. While this may require a resourceful search for Gatorade, it is preferable to expending the required large volumes into multiple intravenous sites. The mechanism of repletion holds for E. coli, Clostridial and Shigella diarrheas, as well as for a large number of other infectious and humoral causes. The large quantities of relatively colorless stool produced must be replaced volume for volume or dehydration, shock, and cachexia supervene. Death has been reported in less than 4 hrs in some untreated cases. The ideal solution for therapy should contain sodium, potassium, bicarbonate, chloride, and glucose and is marketed as balanced electrolyte solution. The patient's close contacts should receive oral Tetracycline prophylaxis. In the case of V. parahaemolyticus, all those who participated in the seafood repast causing the index case should receive prophylaxis.

VI. HEPATITIS

A. INTRODUCTION

Hepatitis has been a constant companion of civilization since the dawn of medical history. There are numerous historical

accounts of carefully detailed outbreaks in descriptions of
great pandemics. Wherever sanitation is compromised and
large groups of people gather, the danger of epidemic exists.
Modern water supplies have done much to reduce waterborne
type A hepatitis, while the development of newer vaccines herald an era of protection from the ravages of type B. Certainly
there are other causes of hepatitis such as yellow fever, lepto-
spirosis, louse-born relapsing fever, cytonegalic virus and
others; however, the classical viral hepatitis remains the most
likely threat to large groups traveling in a tropical environment.

B. PRESENTATION

The Hippocratic description of the onset of classical hepatitis
has changed little over the centuries. Onset with chills, fever,
and weakness, followed by dark urine and jaundice are symptoms not usually missed at presentation. This is especially
true when cases appear in clusters because patients have con-
tracted the disease from a common source. Type A hepatitis is
endemic among school age children and among young adults in
the United States and around the world. Propagation by person-
to-person transmission is fortunately limited to the prodromal
period with rapid dimunition of infectivity once the onset of
jaundice occurs. Fecal-oral remains a primary route of propagation. Type B is not dependent on fecal-oral transmission.
Other modes include saliva, sexual contact, parturition, and
inoculation.
    The laboratory findings are characteristic. The SGOT
(serum glutamic-pyruvate transaminase) is usually over 500
units. Lower values should suggest a search for other etiolo-
gies. The serum bilirubin may reach 20 mg/100 ml. High bilirubin values are seen in G6PD (glucose 6-phosphate dehydro-
genase) deficiency or sickle cell disease in which profound hemolysis may be triggered. High alkaline phosphatase, above 15
Bodansky units, should provoke a search for obstructive causes
for jaundice. The key laboratory test remains the prothrombin
time. In uncomplicated viral hepatitis, this test should be normal. Elevations of prothrombin time should be viewed with
serious concern as this may herald the onset of a fulminant
course.

C. COMPLICATIONS

Extra hepatic manifestations of viral hepatitis have usually been
described with type B hepatitis; however, they do occur with
non-B types. A prodrome similar to serum sickness may occur;

it is characterized by rash, urticaria, polyarthralgia, and in 10-20% of patients, a frank arthritis. Circulating immune complexes have been demonstrated and complement is low.

A second syndrome is that of polyarteritis nodosa, which occurs with type B infection. Actual fibrinoid necrosis and perivascular inflammation of small arteries and arterioles can be demonstrated. Immune complex and complement are deposited in the vessels.

Hepatitis B glomerulonephritis has been noted mainly in the chronic form of the disease. Most often it is membranous or membranoproliferative. Deposits on the basement membrane are nodular.

Fulminant hepatitis occurs in 1-2.4% of patients hospitalized with the disease. It is infrequent in children. Mortality is high despite treatment.

Chronic hepatitis may occur in up to 10% of type B patients and rarely in type A. The basic forms are chronic persistent (mainly chemical abnormality with little histologic change) and chronic active in which significant histologic alteration is present. Therapy is required for patients with chronic active disease.

D. THERAPY

Therapy in this disease involves an appreciation of triage principles in the management of large numbers of patients who may present at one time. Since preventive inoculation is not yet universal, it remains likely that common source cases may begin arriving at the physician in clusters. Military experiences in Korea and Vietnam have clearly indicated that in the absence of loss of appetite, elevated prothrombin time, or complication of immune complex type, both bed rest and strict isolation are generally unnecessary. These patients can be managed without hospitalization, thereby relieving the intense pressure on hospital staffs when large numbers present concurrently. For those selected for hospitalization, limited laboratory studies and enforcing of handwashing is all that is required. Beyond these precautions, the impact of large numbers can be blunted by the intelligent application of medical knowledge of the disease. Almost everyone gets well. Those who don't can be evaluated for persistence at a later time when the press of large numbers is removed. Medical resources do not need to be utilized for care of hepatitis patients who are uncomplicated. They are largely ambulatory self-care in hospital or ambulatory care in their home environment. When hospitalized, the nursing staff needs to be assured that the jaundiced patient is not contagious

by nonparenteral routes given good handwashing technique.
They must be taught to assure that the patient's appetite remains good and that the prothrombin time is normal. Time
spent watching daily or weekly fluctuations of a myriad of laboratory tests is generally nonproductive and expensive. Bed
rest is never required in the uncomplicated patient.

VII. CONCLUSION

During a disaster relief operation in a tropical area, recognition and management of tropical diseases will be as important
as the triage and treatment of multiple casualties. The number
of tropical diseases is large. The occurrence of a particular
disease depends on the incidence of disorders in a given location; this varies considerably. Some common tropical diseases
have been reviewed here. When actually involved in a disaster
relief effort originating in a tropical environment, the physician must review the specific diseases endemic in the impact
area or refugee group.

SUGGESTED READING

Benenson, A. S. : The control of cholera. In Symposium on
Cholera. Bulletin. N Y Acad Med 47:1204-1210, 1971.

Cluff, L. E. , and Johnson, J. E. : Clinical Concepts of Infectious
Diseases. 2d ed. Baltimore, Williams & Wilkins, 1978.

Conrad, M. E. : Pathophysiology of malaria. Hematologic observations in human and animal studies. Ann Intern Med 70:
134-141, 1969.

Daroff, R. B. , Keller, J. J. , Jr. , Kastl, A. J. , Jr. , and
Blocker, W. W. , Jr. : Cerebral malaria. JAMA 202:679-682,
1967.

Everett, E. D. : Metronidazole and amebiasis. Am J Digest Dis
19:626-636, 1974.

Hoeprich, P. D. , ed. : Infectious Diseases. A Modern Treatise
of Infectious Processes. 2d ed. Philadelphia, Harper and Row
Publishers, Inc. , 1977.

Hornick, R. B. , Greisman, S. E. , Woodward, T. E. , DuPont, H. L. , Dawkins, A. T. , and Snyder, M. J. : Typhoid fever: Pathogenesis and immunologic control. Part I. N Engl J Med 283:686-691, 1970.

Juniper, K. , Jr. : Amebiasis in the United States. Bulletin. N Y Acad Med 47:448-461, 1971.

Mandell, G. L. , Douglas, R. G. , Jr. , and Bennett, J. E. , eds. : Principles and Practice of Infectious Disease. New York, John Wiley & Sons, Inc. , 1979.

Southam, C. M. : Serologic studies of encephalitis in Japan. II. Inapparent infections of Japanese B encephalitis virus. J Infect Dis 99:163-169, 1956.

Velimirovic, B. : Plague in South-East Asia. A brief historical summary and present geographical distribution. Trans R Soc Trop Med Hyg 66:479-504, 1972.

Weaver, O. M. , Haymaker, W. , Pieper, S. , and Kurland, R. : Sequelae of the arthropod-borne encephalitides. V. Japanese encephalitis. Neurology 8:887-889, 1958.

WHO (World Health Organization): Pathogenic mechanisms in dengue hemorrhagic fever: Report of an international collaborative study. Bulletin. WHO 48:117-133, 1973.

Chapter 17

PEDIATRIC CASUALTIES
Frederick M. Burkle, Jr. , M. D. , M. P. H.

I. GENERAL

Little attention is given in the disaster-related literature to the
particulars of the pediatric victim. Prehospital care of the
critically ill child has received scant attention by the Emergency
Medical Services Systems Act and the programs it supports. [1]
Advanced Cardiac Life Support (ACLS) and Advanced Trauma
Life Support (ATLS) courses emphasize the adult. [2,3] Hospital
and community triage simulations and disaster drills are frequently oriented toward adult casualties. Natural and manmade
disasters, however, do not select out the pediatric population.
One of the greatest tragedies of disaster medicine is witnessing
the unfortunate toll of innocent pediatric victims.

Health care personnel called upon to assist in disaster care
come from the ranks of individuals who see only occasional
pediatric trauma, little of it being multiple trauma. Physicians
who cared for children during the Vietnam War will attest to
the frequency of pediatric casualties resulting from weapons
that recognize neither a sex nor an age distinction. Physicians
returning from refugee or disaster-related care in foreign
lands frequently state they would have fared better with improved knowledge of pediatrics and pediatric resuscitation
skills.

This chapter contains reminders of the practical skills required in dealing with triage and the multiple trauma of
disaster-related pediatric casualties.

II. HYPOVOLEMIA

A. Signs of hypotension independent of age are cool, clammy
skin, thready pulse, weakness, fatigue, thirst, dizziness,
and poor capillary filling. Impaired mental status, frequently the earliest sign of shock, is easily missed in children
because it is passed over as the behavior of a frightened
child. Postdisaster injured children are frequently stoically

quiet and overwhelmed by the surrounding events. A child who is agitated and thrashing is exhibiting a mental status change.

B. Blood pressure in children is age-dependent. The BP cuff must be one-half to three-quarters the size of the child's arm.
   1. Significant hypotension
      a) Less than 6 years: Systolic BP 60 or less
      b) More than 6 years: Systolic BP 70 or less[4]
   2. A formula utilized for the specific determination of normal age-related BP is:

$$\text{Systolic BP} = 80 + 2 \times \text{age in years}$$
$$\text{Diastolic BP} = 2/3 \text{ systolic}$$

C. Treatment
   1. Attention to the ABCs, cervical collar, backboard, splints, and control of bleeding are basic. Pitfalls in pediatric resuscitation are discussed below.
   2. Antishock trousers (mast suit) use may be critical in the pediatric hypovolemic patient who needs only to lose a relatively small volume of blood to become hypotensive.
      a) Antishock trousers do the following:
         (1) Provide an increase in peripheral vascular resistance necessary to maintain adequate blood pressure.
         (2) May return one-tenth to one-fifth of blood volume to the central circulation within 2 min.[4]
         (3) Control hemorrhage by direct tamponading effect.
         (4) Provide the venous filling necessary to recognize and cannulate veins for IV fluids.
      b) In disaster situations, if pediatric antishock trousers are not available, both of the child's lower extremities may be placed in one adult antishock trouser leg. Since trouser legs are independently inflatable, two children may be facilitated by one adult antishock suit; the second child's legs are placed in the distal end of the remaining trouser leg. Obviously, these are temporizing and lifesaving procedures that demand both creativity and risk-taking.
   3. Vertical elevation of the legs by using Ace elastic wrappings or air splints (one adult arm air splint fits a child's leg well) may also add lifesaving volume replacement to the central circulation and maintain peripheral vascular resistance.

4. IV fluids and blood
   a) Assume a normal blood volume of 80-90 ml/kg. Use
      the following formulae which is based on a 25 kg
      child:

> Class I hemorrhage: Up to 15% = 300 ml
> Class II hemorrhage: 20-25% = 400-500 ml
> Class III hemorrhage: 30-35% = 600-700 ml
> Class IV hemorrhage: 40-50% = 800-1000 ml
> Class III and IV require both crystalloids and
> blood for resuscitation. [3]

   b) Due to compensatory mechanisms, the detection of
      early or impending shock states is difficult. In a
      disaster situation, little time is given to debate or
      consultation. With the earliest suspicions of shock, a
      fluid challenge of either normal saline or Ringer's
      lactate of 10 ml/kg should be given rapidly. Repeat
      10 ml/kg if signs are not reversed. The diagnosis is,
      therefore, established.
   c) Patients recognized to be in shock are given 15-20
      ml/kg over 15-30 min (neonates: 45-60 min). [5] Some
      patients may require 35-40 ml/kg in the first hour
      before preoperative stabilization is achieved. [6] If
      signs of shock persist, give 5% albumin 10 ml/kg
      over 45 min, [7] or crossmatched blood 20 ml/kg, or
      plasma or plasmanate 10-20 ml/kg over 20-30 min.
      Blood is administered through the largest needle pos-
      sible, preferably 18-gauge or larger. In children
      this may not be possible. Whole blood transfusion
      can be done through a 21-gauge needle without hemo-
      lysis. [8] In desperate situations and in infants, small
      volumes of blood may be encouraged, but not forced,
      through a smaller needle if mixed with a small
      amount of normal saline. Clysis and tibial bone mar-
      row infusions may prove lifesaving.
   d) After fluid load, resuscitation is continued with D5
      lactated Ringer's at 2-3 times maintenance. In non-
      traumatic resuscitation, add potassium 5-10 mEq/
      500 ml as soon as the child passes urine. [6] Caution is
      necessary where large amounts of potassium are
      liberated from tissues in multiple trauma.
   e) Children should go to the OR when urine volumes
      (minimum 1 ml/kg/hr) are adequate; ideally when
      specific gravity of less than 1.020 (less than 1.015 in
      infants) is attained. [6]

f) With children who are in severe shock with a history of 8-10 hrs of anuria (as with prolonged entrapment), the initial fluid is 5% albumin 10 ml/kg over 30 min followed by normal saline, 25-30 ml/kg in 1 hr. [6] The child is catheterized; with strict intake and output recordings; and frequent EKG, serum potassium, and calcium evaluations.

g) Maintenance fluid determination is simplified by the following table:[9]

Weight Range	Fluid Requirements
2. 5-10 kg	100 ml/kg
10-20 kg	1000 ml + 50 ml/kg over 10 kg
Over 20 kg	1500 ml + 20 ml/kg over 20 kg

5. Medication assistance (shock not due to hypovolemia)
   a) Dopamine: Mix 200 mg in 250 ml D5W. Begin with 1-5 μg/kg/min.
   b) Isoproterenol: Mix 1 mg in 250 ml D5W. Begin with 0.1 μg/kg/min and titrate to effect.

III. PITFALLS IN CPR

A. Rather than provide the reader with pediatric CPR procedures, this section will focus on areas in which pediatric resuscitation differs from adult resuscitation.
   1. Pediatric arrests are rarely cardiac in origin, therefore, arrhythmias are infrequent. Bradycardia may be seen in hypotension; electromechanical dissociation may alert one to a cardiac tamponade.
   2. Drug and defibrillation doses are based on body weight in kg as shown in Table 17-1.

Table 17-1. Body Weight Estimates

Years	Weight
1	10 kg
3	15 kg
5	20 kg
8	25 kg
10	30 kg

3. Commonly used medications
   a) Sodium bicarbonate: 1-2 mEq/kg
   b) Epinephrine (1:10,000): 0.01 mg/kg = 0.1 ml/kg = 1 ml/10 kg
   c) Atropine: 0.03 mg/kg
   d) Lidocaine: 1 mg/kg
   e) Bretylium: 5 mg/kg
   f) Calcium chloride (10% solution): 0.2 ml/kg
   g) Decadron: 0.5 mg/kg
   h) Mannitol: 1 g/kg
   i) Defibrillation: 2-3 watt-sec (joules)/kg
4. Airway maintenance
   a) Avoid hyperextension of the neck. Hyperextension will narrow the airway in the area of cricoid ring in children under age five.
   b) Endotracheal and nasotracheal intubation may be a difficult procedure for the inexperienced. Bag-mask-valve ventilation in children provides adequate ventilatory function that may not be equally true in adults.
   c) Estimate endotracheal tube size by the size of the distal phalanx of the fifth digit or by the size of the external nares.
   d) Universal ET tube for infants is 3.5 mm.
   e) Use noncuffed ET tubes below age eight.
   f) Esophageal obturator airways are not indicated at this time in children under age 16.

IV. CHEST AND ABDOMINAL TRAUMA

A. Evaluation of chest trauma in children is similar to that seen in adults. Pneumothorax and hemothorax require chest tube drainage. A pneumothorax in children may not be appreciated on physical examination due to transmission of breath sounds across the mediastinum from the normal side.
   1. The chest tube size is 8-10 French in a premature infant up to 28 French for adolescents. [10] The location is the fourth ICS using the axillary approach. The anterior approach is to be avoided, especially in infants where the large thymus broadens the upper mediastinum.
   2. Thoracotomy may be necessary if blood drainage from the chest tube is more than 3-5 ml/kg/hr for 2 consecutive hrs or 1.5 ml/kg/hr for more than 4-6 hrs. [11]

B. The liver is larger and more vulnerable in the infant. Liver and spleen lacerations occur commonly without rib fractures. The pliable ribs in children ordinarily do not fracture.

V. HEAD TRAUMA

A. Hyperventilation is the most rapid means of lowering increased intracranial pressure. Hyperventilation at a rate of 18-21 times/min will provide for a $PaCO_2$ of 24-28 mmHg. Check ventilatory rate against blood gas results as soon as triage demands allow.

B. Furosemide (Lasix) 1 mg/kg given before mannitol 1 g/kg will prevent the transient increase in ICP seen with mannitol treatment alone, and will lower ICP at a more rapid rate. Strict attention to intake and output and to electrolyte balance is necessary. Be alert to mannitol-induced pulmonary edema. Head trauma in children may provoke hyperemia, not cerebral edema. Mannitol will cause increased ICP in these situations. CAT scans, if available, will make the clinical distinction possible. [12]

C. Elevation of head 45° will lower ICP 7-13 mmHg. [13]

D. Suctioning the child will increase ICP for up to 30 min.

VI. ORTHOPEDIC TRAUMA

A. Due to cartilaginous epiphyses and thicker periosteums, children's bones are more resilient to trauma. They may sustain a fracture without exhibiting early radiologic evidence. Sensitivity to palpation or weight bearing must be treated as a fracture with appropriate splinting.

B. Numerous incidents are recorded of children surviving crush injuries from earthquake disasters. Little is noted on x-ray although numerous cortical fractures may exist. Extensive soft tissue and muscle damage with risk of acute renal failure is assumed despite early evidence to the contrary. Due to anticipated swelling, extremities are splinted, not casted. Frequent neurovascular checks of the distal extremity are necessary. Early hyperkalemia requires urgent care. Consider emergency hemodialysis.

C. In disasters, where massive trauma and treatment delays predominate, gangrene, and disseminated intravascular coagulation (DIC) will threaten care. Controversy remains on

the best treatment management of DIC. Fresh whole blood,
fresh frozen plasma (10-15 ml/kg), and platelet and factor
concentrates are accepted approaches. Availability of concentrates in disaster situations limits their applicability. If
bleeding persists and time dictates urgency, IV heparin at a
starting dose of 100 units/kg is attempted. [14]

VII. BURNS

A. Due to the deep inhalations of a crying child, the initial inspiration of gases in smoke and chemical exposures may be
more injurious. As in the adult, a delay occurs between exposure and onset of pulmonary edema. Due to sparse nasal,
eyebrow, and facial hairs, singed hairs may not give clues
to airway burns. Inhaled burns require urgent intubation.
All children must be admitted for 24-48 hrs.

B. Judging burn depth is difficult in children. Burns which are
usually superficial in adults frequently are, or progress to,
full-thickness in children.

C. Determine the size of the burn by means of the following:[15]
  1. Head: 19% (Subtract 1% each year over one year till age
       nine.)
  2. Posterior trunk: 18%
  3. Anterior trunk and perineum: 18%
  4. Upper extremities: 9%
  5. Lower extremities: 13% (Add 1/2% to each lower limb
                              for each year over one year till age
                              15.)

D. Fluid therapy for children is based on 3 ml x % BSA x
weight in kg, with half infused in the first 8 hrs and the remainder over the next 16 hrs plus maintenance. [3]

VIII. TRIAGE OF PEDIATRIC CASUALTIES

A. In a field situation, the general principles of triage for
adults also apply to children. A crying child may be lost,
not injured.

B. In a hospital setting, urgent pediatric casualties go immediately to the emergency room. Other pediatric casualties go
to pediatric units where pediatricians and nurses familiar
with the demands of pediatric care continue stabilization
and evaluation.

C. In disaster situations where all physicians are likely to be
    pressed into service, pediatricians and generalists should
    take special interest in managing the following:[16]
    1. Nutritional and electrolyte requirements of prolonged
        entrapment or multiple trauma.
    2. Provision of blood and blood products.
    3. Screening, early recognition, and treatment of crush-
        related hyperkalemia and renal failure.
    4. Treatment of progressive hypoxemic respiratory failure
        and pulmonary edema from trauma or smoke inhalation.
    5. Treatment of sepsis from contaminated wounds and com-
        plications of trauma, i. e. , pulmonary sepsis.
    6. Treatment of hypothermia and hyperthermia.

D. Due to their public health orientation, pediatricians should
    be triaged to anticipate and deal with outbreaks of commun-
    icable disease.

REFERENCES

1. Holbrook, P. E. : Prehospital care of critically ill children.
    Crit Care Med 8(10):537-540, 1980.
2. McIntyre, K. M. , Lewis, A. J. , eds. : Textbook of Ad-
    vanced Cardiac Life Support. American Heart Association,
    1981.
3. American College of Surgeons, Committee on Trauma: Ad-
    vanced Trauma Life Support, 1980.
4. Los Angeles Pediatric Society: Prehospital Care of Pedi-
    atric Emergencies, Management Guidelines. American
    Academy of Pediatrics, 1980.
5. Mathewson, J. : Problems in detection and management of
    pediatric shock. ER Reports 2(8):31-36, 1981.
6. Pringle, K. , et al. : Preoperative and postoperative care
    of the pediatric surgical patient. Crit Care Med 8(10):554-
    558, 1980.
7. Dube, S. V. : Cardiopulmonary Emergencies. In Dube, S. V.
    (ed.) Immediate Care of the Sick and Injured Child. Saint
    Louis, C. V. Mosby Co. , 1978.
8. Buchanan, G. R. , and Hartwig, R. : Blood Product Trans-
    fusions. In Levin, D. L. (ed.): A Practical Guide to Pedi-
    atric Intensive Care. St. Louis, C. V. Mosby Co. , 1979.
9. Olness, K. : Practical Pediatrics in Less-Developed Coun-
    tries. Eden Prairie, Minn. , The Garden, 1980.
10. Moore, G. C. , et al. : Thoracentesis and Chest Tube Inser-
    tion. In Levin, D. L. (ed.): A Practical Guide to Pediatric
    Intensive Care. St. Louis, C. V. Mosby Co. , 1979.

11. Singh, R. P. : Chest Trauma. In Dube, S. V. (ed.): <u>Immedi-</u>
<u>ate Care of the Sick and Injured Child</u>. St. Louis, C. V.
Mosby Co. , 1978.
12. Bruce, D. A. , et al. : Resuscitation from coma due to head
injury. Crit Care Med 6(4):254-269, 1978.
13. Kenning, J. A. , et al. : Upright patient positioning in the
management of intracranial hypertension. Surg Neurol
15(2):148, 1981.
14. Hardaway, R. M. : A new look at disseminated intravascular coagulation. ER Reports 2(9):37-40, 1981.
15. Touloukian, R. J. , and Krizek, T. J. : <u>Diagnosis and Early</u>
<u>Management of Trauma Emergencies</u>. Springfield, Illinois,
Charles C Thomas Co. , 1974.
16. King, E. G. : The Moorgate disaster: Lessons for the internist. Ann Intern Med 84(3):333-334, 1976.

TRAUMA MANAGEMENT IN DISASTER MEDICINE

THE REALITIES OF TRAUMA IN DISASTER MEDICINE: AN INTRODUCTION

Frederick M. Burkle, Jr., M.D., M.P.H.

Section III concerns itself with specific areas of trauma management. The chapters include the traditional approaches to trauma written by those versed in trauma life support protocols and practiced in major medical centers. They have been included as necessary reminders of expected standards in an ideal situation. However, those readers who have experienced the grizzly realities of disaster medicine will quickly recognize the contradictions that these chapters provoke. The ideal situation never exists in disaster medicine.

If everything proceeds as planned and all patients receive the full benefit of standard procedures commonly practiced in tertiary care trauma centers, one should clearly question if a disaster was in actuality occurring. In realistic terms, injuries not immediately responsive to traditional and sometimes creative efforts to insure an airway, provide lung expansion, maintain circulation or control hemorrhage, should never enter the triage or evacuation system. This grim fact is rarely appreciated by those not experienced in the decision demands that make disaster medicine what it is.

Indeed, improved organization and rapid and efficient attempts at correcting the ABCs by trained personnel with appropriate stabilization will improve any victim's chance at survival. The instinctive knowledge of trauma life support protocols should be the basic bottom line standard for anyone involved in disaster medicine. Students and practitioners of disaster medicine will improve the system and in turn will better the overall percentages. Despite this, many victims will not survive. The earlier this fact is realized the more rapidly physicians will divert their attention to those having a better chance at survival. This may be dictated by the triage officer. If standard procedures fail, victims need to be supported in their death. Spiritual support with clergy as essential members of any triage team has been well realized historically by the military. The grieving process is shared by the victim and physician alike. It is a lonely and desperate time for both. Physicians may live with the consequent dilemma for a lifetime, wondering what might have been.

Expressed leadership, decisiveness, and temporary suppression of emotional input are the hallmarks of good clinical judgment in disaster medicine. We will all be fortunate if these disturbing realities are rarely practiced in our lifetimes.

As you read these chapters, approach the ideal if you can. Do not, however, forget that those skills may not be practiced on everyone, nor should they be. If triage, as well as standard procedures and evacuation principles, are appropriately practiced, the greatest number of lives will be saved.

Chapter 18

THE NATURE OF WOUNDS AND THEIR TREATMENT
Jack B. Peacock, M.D.

I. INTRODUCTION

This chapter will describe the variety and types of injuries
commonly associated with specific wounding agents and will not
deal with specific organ systems injuries. The epidemiology,
physical aspects, and local and systemic effects of wounds produced by particular agents will be described to provide background for discussion of field treatment, triage, and resource
management in both military and civilian disaster situations.

The types of wounds to be considered include burns, missile wounds, blast injuries, and crash injuries. It should be
remembered that while there are similarities between civilian
and military wounds, wounding agents may differ in some degree. For example, armaments utilized by the military may,
because of higher muzzle velocities, produce more severe
wounds than are generally seen in civilian practice.

II. BURNS

A. EPIDEMIOLOGY

Burn wounds result from the application of energy or corrosive substances to tissues. Some of the types of energy which
cause burns are heat (in the form of radiant energy), hot liquids
or metals, and electrical energy (in the form of high voltage
electrical current). Acids and alkalis are among the most common forms of corrosive substances that cause burns. Table
18-1 illustrates the three main types of burns.

In the civilized world, burns result most often from con-
flagrations, electrical injuries, and chemical exposures. They
may be seen in association with explosions and with exposure to
ionizing irradiation following the detonation of thermonuclear
devices.

Table 18-1   Types of Burns
_____

Thermal: Fire, hot liquids or metals, radiant energy,
              direct application of heat

Chemical: Contact with corrosives

Electrical: High voltage current

_____

B. PATHOLOGY

Whatever the nature of the wounding agent, burn wounds result
from the denaturation of cellular protein after contact with the
agent, which then results in coagulation necrosis. The depth
and extent of the wound is determined by the intensity and duration of tissue contact with the wounding agent.

For cutaneous burns, the morbidity and mortality resulting
from the burn are in proportion to both the extent of the wound
and the depth of the injury. However, the nature of the wounding
agent itself plays an important role in determining both the
severity of the injury and, to some extent, the outcome.

The depth of the burn wound is referred to as the degree of
the burn; burns are generally classified as first, second, or
third degree as shown in Table 18-2.

Rapid healing is normally observed in first degree burns.
Second degree burns retain viable epithelial elements from
which epithelialization can occur. Third degree burns, where
no epithelial elements are preserved, heal by deposition of
scar tissue or require skin grafting.

First degree burns are of little clinical or physiological
significance. Second and third degree burns, however, result
in loss of the water barrier and thermal regulating functions of
the involved skin; they also treat open wounds which have the
potential for infection.

Table 18-2.   Classification of Burn Depth
_____

First Degree: Involves only the superficial epidermis

Second Degree: Involves the dermis but with preservation of
                  viable epithelial elements

Third Degree: Involves destruction of all cutaneous elements
                  of the skin

_____

C. SPECIFIC FIELD TREATMENT

1. Resuscitation

Any important, immediate, physiologic effects which result are from the rapid losses of intravascular water and protein into both the burn injury and the interstitial space; these cause hypovolemic shock. The magnitude of fluid loss is proportional to the extent of the burn, whether it be second degree, or third, or both. The extent of the burn wound is defined in terms of the percent of body surface area involved. The rule of nines (Figure 18-1) is helpful in determining extent; but for greater precision, a standard burn chart is useful.

Prevention of burn shock requires rapid restoration of intravascular volume in the 24-hr period immediately following injury. Volume restoration is most easily accomplished by the intravenous infusion of balanced salt solution (Ringer's lactate) in volumes sufficient to normalize cardiovascular function. Estimates of the volumes of crystalloid required are based on the extent of the injury and can be readily calculated using standard formulas as shown in Table 18-3.

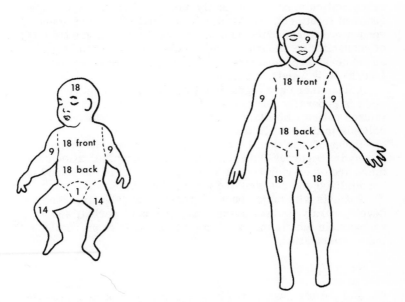

Figure 18-1. Rule of Nines

Table 18-3.   Fluid Resuscitation for Burned Patients

First 24 hrs

> Lactated Ringer's (or normal saline): 4 ml/kg body weight x % burn
> Infusion rate: 1/2 the estimated volume in first 8 hrs, 1/4 in second 8 hrs, 1/4 in third 8 hrs

Second 24 hrs

> Glucose in water to replace evaporative water loss and maintain normal saline sodium concentration

It should be emphasized that calculated fluid requirements for resuscitation of burned patients merely represent an estimate of the requirements for the individual patient, and that resuscitation must be constantly monitored to assess the adequacy of treatment. Restoration of normal vital signs, central venous pressure, urine output, and mental status are the goals of resuscitation. Hourly urine outputs in adults in the range of 35-50 cc/hr are considered adequate. In children, an output of 1 cc/kg body weight is adequate.

Unless there are signs of active bleeding, blood replacement is generally unnecessary in the resuscitation of the burn-injured patient. Similarly, the use of plasma expanders or colloids in the first 24 hrs is rarely necessary.

Burns of less than 10-15% body surface area do not generally require vigorous fluid resuscitation or hospitalization unless there are other risk factors involved. Larger burns should be hospitalized and resuscitated appropriately.

Patients with major burns, greater than 20%, frequently develop paralytic ileus in the initial postburn period, and a nasogastric tube is indicated in these patients to prevent vomiting and aspiration.

2. Wound Care

Care of the burn wound requires stopping the burning process and prevention of infection. Removal of clothing is essential. Application of cold or wet packs should be avoided to reduce loss of body heat. The burn wound should be cleansed gently with sterile saline to remove dirt and debris. Loose skin should be debrided, leaving blisters intact for the most part. A topical antibacterial cream, such as Sulfamylon or silver sulfadiazene should be applied to the entire wound, and a dressing or sterile cover applied to prevent further contamination. Dressing changes and reapplication of the topical antibacterial agent should be accomplished at least twice daily. Consideration should be given to early excision and grafting of small full thickness burns.

The use of prophylactic systemic antibiotics in the initial treatment of the burn patient is controversial and probably not essential. Adequacy of tetanus immunization should be assured, however, and tetanus immunization instituted where indicated.

D. SPECIAL PROBLEMS

1. Inhalation Injury

Inhalation injury is the term applied to the family of injuries to the bronchopulmonary tree which is seen in association with burns. It includes direct thermal or chemical injury to the upper airways, which results in mucosal edema and the potential for airway obstruction, as well as the effects of smoke and toxic gas inhalation on the respiratory epithelium and pulmonary gas exchange. Finally, carbon monoxide poisoning, as the result of inhalation, may be considered a part of the syndrome.

Inhalation injury should be suspected in any patient who has been burned in a closed environment. Physical signs include the presence of burns about the head and face, singing of nasal hair, the presence of burns in the mouth and pharynx, the presence of soot in the sputum or upper airways, and signs of respiratory distress or stridor. Neither auscultation of the chest nor chest x-rays are diagnostic early in the process. Finally, clinical signs of hypoxemia, such as tachypnea or alteration of level of consciousness, should be looked for.

Treatment of inhalation injury is aimed at preservation of the airway and maintenance of adequate oxygenation. High concentrations of humidified oxygen should be provided, and, where there is danger of impending upper airway obstruction, endotracheal intubation is indicated.

2. Chemical Burns

Chemical burns differ from thermal burns in that the burning process continues as long as the chemical is in contact with the

patient. Therefore, removal of the agent by copious irrigation
with water is essential. Alkalis are, in general, more resistant
to removal by irrigation than are acids and require prolonged
irrigation in order to stop the burning process. Phosphorous
burns, associated with smoke grenades and incendiary devices,
should be debrided to remove residual phosphorous.

3. Electrical Burns

Patients with electrical injury should be suspected of having
severe damage to underlying muscle, bone, nerve, and other
organs resulting from the passage of high voltage current
through the body, and the extent of such damage may not be reflected by the extent of obvious cutaneous injury. For this
reason, electrical burns require surgical exploration and early
debridement of nonviable tissue, as well as fasciotomy, to prevent development of compartment syndromes in the extremities.

4. Compartment Syndromes

Swelling of tissues deep to the burn wound when confined by
surrounding fascia, as in the case of muscles of the extremities, or by the firm, unyielding eschar of third degree burns,
may compromise the blood supply to the involved muscle and to
the extremity distal to the involved area. The potential for the
development of a compartment syndrome is present where there
is electrical injury and where there are circumferential burns
of the extremities.

The diagnosis of compartment syndrome is based on suspicion and physical findings indicative of vascular compromise,
such as increasing pain, loss of neuromuscular function, or
diminished or absent arterial blood flow distal to the injury.

Treatment is aimed at release of constriction either by
fasciotomy, in the case of electrical burns, or by escharotomy
in circumferential third degree burns. Escharotomy can be
performed without anesthesia or blood replacement by simple
incision through the burn eschar into the subcutaneous fat in a
manner analogous to bivalving a plaster cast (Figure 18-2).

On occasion, ventilation may be compromised as a result
of the presence of circumferential third degree burns of the
thorax which restrict respiratory excursion. Thoracic escharotomy is indicated under these circumstances.

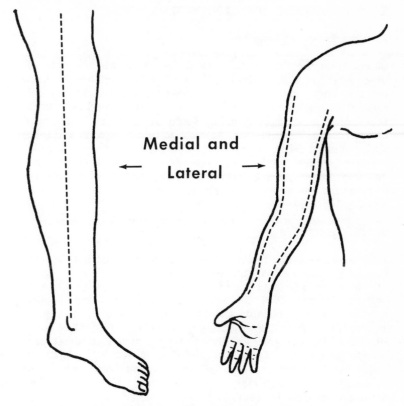

Figure 18-2.   Escharotomy incisions

5. Associated Injuries

Patients with burns may have other injuries sustained at the
time of the burning incident. In general, the other injuries
should be treated in the same manner as if there were no burns
present.

6. Age and Associated Illness

Patients at extremes of age (50 or older, 5 or younger) who are
burned have a higher mortality than young adults. Similarly,
patients with other underlying illness, particularly diabetes or
cardiopulmonary disease, are at greater risk.

E. IMPLICATIONS FOR RESOURCE PLANNING

1. Equipment and Supplies

Supplies for the care of the patient should include adequate volumes of resuscitative fluids (Ringer's lactate or normal saline), intravenous fluids, indwelling bladder catheters and urine collection devices, and dressings. Medications should include topical antibacterial agents (e. g. , Sulfamylon, silver sulfadiazene), and narcotics for injection, as well as tetanus toxoid and tetanus immune globulin. In addition, equipment should be on hand for endotracheal intubation, cardiovascular monitoring, surgical debridement, and escharotomy. The equipment necessary to measure hematologic and electrolyte status, as well as the level of blood gases, should be available.

2. Triage and Transportation

Important decisions in the management of burn patients, particularly in the face of limited resources and personnel, are (1) the need to hospitalize the patient, and (2) the likelihood of patient survival. Patients who are unlikely to survive, regardless of therapy, probably should not be recipients of precious resources. As mentioned earlier, patients who might be included in this category are those who are at the extremes of age or who have severe associated injuries or illnesses. In addition, cutaneous burns in excess of 60-70% body surface area should be considered at high risk, and larger burns should be denied all but supportive therapy.

Burns in the following categories should be considered major burns and will require hospitalization:

1. All burns greater than 15% in adults or greater than 10% in children.
2. Third degree burns greater than 2% body surface area.
3. All burns involving the face, eyes, ears, hands, feet, or perineum.
4. Circumferential burns of the trunk or extremities.
5. All burns with evidence or suspicion of inhalation injury.
6. Electrical and chemical burns.
7. Burns associated with other injuries (fractures, internal injuries) or major illnesses (diabetes, cardiovascular disease).
8. Burns in patients under 2 years of age or over 50 years of age.

III. MISSILE WOUNDS

A. EPIDEMIOLOGY

Missile wounds include wounds produced by firearms, by explosive devices, and by accidental explosions. Civilian weapons in general use today usually do not have the wounding power of military weapons, particularly where firearms are concerned. However, high-powered firearms are gaining increasing popularity in the civilian world, and military weapons appear to be readily available to terrorist groups outside the military.

Explosive devices in use by the military are usually designed to wound through the production of metallic fragments upon explosion; these fragments are hurled in the direction of the adversary. Civilian explosive devices generally wound through the production of blast effects and the creation of secondary fragments (e. g. , glass, wood, masonry) from damaged structural surroundings.

B. PATHOLOGY

1. Wound Ballistics

The wounding power of missiles is proportional to both the mass of the missile and the square of the velocity with which the missile strikes the victim $F = MV^2$. In general, mass is less variable among types of missiles, and velocity appears to play the dominant role in determining wounding power. Velocity at the wound is directly proportional to the velocity of the missile at the point from which it is fired and inversely proportional to the distance between the fire point and impact. The velocity of the missile at the point from which it is fired is termed the muzzle velocity. The amount of kinetic energy which has to be absorbed and dissipated by the tissue, ultimately determines both the amount of damage that results and the depth of penetration of the missile as illustrated in Table 18-4.

Table 18-4.   Muzzle Velocities

Size	Velocity (ft/sec)
22 short	900
25 caliber	800
38 caliber	925
45 caliber	850
30 caliber	1970
7. 62 mm	2750
5. 56 mm (M-16)	3250

When a missile with great kinetic energy strikes solid tissue, the absorption and dissipation of that energy within the tissue results in the formation of a cylindrical region of temporary cavitation about the path of the missile, producing a zone of tissue damage several-fold larger than the size of the missile itself. This is particularly true for high velocity firearms missiles used by the military (M-16, AK-47). Therefore, there may be little relation between the size of the cutaneous entrance wound and the extent of underlying tissue damage along the path of the missile. In addition, upon striking solid tissue such as bone, secondary fragments are produced, adding to the extent of tissue injury. Generally, firearms in use by the civilian populace have lower muzzle velocities and result in tissue destruction which is more nearly limited to the immediate path of the missile.

Fragmentation devices generally have a much greater diminution in wounding power over distance than firearms do. The same is true for shotguns. However, wounds caused by fragmentation devices and shotguns tend to be numerous and may be scattered over several regions of the body, depending on the proximity of the victim to the wounding agent. At close range, both fragmentation devices and shotguns can produce devastating wounds due to the combination of blast effect and concentration of numerous missiles into a small area. Conversely, with increasing distance, the wounding power of fragmentation devices and shotguns diminishes rapidly, and, though the wounds may be widely scattered over the body, penetration is limited.

2. Distribution of Wounds

As should be expected, the extremities are most frequently involved in missile injuries. However, injuries to the head, neck, and trunk are potentially much more lethal as shown in Table 18-5.

Table 18-5. Missile Wounds by Body Area

Site	GSW	Other
Lower extremity	43%	35%
Upper extremity	24%	27%
Head and neck	6%	12%
Chest	9%	9%
Abdomen	9%	5%
Flank, back	9%	12%

In the management of wounds caused by missiles, consideration should be given to the early identification and treatment of life-threatening and limb-threatening injuries as separate from those which are trivial. Wounds which penetrate any of the major body cavities (i.e., cranium, chest, abdomen) should be considered potentially life-threatening. Wounds of the extremities, which are in the region of major vessels, offer the potential for vascular injury and loss of limb. Similarly, wounds of the extremities with massive tissue damage represent a threat both in terms of limb loss and in terms of potential for subsequent development of a life-threatening infection in the damaged tissue (gas gangrene). Finally, superficial wounds, with the exception of potential vascular injuries, are for the most part considered to be trivial in the circumstances of disaster management.

3. Specific Field Management

a) <u>Hemorrhage and Shock.</u> Internal and external hemorrhage and resulting shock represent an immediate threat to the life of the wounded patient. Immediate efforts must be made to identify and control hemorrhage and to restore vascular volume. External hemorrhage, even that from a major vessel, can usually be controlled by direct manual pressure, pressure dressings, or air splints. Tourniquets should not be used except where the extremity distal to the injury is nonviable. Internal hemorrhage will usually require surgical intervention and control. However, the pneumatic antishock garment may be useful in both circumstances to provide temporary tamponade of hemorrhage until blood volume has been restored and operation can be undertaken.

The extent of hemorrhage can be roughly quantitated from the patient's condition on initial presentation as shown in Table 18-6.

Patients with grade I hemorrhage generally are relatively asymptomatic from their blood loss and present without evidence of cardiovascular instability (e.g., hypotension, tachycardia, diminished tissue perfusion). Patients with grade III

Table 18-6. Classification of Hemorrhagic Shock

Grade I : Acute loss of less than 15% of total blood volume

Grade II : Acute loss of 15-30% of total blood volume

Grade III: Acute loss in excess of 30% of total blood volume hemorrhage generally present in extremis with little or no palpable pulse or blood pressure. Those with grade II hemorrhage present with moderate hypotension, tachycardia, and evidence of decreased tissue perfusion.

Recalling that normal blood volume averages about 70 cc/kg body weight or approximately 5 liters in the average adult, one can roughly quantitate the extent of blood loss based on assessment of the patient's cardiovascular function and tissue perfusion on presentation. This estimate can be useful both in gauging the fluid volume required for restoration of blood volume and, later, in comparing that estimate to actual requirements in an effort to determine whether or not there are continuing unrecognized blood losses.

Patients with grade I hemorrhage can usually be completely resuscitated with the use of crystalloid solutions alone and therefore should not require blood transfusion. Patients with grade II and grade III hemorrhage will generally require blood in addition to crystalloid during resuscitation.

Ringer's lactate is the crystalloid solution of choice in the initial resuscitation of the injured patient. Normal saline may be used if the former is not available. Crystalloid requirements for resuscitation approximate three times the amount of blood lost. In grade I hemorrhage, for example, with a 750 cc estimated blood loss, resuscitation with crystalloid will require approximately 2250 cc of solution.

For all patients, fluid resuscitation should be initiated with crystalloid solution infused through large-bore (14-16 gauge) intravenous catheters at rates sufficient to normalize cardiovascular function. Blood, when required, should be crossmatched when possible or at least type-specific. Where time does not permit typing and crossmatching, type O blood should be used.

Essential monitoring during the resuscitation period should include measurement of blood pressure, pulse, urine output, and level of consciousness. The initial hematocrit is of no use in estimating the extent of hemorrhage, although it serves as a useful baseline for comparison to later hematocrit determinations.

b) Cardiopulmonary Complications. Early attention must be given to the identification and correction of cardiopulmonary abnormalities produced by the wound. Specifically, pericardial tamponade, tension pneumothorax, and massive hemothorax require immediate treatment if the patient is to survive. Both because of the potential for ventilatory and circulatory embarrassment in all severely or potentially, severely injured patients, oxygen should be administered at inspired volumes necessary to maintain adequate oxygenation.

c) <u>Recognition of Hidden Injury</u>. Intraabdominal and intra-thoracic injury must be suspected whenever there is a wound of entrance about the trunk. Where firearms missiles are concerned, wounds of the trunk should be assumed to have produced injury within either or both of these body cavities. However, where fragmentation wounds or long-range shotgun wounds are concerned, the presence of a cutaneous injury over the trunk does not necessarily imply internal injury. The classical physical findings of intrathoracic and intraabdominal injury, when present, will confirm the diagnosis. However, where these findings are absent, the physician must resort to either radiographic investigation or continued reexamination in order to establish the presence of internal injury. In general, plain radiographs of the chest or abdomen, taken in two views, PA and lateral, are most useful in determining whether or not there is an intracavitary missile.

Vascular injuries must be suspected when there is a wound in the vicinity of a major vessel, even in the absence of classical signs of hemorrhage from the wound or distal ischemia. Physical examination, documenting the presence or absence of pulses distal to the wound or of vascular bruits, is useful when positive. Findings of bruits, pulselessness, or tissue ischemia distal to the wound are diagnostic. Similarly, the presence of nerve injury should alert one to the possibility of injury to blood vessels in the immediate proximity. However, it is important to remember that a significant number of vascular injuries present without signs of distal ischemia. It is, therefore, essential that the physician maintain a high index of suspicion when assessing wounds in the vicinity of major vascular structures, and limb loss may be avoided by appropriate exploration of such wounds or by angiography to document the presence or absence of vascular injury. Where angiography is not readily available, early exploration may be indicated for limb salvage.

4. Management of Local Injury

The management of specific organ injuries is discussed elsewhere in the text. The management of local soft tissue injuries is directed toward excision of devitalized tissue and prevention of infection. Following treatment of hemorrhagic shock and life- and limb-threatening injuries, all wounds should be surgically explored, and thorough debridement of all devitalized tissue performed. All foreign material, such as clothing, dirt, or wadding from shotgun shells, should be removed. Generally, there is no need to remove the metallic fragments from soft tissues.

Following debridement, the wound should be thoroughly irrigated with sterile isotonic saline. Jet irrigation through the use of a commercial irrigation device (e. g. , Water Pik) or by needle and syringe are superior to merely flushing the wound. All cutaneous wounds should be left open and dressed for later delayed primary closure in order to decrease the incidence of wound infection. Delayed primary closure can be accomplished 3-5 days following operation.

Systemic antibiotics are probably indicated in all missile wounds. Broad-spectrum antibiotic agents, such as a first generation cephalosporin, should be administered parenterally in therapeutic doses as soon after wounding as possible. Delay in the administration of antibiotics much beyond 2 hrs from the time of wounding negates their prophylactic effect in preventing wound infection.

As with all wounds, patients with missile injuries should be adequately immunized against tetanus.

5. Implications for Resource Planning

Adequate volumes of crystalloid solutions and infusions sets for resuscitation from shock are necessary as is oxygen and the equipment for oxygen administration. Further requirements include endotracheal and/or tracheostomy tubes, chest tubes, urinary catheters, nasogastric tubes, and an assortment of drains and suture material, as well as dressing materials. Equipment should include, at the minimum, a portable x-ray machine and the capability of processing radiographs, along with an assortment of general surgical and vascular surgical instruments. Blood for transfusion should be readily available, especially type O. It is extremely valuable to have the capability of collecting blood from noninjured donors in order to ensure a continuing supply of blood.

IV. BLAST INJURIES

A. EPIDEMIOLOGY

Blast injuries occur as a result of accidental or intentional detonation of flammable or explosive materials. In the civilian sector, such injuries are likely to result from industrial accidents or terrorist bombings. In the military, blast injuries result from detonation of antipersonnel explosive weapons, including thermonuclear devices, mines, conventional bombs, mortar shells, artillery rounds, etc.

B. PATHOLOGY

Whatever the cause, the effects of blast injury can be classified into three groups as shown in Table 18-7. The primary effects are due to the direct impact of the sudden variation in environmental (atmospheric or hydrostatic) pressure on tissues. Primary effects are seen in both air and underwater blasts, while secondary and tertiary effects occur only in air explosions. The primary blast can produce perforation of tympanic membranes, resulting in sudden deafness. More important, however, are the effects of the blast on the lungs; the result is pulmonary contusion and laceration. In underwater blasts, injuries to the abdominal contents predominate, and bowel injuries are common.

Secondary effects are due to the creation of secondary missiles from the acceleration of masonry, glass, and other materials created by the blast. These missiles can produce a variety of wounds, depending on where they strike the victim; this is illustrated in Table 18-8. In addition, thermal burns can result from the explosion; they are considered to be secondary injuries.

Tertiary injuries result from acceleration of the victim through space from the force of the explosion. Injuries produced depend on rate of acceleration deceleration and on where the victim strikes stationary objects. Injuries to be anticipated include concussion and craniocerebral injury, injury to solid organs (spleen, liver), bony fractures, and joint dislocations.

Thus, the combined effects of the blast can produce a variety of injuries including compression effects, burns, missile injuries, and blunt (deceleration) injuries as shown in Table 8-9. Life-threatening injuries will include major burns, craniocerebral, chest, and intraabdominal injuries. Of those who survive the explosion initially, the majority will require hospitalization, two-thirds for periods greater than 72 hrs.

Table 18-7.   Biologic Effects of Blast Injury

Primary: Due to sudden variation in environmental pressure

Secondary: Injury produced by secondary missiles

Tertiary: Injury produced by acceleration of the victim

Table 18-8. Distribution of External Injuries

Site	%
Arms	25
Legs	18
Head and neck	38
Trunk	19
Flank, back	20

Nearly half the burn victims will sustain major body surface area burns. A majority of immediate deaths are due to structural collapse and crush injury.

C. SPECIFIC FIELD MANAGEMENT

Because of the protean manifestations of blast injury, all victims should be initially suspected of having sustained potentially serious injuries. Particular attention should be given to early identification and treatment of pulmonary complications and hypovolemic shock, and the physician must be alert to the potential for occult intrathoracic and intraabdominal injuries.

The details of treatment of specific organ systems' injuries are outlined elsewhere in the text. A useful adjunct to diagnosis of occult intraabdominal injuries is the use of peritoneal lavage.

D. IMPLICATIONS FOR RESOURCE PLANNING

A major explosion will require all the resources of an acute care hospital, including diagnostic radiology, operating room, and blood banking facilities. As many as half the patients will require operative treatment, and the requirements for transfusion approximate 1 unit whole blood per victim.

Table 18-9. Distribution of Total Injuries

Injury	%
Craniocerebral	44
Chest	20
Abdominal	10
Extremities	40
Burns	30
Superficial wounds	70

V. CRUSH INJURY

A. EPIDEMIOLOGY

Crush injuries most frequently result from the collapse of occupied structures either as a result of structural fault or as a
result of explosion or earthquake. Occasionally such injuries
are sustained as a result of a vehicular accident, such as the
overturning of a passenger vehicle, or in railway accidents.

A major problem with the management of victims of crush-
ing injuries under these circumstances is gaining access to the
victims in order to effect rescue and initiate treatment.

B. PATHOLOGY

1. Local Effects

The immediate effects of crush injury are those associated with
deformation of the victim's supporting skeleton and solid organs, resulting in fractures, fracture-dislocations, and solid
organ injury. In addition, however, portions of the body
trapped in the wreckage suffer from the combined effects of
tissue hypoxia, due to compromised circulation, and direct
tissue injury, due to pressure and contusion. The effects result
in progressive tissue swelling, leading to lactic acidosis and
cell death.

Where muscle groups of the extremities, in particular, are
injured, expansion of swelling muscle is limited by enveloping
fascia, further compromising muscle cell perfusion and accel-
erating cellular death. Further, major blood vessels of the extremities traversing these muscular compartments may be
progressively occluded by the continued swelling of surrounding
tissues, further aggravating the ischemic state. This combination of effects is often referred to as a compartment syndrome,
and the syndrome can be seen in all muscle compartments of
the extremities. The end result, if unrecognized and untreated,
is not only loss of the affected muscle groups, but also the potential for ischemic necrosis of the entire extremity.

2. Systemic Effects

The systemic effects of crush injury include hypovolemic shock,
ventilatory compromise, and cardiac failure. Shock may be
due to apparent or occult blood loss secondary to internal injuries. However, significant and life-threatening hypovolemia can
also result from the loss of intravascular water into damaged

and hypoxic tissues in the absence of significant hemorrhage.

Pulmonary dysfunction may result from compromised respiratory excursion, and asphyxia, if the victim's thorax is trapped in the wreckage and debris. Direct injury to the thoracic cage and lung, resulting in pulmonary contusions and laceration, pneumothorax, and hemothorax, also occur. In addition, gas exchange can be further impaired as a result of traumatic fat embolism.

Traumatic asphyxia is a misnomer in that it is a constellation of signs that reflect a sudden increase in intrathoracic pressure. Such signs include edema, petechiae, and subcutaneous hemorrhage, which is particularly prominent over the face, eyes, and neck. These findings do not imply that the victim has suffered asphyxia, but they should alert the physician to the possibility of intrathoracic and intraabdominal injuries that may result simultaneously.

Metabolic acidosis and hyperkalemia secondary to prolonged cellular ischemia and tissue necrosis can be profound. These events, however, may not be manifest until the victim has been extricated and perfusion of injured tissues restored. The physician should, therefore, be alert for the development of this complication during the resuscitation phase.

Renal failure may result from the combined effects of hypovolemia, acidosis, and the release of myoglobin from injured muscle.

C. SPECIFIC FIELD MANAGEMENT

1. Shock Management

The management of hypovolemic and hemorrhagic shock are detailed elsewhere in the text; however, large volumes of resuscitative fluids may be required in victims of crush injury, particularly where rescue has been prolonged.

2. Wound Care

Extremity injuries, in particular, should be carefully evaluated for the development of compartment syndromes. The syndrome should be suspected wherever there has been closed injury to muscle groups or prolonged ischemia of an extremity secondary to vascular compromise. Recognition is based on suspicion due to the mechanism of injury and the combined signs of neuromuscular dysfunction, swelling, and vascular insufficiency. Muscle groups should be carefully palpated to estimate whether or not the fascial compartment is tense. Muscular function should also be assessed. Diminished neural function (particularly sensation) distal to the injury and evidence of arterial insufficiency or interference with venous return should alert the examiner to the possible presence of the syndrome. Direct measurement of muscle compartment pressure, while a sensitive index, is probably not practical under disaster circumstances.

Treatment of compartment syndrome is based on operative exploration of the muscle compartments and wide fasciotomy. In circumstances where fasciotomy does not restore circulation, amputation may be indicated.

3. Renal Complications

Brisk diuresis, induced by adequate restoration of intravascular volume and the administration of osmotic diuretics, such as mannitol, is the most effective measure in the prevention of renal failure secondary to myoglobin deposition in the renal tubules. Alkalinization of the urine by restoration of acid-base balance and the administration of bicarbonate is also helpful.

4. Ventilatory Problems

In addition to looking for the obvious injuries which result in ventilatory compromise (e. g. , rib fractures, hemothorax, pneumothorax, flail chest), one should be alert to the development of pulmonary dysfunction secondary to pulmonary contusion and to fat embolism. Both of these entities are characterized by progressive hypoxia and the development of radiographic changes in the lung fields that characteristically appear many hours after the development of the physiologic signs of injury. Oxygen therapy and positive pressure ventilation may be critical to survival in these patients. In addition, fluid overload should be avoided if it is at all possible to do so. Finally, attention should be given to the prevention of pulmonary infection. The use of prophylactic antibiotics is controversial in this situation; however, care should be taken to protect the bronchopulmonary tree from bacterial contamination.

D. IMPLICATIONS FOR RESOURCE PLANNING

Because of delays in rescue, resuscitation may need to be initiated at the scene. Equipment for airway management, oxygen administration, fluid volume resuscitation, and wound coverage are essential under these circumstances. In addition, long back boards, cervical collars, and extremity splints may be helpful at the scene and during extrication.

The definitive management of the seriously injured patient requires the facilities of a full service hospital, including operating room, blood banking, diagnostic radiology, and intensive care services.

Consideration should be given at the scene to the possible necessity for amputation of an extremity to expedite rescue, particularly where rescue efforts are hampered or there is danger of continuing structural collapse or fire. A guillotine amputation with application of a tourniquet can be lifesaving under these circumstances.

Because of the potential for a number of fatal injuries to occur at the scene, resources probably should not be expended on patients who in all likelihood cannot be resuscitated, such as patients with severe neurologic injuries and patients with agonal cardiopulmonary function.

VI. PREVENTION OF WOUND INFECTION

Open wounds and injuries to hollow viscera (e. g. , gastrointestinal, genitourinary, and respiratory tracts) create the potential for the development of wound infection. This potential is further compounded by the occurrence of shock, poor tissue perfusion, and massive contamination of the wound with microorganisms and foreign bodies (e. g. , dirt, clothing, etc.). In addition, there is accumulating evidence that victims of major injury are immunodepressed.

Important considerations in the prevention or development of infection following wounding include those related to wound microbiology, the wound environment, and host defenses.

All open wounds are contaminated with bacteria. The most prevalent contaminating bacteria are the resident flora of the skin and those of the gastrointestinal, genitourinary, and respiratory tracts. Bacterial factors of importance include the numbers of contaminating organisms, their virulence, and bacterial synergism.

Since little can be done at the outset to control bacterial virulence, attention must be given to reducing the numbers of contaminating organisms and to preventing continued contamination. The presence of foreign bodies, devitalized tissue, and fluid collections in the wound potentiate the development of infection, even with minimal bacterial contamination.

Thorough debridement of the wound with removal of obvious foreign material and nonviable tissue are of prime importance in reducing the extent of bacterial contamination. Tissue viability can be assessed by gross inspection, and nonviable tissue should be sharply excised. Jet lavage irrigation is superior to other methods of eliminating organisms and foreign material. Monofilament or absorbable suture material should be used in preference to braided suture. Implantation of foreign bodies, such as vascular prostheses, should be avoided where possible. Cutaneous wounds should be left open and covered with sterile dressings for delayed primary closure 3-5 days after operation.

Host immune defense can be supported by rapid restoration of blood volume and normalization of cardiovascular function. Early attention to nutritional needs of the patient is also important.

The use of antimicrobial agents remains controversial. However, there is good evidence that parenteral administration of appropriate antibiotics is of benefit in the prevention of infections following open wounds of the abdomen and thorax, in wounds of the central nervous system, in open fractures, and in wounds with massive contamination and soft tissue injury. Further, their use in circumstances where treatment is delayed seems appropriate. To be effective, antibiotic agents must be administered within about 2 hrs from the time of wounding.

All open wounds present the potential for the later development of tetanus. The status of the patient's tetanus immunization should be established, and appropriate immunization administered as outlined in Table 18-10.

Table 18-10.   Tetanus Immunization
_____

1. Tetanus immunization in adults requires at least three injections of toxoid followed by administration of a toxoid booster every 10 years thereafter. In children under 7, immunization requires four injections of DPT with a booster dose at 10-year intervals.
2. For previously immunized individuals with the last booster dose within 10 years, administer 0.5 ml absorbed toxoid for tetanus-prone wounds if more than 5 years have elapsed since the last booster.
3. For previously immunized individuals who received the last booster dose more than ten years previously, administer 0.5 ml absorbed toxoid for all wounds.
4. For individuals not adequately immunized:
    a. For nontetanus-prone wounds, give 0.5 ml absorbed toxoid.
    b. For tetanus-prone wounds,
        1) Give 0.5 ml absorbed toxoid AND
        2) Give 250 units (or more) of human tetanus immune globulin.

Use different syringes and injection sites for administration of toxoid and tetanus immune globulin.

3) Consider antibiotic administration.

BIBLIOGRAPHY

American College of Surgery: A Guide to Prophylaxis Against Tetanus in Wound Management. Bulletin. 1979.

Amato, J. J., Billy, L. J., Lawson, N. S., and Rich, N. M.: High velocity missile injury. Am J Surg 127:454-459, 1974.

Brismar, B., and Bergenwald, L.: The terroristic bomb explosion in Bologna, Italy, 1980: An analysis of the effects and injuries sustained. J Trauma 22:216-220, 1982.

Brown, L. L., Shelton, H. T., Bornside, G. H., and Cohn, I.: Evaluation of wound irrigation by pulsatile jet and conventional methods. Ann Surg 187:170-173, 1978.

American College of Surgery: Field Categorization of Trauma Patients and Hospital Trauma Index. Bulletin. Feb., 1980, pp. 28-31.

Moylan, J. A., Peters, C. R., and Filston, H. C.: Burn therapy updated. N C Med J 38:594-596, 1977.

Rich, N. M., and Johnson, E. V.: Wounding power of missiles used in Vietnam. JAMA 199:157; 160-161; 168, 1967.

Stephenson, S. F., Esrig, B. C., Polk, H. C., and Fulton, R. L.: The pathophysiology of smoke inhalation injury. Ann Surg 1182:652-659, 1975.

Waterworth, T. A., and Carr, M. J. T.: Report on injuries sustained by patients treated at the Birmingham General Hospital following the recent bomb explosions. Br Med J 2:25-27, 1975.

Chapter 19

MULTIPLE TRAUMA
Valeriy Moysaenko, M. D.

I. INTRODUCTION

The Vietnam and Korean Wars allowed rapid evacuation of the
injured by air transport. Casualties arrived at well-staffed,
well-equipped definitive care hospitals usually within an hour
after injury. The treatment logistics of this type of mass casualty situation is well described in the medical literature of the
Vietnam and Korean Wars and of civilian disasters. This chapter will attempt to provide an overview to the management of
multiple trauma casualties during adverse conditions as might
be encountered on a battlefield or in a civilian disaster when
rapid evacuation is unavailable.

II. SITUATION

The protocol described is for the worst possible situation. Assume that resources will be limited for 36 hrs. The limitations
are as follows:

1. One physician
2. No surgeon
3. No surgical facilities
4. Limited supplies

The demands will be exorbitant:

1. Mass casualty
2. Multiple trauma

Some of the obvious consequences of this situation are:

1. Patients with severe injuries requiring immediate life-
saving surgery will be lost.
2. Patients with injuries requiring an inordinate amount of
care or supplies will be lost. In the first case, the loss will

occur because facilities and expertise are not available. In the
second case, if supplies and personnel are diverted for this
type of care, other more salvageable patients might be lost.
Obviously, decisions will need to be made in a rational manner.
The goal is to save as many patients as possible, not to save a
few difficult cases. The physician must function in the real
situation and not become entangled by seductive heroic ideals.

III. PERSPECTIVES

A. INTRODUCTION

At first consideration, one may find the above situation untenable; however, this type of response is inappropriate and is the
result of ignorance.
   Table 19-1 shows that 63% of injuries in this mass casualty
situation are to extremities. These injuries can and should be
easily managed.
   Table 19-2, viewed in conjunction with Table 19-1, supports
the logical assumption that extremity injuries, although frequent,
are rarely lethal and should probably not be lethal. Scrutiny of
the literature indicates that a common cause of death in these
injuries is hemorrhage, which can be prevented easily by controlled pressure.

B. PENETRATING HEAD INJURIES

Table 19-2 shows that the most common cause of death is head
injury, usually a penetrating missile injury. Closed head
trauma is discussed in Chapter 25.
   Table 19-3 indicates that 34/70 cases with penetrating injury who arrived at the hospital alive were stable (Group I). In

Table 19-1.   7869 Hospital Admissions (Vietnam)*

Location	%
Head and neck	12. 0
Thorax	7. 2
Abdomen	7. 1
Upper extremity	22. 4
Lower extremity	40. 6
Other (flank, back, buttocks, genitalia, unidentified)	10. 7

*Heaton, L. D., Rosegay, H., Hughes, C. W., Fisher, G. W.,
and Feighny, R. E.: Military surgical practices of the United
States Army in Vietnam. 1:1-59, Nov., 1966.

Table 19-2. 2600 Casualties Killed in Action in Vietnam
Conflict, January-June, 1968*

Region	%
Head	39. 3
Thorax	37. 0
Abdomen	9. 0
Neck	7. 3
Lower extremity	5. 7
Upper extremity	1. 7

*Maughon, J. S. : An inquiry into the nature of wounds resulting
in killed in action in Vietnam. Milit Med 135:8-13, 1970.

the scenario described, i. e. , no help for 36 hrs, these patients
will survive 36 hrs until reaching a hospital for definitive care
if they are treated with appropriate wound care, fluids, and antibiotics. If the worst case is assumed, Groups II and III will
die. The increase in mortality has gone from 31-52% in patients
with penetrating head injury who have reached a medical facility
alive. Conclusion: appropriate conservative management will
resuscitate approximately 50% of penetrating head injuries.

Table 19-3. Neurological Condition of 70 Patients with
Penetrating Head Wounds on Admission to the
Third Field Hospital (Saigon, Vietnam),
November, 1966*

Group	No. of Cases	Operated	Death
I : Conscious; moderate to no deficit (paresis, hemianopsia)	34	34	0%
II : Stuporous; severe	18	18	22%
III: Moribund and comatose; bilateral dilated, fixed pupils; slow, irregular, or labored respirations	18	0	100%

*Heaton, L.D. , Rosegay, H. , Hughes, C.W. , Fisher, G.W. ,
and Feighny, R.E.: Military surgical practices of the United
States Army in Vietnam. Curr Probl Surg 1:1-59, 1966.

Suggested Management of Head Injuries

1. Stable head injuries can be delayed for evacuation
2. Head injuries with progressing neurological deficits will have priority for evacuation to definitive care.
3. Open head wounds should be washed copiously and gently with sterile saline, and a sterile dressing applied.

C. THORACIC

As shown in Table 19-2, the next large group of lethal injuries are to the thorax. What are some of the characteristics of these injuries? They are usually lethal, not in the wound itself, but in the effects on cardiopulmonary function due to:

1. Airway obstruction
2. Tension pneumothorax
3. Flail chest
4. Open pneumothorax
5. Hemothorax
6. Cardiac tamponade

Airway obstruction may be relieved by head/jaw repositioning, clearing the upper airway, manual thrust maneuvers, or cricothyroidotomy. Chest tube placement will relieve above-numbered problems 2-5, and pericardiocentesis will relieve problem 6.

Conservative treatment consists of chest tube placement, humidification of air, clearing of tracheobronchial secretions, tracheostomy to reduce dead space, volume replacement to correct shock, wound debridement, and dressings. Most very severe thoracic injuries will not reach medical care alive. Table 19-4 shows examples of the types of salvageable chest injuries.

D. ABDOMINAL INJURIES

The third major group of lethal injuries are abdominal injuries. Severe abdominal injuries (major vessel or solid organ destruction) will usually not reach medical care; even if they do, they often expire within 24 hrs despite definitive therapy attempts. The percentage of such patients is small as illustrated in Table 19-5.

Most penetrating abdominal injuries perforate hollow viscera such as small bowel, colon, stomach, etc. , resulting in contamination of the peritoneum. These types of injuries alone

Table 19-4.   Chest Casualties Salvaged Second Mobile Army
              Surgical Hospital (Vietnam), October 1, 1966 -
              July 31, 1967[a,b]

No. of Cases	Type of Injury
165	Total chest cases
107	Chest wall injuries
48	Penetrating injuries treated conservatively
10	Penetrating injuries requiring thoracotomy

[a]Heaton, L. D., Rosegay, H., Hughes, C. W., Fisher, G. W.,
and Feighny, R. E.: Military surgical practices of the United
States Army in Vietnam. Curr Probl Surg 1:1-59, 1966.
[b]Feltis, J. M.: Surgical experience in combat zone. Am J Surg
119:275-278, 1970.

are not immediately life-threatening, and, therefore, these
casualties are not a problem for resuscitation. Definitive surgical treatment within 6 hrs of injury will reduce morbidity and
mortality. Surgical treatment delayed beyond 12 hrs of injury
will not appreciably improve the morbidity or mortality. Such a
delay will still allow salvage of 60% of stable patients with GI
tract injury.[1-3]
    The above information means:

    1. If an abdominal injury can be given definitive surgical
care in 6 hrs, the patient will do very well.
    2. If definitive surgical care is not available for more than
12 hrs, then this casualty is not a priority.

    Abdominal injuries can be maintained conservatively with
IVs, antibiotics, pulmonary care, GI tract decompression and
Foley catheterization. Keep wounds open and clean.

Table 19-5.   Hospital Mortality Rate of Combat Wounded in
              Vietnam (Oct. 1965-June 30, 1966)*

Total abdominal injuries	556
Died within 24 hrs	24 (5%)

*Heaton, L. D., Rosegay, H., Hughes, C. W., Fisher, G. W.,
and Feighny, R. E.: Military surgical practices of the United
States Army in Vietnam. Curr Probl Surg 1:1-59, 1966.

E. PENETRATING NECK INJURIES

Neck injuries, according to Table 19-2, comprise 7% of lethal injuries. High velocity missile injuries to this area cause rapid death because of airway disruption (e. g. , tracheal injury) and/or exsanguinating hemorrhage (e. g. , carotid or jugular injury). If such an injury reaches primary medical care, survival is a possibility if airway control is obtained through a tracheostomy and if hemorrhage control is achieved through pressure or ligature.

F. EXTREMITY VASCULAR INJURIES

Extremity vascular injuries should not present a life-or-death situation. Hemorrhage should be easily controlled by pressure or ligature. The concern here is limb salvage. If the major vascular trunk to an extremity is destroyed and no surgical help is available for more than 10 hrs, ligation of the major limb vessel will result in limb loss in approximately 50% of cases. [4] If definitive surgical help (vessel reconstruction) can be obtained in less than 6-12 hrs, the probability of limb salvage is excellent for isolate vessel injury. Conclusion:

1. A vascular injury less than 6-12 hrs old is a priority for evacuation.
2. A vascular injury greater than 12 hrs old has less priority for definitive care.

G. CONCLUSIONS

Based on information from Vietnam, life-threatening injuries are easily and quickly remedied even with limited resources and personnel. Lives can be saved and sustained with conservative measures until definitive therapy is available. Also, in the majority of cases, these types of injuries can tolerate a significant delay before receiving definitive treatment. When considering a combination of injuries in the multiple trauma victim, it will be the injury least amenable to these conservative measures that will determine triage and evacuation priority as well as ultimate morbidity and mortality.

IV. FUNCTION OF PHYSICIAN IN CHARGE

A. PLANNING

At times, the physician may be able to anticipate involvement in a mass casualty situation well in advance of the event. For example, the physician may practice in an area prone to natural disasters such as tornadoes or floods. Long-term preparation for mass casualty care includes the following:

1. Acquire knowledge of the type of battle or disaster. This will modify the type of preparation required. For example, chemical warfare will require decontamination equipment. After a tornado, many penetrating missile injuries can be anticipated from flying debris.

2. Lay aside a cache of supplies:
   a) Blood pressure cuff, stethoscope
   b) Intravenous fluids and equipment
   c) Medication (e. g. , morphine, lidocaine, antibiotics, diuretics, steroids, etc.)
   d) Oropharyngeal, endotracheal, and nasopharyngeal tubes
   e) Chest tubes, chest bottles, one-way valves
   f) Surgical trays for cricothyroidotomy, chest tubes, and wound debridement
   g) Dressings
   h) Monitors: EKG, CVP (if available)
   i) Cervical collar, back boards, cervical tongs
   j) Laryngoscope (bag-valve-masks)
   k) Ventilator, oxygen
   l) N/G tubes, Foley catheters

3. Obtain training in mass casualty management for yourself and your personnel.

4. Often organization must occur just prior to the arrival of casualties. This involves:
   a) Assigning personnel specific duties
   b) Laying out supplies according to triage areas and individual patient stations

V. ORGANIZATION OF PERSONNEL IN MULTIPLE TRAUMA

Triage principles for multiple trauma are discussed in Chapter 4. The purpose of triage is to save lives by recognizing lethal injuries, by resuscitating and stabilizing the patient, and by giving disposition. If these facets of triage are not well organized, a delay occurs and people die.

What causes delays?

1. Slow response
2. Poor organization
3. Poor clinical acumen (not recognizing the immediate class of injury)

4. Poor resuscitative skills
5. Unwarranted assumptions:
   a) That "someone" in the immediate area will recognize the new patient just brought into his area and start resuscitation
   b) That "someone" in the immediate area has the skills for adequate resuscitation
   c) That "someone" in x-ray will appropriately monitor and handle the patient
   d) That "someone" has written the accurate diagnosis and treatment on the patient card

The person in charge must periodically check the function of his organization and the abilities of his personnel to be sure everything is ready. In the actual situation, he must be sure that people are assigned specific duties so that the above assumptions are not made.

VI. ESTABLISHING EVACUATION PRIORITIES IN MULTIPLE TRAUMA

If the patient can receive definitive surgery in less than 6-12 hrs from injury, he/she should have priority evacuation consideration. If the patient is more than 12 hrs from injury, urgent surgery will be of decreased value, especially in vascular and abdominal injuries.

Evacuation Decisions. First priority for evacuation:

1. Progressive neurological deficit in head injury
2. Abdominal injuries less than 6-12 hrs old
3. Thoracic injuries with continuing hemorrhage, major progressive pulmonary failure, and cardiac tamponade
4. Limbs with vascular injuries less than 6-12 hrs old

The above group will benefit from early definitive surgical care. Beyond the described time periods these groups will not have dramatic benefits from surgical treatment; therefore, they fall into the class of stable delayed injuries and the triage physician will need to make individual judgments on evacuation to definitive care.

After all of the above is complete, personnel are directed in wound debridement, wound care, and other aspects of medical care.

VIII. SUMMARY

Caring for a single multiple trauma victim is complex even in a well-equipped trauma center. Caring for many such patients in a mass casualty situation with limited personnel and resources and no immediate surgical support is an even more imposing and stressful task. The situation is not untenable, however. Based on the data presented here, one can see that casualties with potentially lethal injuries can often be stabilized with simple conservatives such as a chest tube, IV fluids, wound cleansing, and debridement. Once stabilized, these patients can frequently tolerate a significant delay before receiving definitive treatment. Initial triage decisions are based on what you observe in the abbreviated primary assessment. With multiple injuries, the least easily correctable lesion will often decide the triage and evacuation category. Review of the data from previous manmade and natural disasters will assist in assignment of evacuation priorities.

REFERENCES

1. Bowers, W. F. , and Hughes, C. W. : Surgical Philosophy in Mass Casualty Management. Springfield, Illinois, Charles C. Thomas Publishers, 1960.
2. Howard, I. M. , and DeBakey, M. E. : Cost of delayed medical care. Milit Med 118:343-357, 1956.
3. Lippincott, J. B. , and Co. (Pub.):Handling of abdominal wounds under mass casualty conditions. Surg Forum VIII:168-172, 1956.
4. DeBakey, M. E. , Simeone, F. A. : Battle injuries of the arteries in World War II: An analysis of 2471 cases. Ann Surg 123:534-579, 1946.

BIBLIOGRAPHY

Oglesby, J. E. : Twenty-two months of war surgery. Arch Surg 102:607-613, 1971.

Jones, E. L. , et al. : Early management of battle casualties in Vietnam. Arch Surg 97:1-15, 1968.

U. S. Government Printing Office: Emergency War Surgery. First United States Revision of the Emergency War Surgery NATO Handbook. Washington, D. C. , 1975.

Chapter 20

SHOCK AND ITS TREATMENT IN FIELD SITUATIONS
Earl W. Ferguson, M.D., Ph.D.

I. INTRODUCTION

Many factors have been credited with the marked reduction of mortality rates in U.S. armed conflicts since World War II. One of the important factors has been the continuous availability of blood for the treatment and prevention of shock in these mass casualty situations. Future conflicts, because of their magnitude or because of interdiction of supply or evacuation routes, may require the treatment of shock in the field without adequate supplies of blood and/or other resuscitative fluids. Likewise, in unexpected civilian mass casualty situations, adequate blood and fluids may not be available.

Treatment of shock using only those supplies which are available at the time of a disaster may tax not only those resources, but also the imagination and resourcefulness of physicians and paramedical providers who find themselves confronted with the unexpected, unthinkable event.

This chapter presents a basic, simplified scheme of evaluating and handling hemorrhagic shock based largely on the approach taught by the American College of Surgeons' Committee on Trauma in the Advanced Trauma Life Support Course.

II. DEFINITION OF PROBLEM

Hemorrhagic or hypovolemic shock may be the most serious problem to consider in planning for and managing a mass casualty disaster. Shock will not only be one of the major life-threatening emergencies, it will be one of the emergencies most likely to tax resources to their limits. Shock must be treated immediately, since any delay in treatment may result in the death of the patient or permanent damage to vital organs.

Since hemorrhagic or hypovolemic shock in previously healthy individuals will be the major type of shock encountered in the first 36 hrs of a mass casualty disaster, this chapter will focus primarily on hemorrhagic/hypovolemic shock. Because of the nature of mass casualty disasters, strategies for the management of a large number of cases of shock in a brief period of time (i. e. , the group management of shock), as well as for management of the individual patient with shock will be discussed.

III. CLASSIFICATION OF HEMORRHAGIC SHOCK

A. INTRODUCTION

Since an adult's blood volume represents approximately 7% of his/her total body weight, a 70 kg man has a blood volume of approximately 5 liters. The following classification of hemorrhagic shock is based on percent blood volume loss, but values of absolute volume loss for a 70 kg man are also included. It is often easier, especially in an emergency situation, to remember classes of shock based on absolute volume losses for a 70 kg man and then to make adjustments according to patient weight. For simplicity, only three classes of hemorrhage will be used; mild, moderate and severe.

B. MILD HEMORRHAGE

1. Definition

A mild hemorrhage is an acute blood loss of less than 20% of blood volume or less than 1 liter in a 70 kg man.

2. Signs and Symptoms

   a) General Status. Alert and normal (apprehensive mental status)
   b) Pulse Rate. Minimally increased
   c) Blood Pressure. Normal
   d) Respirations. Normal
   e) Capillary Blanch Test. Normal (Blood compressed from a fingernail bed or thenar eminence returns within two seconds.)
   f) Tilt Test. Normal (Systolic pressure drop less than 20 mmHg and pulse rate increase less than 20 beats/min from supine to upright posture.)

3. Treatment

   a) Intravenous Crystalloid. Every ml of blood loss must be replaced with 3 ml of crystalloid (3 for 1 rule) since only one-third of the infused crystalloid will remain in the vascular space.
   b) Blood. Not required

C. MODERATE HEMORRHAGE

1. Definition

A moderate hemorrhage is the acute loss of 20-30% of blood volume (1-1. 5 liters in 70 kg man).

2. Signs and Symptoms

  a) General Status. Alert and apprehensive
  b) Pulse Rate. Greater than 100 beats/min
  c) Blood Pressure
      (1) Decreased systolic pressure
      (2) Increased diastolic pressure
      (3) Decreased pulse pressure
  d) Respirations. Greater than 20 breaths/min
  e) Capillary Blanch Test. Abnormal (greater than 2 sec)
  f) Tilt Test. Positive (Systolic pressure drops more than 20 mmHg and pulse rate increases more than 20 beats/min from supine to upright posture.)

3. Treatment

  a) Intravenous crystalloid (3 for 1 rule)
  b) Blood not necessarily required

D. SEVERE HEMORRHAGE

1. Definition

A severe hemorrhage is the acute loss of greater than 30% of the blood volume (more than 1. 5 liters in a 70 kg man).

2. Signs and Symptoms

  a) General Status. Confused, pale, sweating, and obviously in acute distress
  b) Pulse Rate. Greater than 120 beats/min
  c) Blood Pressure. Systolic pressure less than 90 mmHg
  d) Respirations. Greater than 30 breaths/min
  e) Capillary Blanch Test. Positive
  f) Tilt Test. Positive

3. Treatment

  a) Intravenous Crystalloid. 3 for 1 rule
  b) Whole Blood Replacement

Table 20-1. Summary of Hemorrhagic Shock Classes*

Sign	Mild	Moderate	Severe
Blood loss	20%	20-30%	>30%
Blood loss (70 kg man)	1 liter	1-1.5 liters	>1.5 liters
Mental status	Normal	Anxious	Lethargic
Pulse rate	100	100	>120
Blood pressure	Normal	Pulse press	<90 systolic
Capillary blanch test	Normal	Positive	Positive
Respiratory rate	Normal	20	>30
Fluid replacement	Crystalloid	Crystalloid	Crystalloid + blood

*Table modified from Advanced Trauma Life Support Course, Student Manual. Committee on Trauma, American College of Surgeons, 1981.

F. HEMORRHAGIC SHOCK CLASSES (see Table 20-1)

IV. INDIVIDUAL PATIENT ASSESSMENT AND MANAGEMENT

A. GENERAL PRINCIPLES

Rapid diagnosis of shock followed simultaneously by institution of volume replacement and other supportive measures and by determination of and elimination or alleviation of the precipitating cause of shock are the keys to successful shock management. Bleeding must be controlled as effectively and quickly as possible, first by direct pressure and then by pressure dressings and ligation or repair of significant bleeders. Military antishock trousers or air splints may be useful for tamponade of bleeding sites. Tourniquets should be used only as a last resort.

B. REPLACEMENT OF CENTRAL BLOOD VOLUME AND
   OXYGEN CARRYING CAPACITY

1. Trendelenburg Position

2. Central Intravenous Line

The site should depend largely on the experience and expertise
of the individual placing the line (possibilities are internal jugular, subclavian, femoral, or more peripheral cut down) and
on the time constraints demanded by the situation.

3. Volume Infusion

   a) Crystalloid. Because only one-third of the volume of infused crystalloid will remain within the vascular space, at
least three times the estimated blood loss must be infused. If
an accurate estimate of blood loss cannot be made or if blood
loss is continuing during replacement of volume, replacement
must be guided by the clinical response of the patient (i. e. ,
general status, pulse rate, blood pressure, urine output, etc.)
and by more sophisticated monitoring techniques, if available.
      (1) Central Venous Pressure (CVP) Monitoring. The
CVP should be raised to, and maintained at, 10-15 cm of water
by volume infusion.
      (2) Pulmonary Wedge Pressure. The pulmonary wedge
pressure should be raised to, and maintained at, 15-20 mmHg.
      (3) Fluid Challenge. Once the patient has shown a sig-
nificant clinical response and monitored variables are returning to or have returned to the normal range, adjustments in the
rate of infusion must be made. In a sense, the rapid initial replacement of fluids while closely monitoring the patient's response has been the first fluid challenge. However, once the
patient is relatively stable, another fluid challenge (such as an
additional 200-300 ml in 10-15 min) above the maintenance level
of infusion will give additional useful data for patient management. If the CVP rises more than 5 cm or exceeds 15 cm, or if
the wedge pressure rises more than 5 mm or exceeds 20 mm,
the rate of infusion before the fluid challenge should be maintained. If the CVP and/or the wedge pressure remains high or
continues to increase, the maintenance level of infusion should
be decreased. If, however, there is a minimal increase in CVP
or wedge pressure with the fluid challenge, the maintenance
level of infusion should be increased. General principles of
common sense and careful monitoring of patient responses
should be used to guide fluid therapy rather than hard and fast

rules. Rules are no substitute for good clinical judgment. Even if CVP monitoring is not available, clinical response can be closely monitored by observing for jugular venous distention, listening for pulmonary rales and gallops, and following the urine output.

b) <u>Blood</u>. Packed red blood cells or whole blood should be infused when large volumes of blood are lost (e. g. , severe hemorrhage, greater than 1. 5 liters or 30% of blood volume) or when the decreased oxygen-carrying capacity of the blood is preventing an adequate recovery from shock, despite volume replacement. Generally, maintenance of an adequate volume, as reflected by urine output, and a hematocrit above 30% will allow recovery in previously healthy individuals; if the hematocrit drops below that level and the patient remains unstable, replacement of red cells should be initiated.

(1) <u>Blood Typing and Crossmatching</u>. Blood should be typed and crossmatched except in extreme emergencies, in which type specific uncrossmatched blood or either O positive (males) or O negative (females of childbearing age) blood should be employed.

(2) <u>Blood Warming</u>. Blood warmers should be used to prevent hypothermia and dysrhythmias when large volumes of blood must be infused. If blood warmers are not available, they can be easily improvised. Coils of IV tubing can be run through a pan of warm water (39-40°C) and units of blood can be pre-warmed in a similar manner.

(3) <u>Blood Filters</u>. Blood filters should also be used to remove platelet and fibrin aggregates.

(4) <u>Depletion of Clotting Factors in Massive Transfusions</u>. Blood bank blood is often deficient in certain labile clotting factors. With massive transfusions of blood bank blood (more than 10 units), bleeding may occur because of this deficiency in clotting factors. This problem is easily corrected by transfusion with fresh whole blood or fresh frozen plasma to replace the clotting factors. The problem can be avoided by giving a unit of fresh whole or fresh frozen plasma with every 5-10 units of blood bank blood.

(5) <u>Consumption Coagulopathy</u>. An added complication of traumatic hemorrhagic shock may be consumption coagulopathy. Platelets and clotting factors may be rapidly consumed by the activation of the clotting mechanisms because of extensive tissue damage. Eventual depletion of platelets and clotting factors by clotting paradoxically leads to bleeding. If this occurs, fresh whole blood or fresh frozen plasma and platelet packs should be given.

C. TREATMENT OF TISSUE HYPOXIA AND ACIDOSIS

Rapid reestablishment of adequate circulating blood volume and oxygen-carrying capacity are the most important steps to reestablish adequate tissue perfusion and aerobic metabolism and to correct tissue acidosis.

Increasing the oxygen content of inspired air by the administration of oxygen is a useful adjunct to therapy and oxygen should be administered as soon as possible. Oxygen by 40% ventimask at a flow rate of 6-8 liters/min is more than adequate for those patients who do not have compromised pulmonary function. Endotracheal intubation and mechanical ventilation should be initiated rapidly in patients who are inadequately ventilated. It should be remembered that increasing the oxygen-carrying capacity of the blood and reestablishing adequate tissue perfusion is more important than giving oxygen to a patient who is ventilating well on room air.

For example, increasing the arterial oxygen tension from 60 or 70 mmHg to 150 mmHg may increase hemoglobin saturation from 90% to more than 99%, but the increase in oxygen content of the blood is minimal compared with the increase generated by increasing the hematocrit from 20-40%. Likewise, administration of sodium bicarbonate to correct severe metabolic acidosis (pH less than 7.25) may be of value, but reestablishment of aerobic metabolism in the tissues is the key to successful management of shock.

D. DRUGS

1. Sympathomimetic Drugs. Catecholamines and other sympathomimetic drugs should generally be avoided in shock. Dopamine or dobutamine may be of limited value if shock persists after adequate volume replacement. However, use of these drugs requires careful monitoring. They should probably not be used in a mass casualty/field setting.

2. Vasodilators. Vasodilators such as sodium nitroprusside are of uncertain value in hemorrhagic shock. If, after adequate volume replacement, tissue acidosis and shock continue, they may be of limited value. However, their administration must be carefully monitored and they are probably of no value in the management of shock in a field setting.

3. Corticosteroids. Corticosteroids may be of value in severe hemorrhagic shock largely because of their potential usefulness in the prevention of adult respiratory distress syndrome (i. e. , ARDS, shock lung). Methylprednisone (30 mg/kg) should be given initially and repeated in 4 hrs in cases of severe shock.

V. MILITARY ANTISHOCK TROUSERS (MAST)

MAST are pneumatic garments designed to displace blood from the lower extremities and the abdomen into the central blood volume. They are particularly useful in profound shock when adequate volume replacement cannot be rapidly initiated. They effectively reduce the volume of blood necessary to perfuse the vital organs by decreasing the perfusion of the lower extremities and by preventing the pooling of blood in the abdomen.

A. INDICATIONS

1. Inability to restore circulating blood volume rapidly in shock.
2. Adjunct for control of hemorrhage from lower extremities and abdomen and for splinting of lower extremities and pelvis.

B. ABSOLUTE CONTRAINDICATIONS

Pulmonary edema absolutely contraindicates the use of MAST.

C. APPLICATION AND USE

1. MAST should be applied by sliding them under the patient and securing them in the following sequence: around the left leg, then the right leg, and finally the abdomen.
2. After all air hoses have been connected and while the patient's vital signs are being monitored, the legs of the pants should be inflated. The amount of inflation should be determined by the patient's blood pressure response. Inflation of the pants should be discontinued when the patient's systolic blood reaches 100 mmHg or when the legs are inflated to their maximum pressure (usually 80-100 mmHg).
3. If, after complete inflation of the legs of the pants, the patient's blood pressure remains below 100 mmHg, the abdominal portion of the trousers should be inflated. Again, the rate of inflation of the trousers should be determined by the systolic response. If the patient's systolic blood pressure remains below 100 mmHg, the trousers should be left maximally inflated while volume replacement continues.
4. As the systolic pressure increases above 100 mmHg with volume replacement, the MAST can be deflated cautiously, deflating first the abdomen and then the legs. Deflation should be slow and should be done with constant monitoring of the blood pressure. If the systolic pressure drops more than 5 mmHg, deflation should be discontinued and volume replacement given

until the pressure again increases above 100 mmHg. Should the pressure fall suddenly, the trousers should be reinflated to maintain a systolic pressure above 100 mmHg.

5. MAST decrease perfusion of the lower extremities and, therefore, accentuate anaerobic metabolism and lactate production in those tissues. This can be a problem, particularly during deflation of the trousers. The problem can be avoided by restoring blood volume and decreasing the pressure in the pants as soon as possible and by being alert for, and treating, any metabolic acidosis that does occur during MAST use.

D. MAST

MAST are particularly suited for the field management of shock casualties. They are of value when definitive treatment of shock (i. e. , volume and blood replacement) cannot be immediately initiated. They may allow stabilization and transport of shock cases to facilities where such care is available.

VI. RESOURCE MANAGEMENT DURING A MASS CASUALTY DISASTER

The management of a group of shock casualties in a mass casualty disaster may be quite different from the management of a single patient. If there is an adequate supply of intravenous fluids, blood, and trained personnel, and if patients can be rapidly transported to an intensive care facility, management may be no different than what we currently consider optimal care for shock. However, if supplies are inadequate and/or if treatment must be rendered under field conditions, patient management must be quite different.

The strategies for optimizing the critical care for individuals with shock under conditions of limited resources will vary according to what resources are limited and to what extent they are limited. These strategies can be grouped around three major management casualties: First, there must be adequate fluids and equipment for the replacement of depleted intravascular volume. Second, there must be adequate red cells for replacement of depleted oxygen-carrying capacity of the blood. Third, there must be an adequate number of trained personnel to administer treatment.

A. WHAT IF INTRAVENOUS FLUIDS AND EQUIPMENT FOR THE REPLACEMENT OF DEPLETED INTRAVASCULAR VOLUME ARE LIMITED?

In evaluating the management of shock in the face of limitations in the ability to replace intravascular volume, it is best to reduce the pathophysiological problems of shock management to the basic problem—restoration of the <u>central blood volume</u> in order to provide enough blood to perfuse the heart, lungs, and brain. The solution of other problems in shock management build on the solution of that basic problem.

If central blood volume cannot be restored by intravenous fluids, it must be restored, if possible, by other means. The immediate, obvious step in increasing venous return and central blood volume in any patient is to place him in the Trendelenburg position. Arresting further bleeding and applying general supportive measures may allow recovery from even a moderate hemorrhage (1-0. 5 liter) in situations where intravenous fluids are not available. In this situation, physiologic stabilization of the patient and cautious administration of oral fluids (e. g. , water, clear liquids) may be adequate for recovery.

In more severe cases of hemorrhagic shock, MAST may be utilized to further decrease pooling in the extremities and the abdomen, as well as to decrease perfusion of the lower extremities, thus shunting more blood to the brain and other vital organs. The use of MAST may allow the patient to survive severe hemorrhagic shock long enough to get more definitive care. Air splints and ace wraps may be used as substitutes for MAST in an emergency situation. Oral fluids will probably be of no value in these patients because of decreased splanchnic perfusion and poor uptake of liquids in the gut; they are also dangerous because of the patient's compromised mental status and risk of aspiration.

B. WHAT IF INTRAVENOUS FLUIDS ARE AVAILABLE, BUT BLOOD IS NOT READILY AVAILABLE?

For mild to moderate hemorrhages, this is not a problem. However, for severe hemorrhages, management will be affected. Here, the basic pathophysiological problem is not just restoration of blood volume and tissue perfusion, but the restoration of an adequate number of red blood cells to carry an adequate supply of oxygen to tissues once they are adequately perfused. If blood is not readily available from blood banking facilities, it must be obtained elsewhere. The most obvious

place is from the "walking blood bank. " In the military, all individuals have their blood type determined when they enter the
service and their blood type is printed on both their military
identification card and on their "dog tags. " In an emergency,
donors with type specific or type O blood can be readily identified. A similar pool of donors is available in the civilian community, although identifying donors with the correct blood type
will be more difficult.

   Another initially less obvious source of red blood cells,
especially under extreme mass casualty conditions where walking blood bank donors may be insufficient, is fresh or stored
cadaver blood. Russian investigators in the 1930s observed that
blood clotted and lysed immediately after death and that the re-
liquified blood could be stored and used for transfusions without
adding anticoagulants. The red cell survival and metabolic and
oxygen-carrying capacity of red blood cells from both cadaveric
donors and live donors have been shown to be similar. Previously healthy individuals who die suddenly from trauma may
thus be an extremely important cadaver blood bank under emergency mass casualty field conditions. This source of blood
should not be overlooked, nor should one hesitate to use it to
save the living. Blood can be easily collected from cadaver
donors by placing them in the Trendelenburg position and can-
nulating the internal jugular. Cadaver blood should be obtained
several hours after death. Cadaver blood should be kept cool to
decrease autolysis and cultures of cadaver blood should be obtained. Stroma-free hemoglobin and synthetic oxygen carriers
may also soon be available for use in emergency situations
where red cells are not available.

C. WHAT IF TRAINED PERSONNEL ARE LIMITED?

When trained personnel are limited, patients must be triaged.
The real question in shock management is: What are the priorities given shock in the triage of patients? Uncomplicated hemorrhagic shock, where bleeding can be readily arrested, should
always be triaged in the immediate category. Whether or not
more complicated cases of shock should be placed in the immediate category must depend on the situation. In general,
cases of shock should be in the immediate category, since delay in its treatment can rapidly lead to death or permanent tissue damage (e. g. , renal failure). However, within the immediate category, the ABCs of cardiopulmonary resuscitation should
apply. Establishing and maintaining a patent airway and breathing must come before circulation and restoration of blood volume.

VII. PLANNING FROM THE EYE OF THE STORM

Planning for the treatment of shock in a mass casualty disaster after the disaster has occurred requires quick thinking and fast footwork. The nature of the disaster will influence the nature and number of casualties that will be, or are already, arriving at the doorstep. However, in all likelihood, hypovolemic/hemorrhagic shock will be a major problem to contend with; therefore, the following questions must be answered rapidly.

A. INTRAVENOUS FLUIDS

1. What intravenous fluids are immediately available?
2. Where and how rapidly can more be obtained?

B. BLOOD

1. How much blood is immediately available?
2. What are the blood types?
3. How rapidly can more blood be obtained?
4. What donors of type O blood are immediately available?
5. What other donors are available?

C. EQUIPMENT AND SUPPLIES

1. What equipment and supplies are on board for the treatment of shock?
2. How many MAST are available?

D. PERSONNEL

1. What personnel are immediately available?
2. How rapidly can more get here?
3. What is the level of training of the personnel available?

Hopefully, uncovering and highlighting deficiencies by a quick assessment of the resources for shock management will allow a rapid formulation of a game plan for correcting or dealing with these deficiencies.

VIII. SUMMARY

Hemorrhagic shock can be managed effectively in a field setting even when minimal resources are available. The keys to its management are rapid recognition and appropriate treatment based on sound physiological principles and common sense adjustments to the realities of the field situation, as well as to the need of the patient. In a field situation with limited supplies, mild hemorrhages (less than one liter) and even moderate hemorrhages (1-1 1/2 liters) can be managed under these conditions using MAST or MAST substitutes (e. g. , air splints, ace wraps), even if whole blood is not available. Whole blood, for treatment of severe hemorrhage can be readily obtained from walking donors as well as cadaveric donors, when it cannot be readily obtained elsewhere.

Shock can be managed under field conditions in a mass casualty disaster with minimal resources. It requires a thorough understanding of the basic physiological problem—inadequate central blood volume to maintain adequate time perfusion—and original thinking in terms of how that problem must be managed as the demands of the situation change.

BIBLIOGRAPHY

American College of Surgeons, Committee on Trauma: Advanced Trauma Life Support Course, 1981.

Emminizer, S. , et al. : Autotransfusion: Current status. Heart Lung 10, 1:83-87, 1981.

Hoffman, J. R. : External counterpressure and the MAST suit: Current and future roles. Ann Emerg Med 9, 8:419-421, 1980.

Houston, M. D. : Diagnosis and treatment of shock. South Med J 73, 4:477-484, 1980.

Jameson, G. A. , and Greenwalt, T. J. , eds. : Blood Substitutes and Plasma Expanders. New York, Alan R. Liss, Inc. , 1978.

Kevorkian, J. , and Bylsma, G. W. : Transfusion of postmortem human blood. Am J Clin Pathol 35, 5:413-419, 1961.

Mendelson, J. A. : Choice of fluids for resuscitation in trauma. Milit Med 146:677-681, 1981.

Shamow, W. N. : The transfusion of stored cadaver blood. Lancet II:306, 1937.

Yudin, S. : Blood for transfusion. JAMA 106:997, 1936.

Chapter 21

ANESTHESIA IN FIELD SITUATIONS
Roger S. Mecca, M.D.

I. INTRODUCTION

The administration of analgesia and anesthesia to victims of
trauma is complex and hazardous, even in a well-equipped medical center staffed with trained anesthesiologists. These patients may have multiple life-threatening injuries which severely interfere with cardiovascular and respiratory function. The
emergent nature of their care often precludes complete evaluation, forcing the physician to rely on clinical acumen and monitoring to diagnose serious unrecognized injuries. Adequate history is seldom obtainable, while full stomachs, compromised
airways, and hypovolemia are the rule.

In a field or disaster setting, these problems will be greatly compounded. Large numbers of critically injured patients
may require simultaneous treatment, necessitating triage and
rapid on the spot interventions. The lack of diagnostic equipment and support personnel will force the physician to make
important therapeutic decisions based on scanty clinical data.
Medical equipment, drugs, and trained personnel may be
scarce or nonexistent. Manpower shortages will mandate careful planning and organization of therapy to ensure long-term patient stability with minimal observation and care. All of these
tasks will need to be accomplished amid fear, confusion, and
fatigue, in a potentially dangerous, contaminated, or inclement
environment.

Surgical interventions which require analgesia or anesthesia
in the field will probably be limited to either minor procedures
(e.g., debridement, closure of lacerations, etc.), or life or
limb-saving interventions (e.g., chest tube placement, arterial
explorations, emergency amputations, etc.). The lack of manpower, facilities, and equipment will require patient stabilization and deferral of most surgical procedures.

II. INITIAL ASSESSMENT

Rapid assessment of airway, breathing, and circulation must
be performed prior to administration of analgesia/anesthesia.
Due to the complex nature of disaster-related injuries and the
inherent limitations placed on the physician, analgesia/anes-
thesia choices will be made under desperate circumstances. A
disaster victim is an unstable victim; analgesia/anesthesia, although necessary, will compound this instability. Once the decision has been made, however, and the procedure is underway,
the ABCs must be constantly reassessed and maintained.

III. HISTORY

If possible, a brief pertinent history should be recorded and
tagged to the patient. This summary should include name,
blood type, allergies, time and nature of injury, time of last
oral intake, previous emergency therapy and medications,
chronic medications, and history of cardiac or respiratory illness.

IV. REGIONAL ANESTHESIA

A. LOCAL ANESTHESIA

Local anesthesia is useful for minor superficial surgical procedures in a disaster setting. Liberal infiltration of prepared skin
and subcutaneous tissue with 1% lidocaine or 0. 5% bupivicaine
with epinephrine will anesthetize peripheral nerve endings and
allow limited dissection. (The use of epinephrine is contraindicated in circumferential blocks of fingers, toes, or extremities
since alpha-adrenergic arteriolar constriction may result in
ischemia and tissue necrosis. Circumferential infiltration
should be avoided even when only plain local anesthetic solution
is used. Unfortunately, local anesthesia is often inadequate in
deeper muscle or bone dissections. The morbidity of local anesthesia is low, since systemic uptake of anesthetic is minimal.
The procedure is simple to perform, and yields a high percentage of successful anesthetics. Little monitoring of the patient
is required once the anesthetic is set.

B. NERVE BLOCKS

Nerve blocks require the placement of larger amounts of local
anesthetic around nerve trunks which supply a given region of
the body. Since major peripheral nerves are in close continuity

with large arteries and veins, careful aspiration before injection is essential to avoid intravascular injection and systemic
local anesthetic toxicity. Eliciting a mild paresthesia with the
needle is often helpful in locating the nerve to be blocked. However, severe pain or burning with injection usually indicates
intraneural placement of anesthetic, and necessitates repositioning of the needle tip. Some nerve blocks are relatively simple to perform, yield high success rates, and have low morbidity. These straightforward blocks may be useful for more involved procedures on the hands, feet, and chest wall.

For ankle blocks of the nerves supplying the foot, an injection of 5-10 cc of lidocaine or bupivicaine solution is required
for each block. An injection lateral to the posterior tibial artery on the posterior surface of the medial malleolus will anesthetize the tibial nerve, while an injection lateral to the Achilles
tendon in a fan pattern over the posterior lateral malleolus will
anesthetize the sural nerve. Combining these two blocks yields
anesthesia of the plantar surface of the foot and of the heel.
Subcutaneous infiltration from the anterior border of the tibia
to the lateral malleolus will block the superficial peroneal
nerve. Injection between the tendons of the anterior tibial and
the extensor hallicus longus muscles toward the tibia blocks
the deep peroneal nerve. Subcutaneous infiltration around the
saphenous vein superior to the medial malleolus will anesthetize the saphenous nerve. (This block carries a high risk of intravascular injection.) Combining these three blocks yields anesthesia of the dorsum of the foot. Blocking all five nerves will
yield complete anesthesia of the foot, but requires circumferential injections around the ankle. To avoid this problem, the
saphenous nerve can be blocked at the knee.

Nerve blocks can also be safely done for anesthesia of the
forearm, wrist, and hand. The median nerve can be blocked
with 5 cc lidocaine or bupivicaine, either at the elbow by injecting 0. 5-0. 75 cm medial to the brachial artery on a line between the epicondyles, or at the wrist by injecting between the
tendons of the flexor palmaris longus and the flexor carpi radi-
alis at the proximal crease. The ulnar nerve is anesthetized by
injection of 5-10 cc of lidocaine or bupivicaine solution on the
posterior aspect of the medial epicondyle of the humerus or by
injection of 2-4 cc between the flexor carpi ulnaris and the ulnar artery, with an additional injection of 5 cc subcutaneously
around the ulnar aspect of the wrist. Injection of 5-10 cc between the brachioradialis and biceps tendons on the anterior
outer surface of the lateral epicondyle of the humerus will block
the radial and lateral cutaneous nerves of the forearm, while
injection of 5 cc subcutaneously on the radial border of the

wrist, dorsal to the styloid process, will anesthetize the <u>distal radial nerve</u>.

For limited procedures on the chest wall, injection of 3-4 cc of lidocaine or bupivicaine solution under the inferior border of the rib, medial to the posterior axillary line, will anesthetize the <u>intercostal nerve</u> and yield a bank of analgesia in the nerve's distribution on the chest wall. Aspiration for air or blood is essential, since the risk of pneumothorax or rapid intravenous uptake is high with intercostal blocks. Since intercostal dermatomes exhibit significant overlap, blocking a segment above or below the desired distribution will usually yield satisfactory analgesia.

Blocks of larger nerves which innervate whole extremities (e. g. , axillary block, interscalene block, femoral-sciatic block) are more difficult to perform, carry a relatively high morbidity, and have a low success rate in inexperienced hands. Performing these blocks with less than strict asepsis will introduce a high risk of serious infections. The risk of intravascular injection of large, local anesthetic volumes is significant with these more complex nerve blocks. The resulting seizures, coma, respiratory arrest, or cardiovascular collapse from local anesthetic toxicity would be difficult to manage in the field. These sophisticated blocks should only be performed by an experienced individual well-equipped to deal with life-threatening complications. For more detail in individual blocks, the reader is referred to texts by Moore or Erikson.

C. EPIDURAL AND SPINAL ANESTHESIA

These types of anesthesia involve injection of local anesthetic around or into subarachnoid space, respectively. These anesthetics are contraindicated in hypovolemic patients and require strict asepsis with the availability of equipment and drugs for complete support of ventilation and circulation. The patient must be closely monitored throughout the anesthetic. Although reliable anesthesia is usually achieved, acute complications and side effects (e. g. , severe hypotension, total spinal anesthesia with respiratory paralysis) render these techniques unacceptable for field use in a disaster.

V. INTRAVENOUS ANALGESIA AND ANESTHESIA

A. GENERAL CONSIDERATIONS

The fundamental goal of alleviating pain must be tempered with realism in the disaster setting. Pain may be an effective ally in maintaining cardiovascular and respiratory stability in the multiple trauma patient. Painful stimuli and hypovolemia elicit a profound sympathetic nervous system response, which causes local release of norepinephrine from the postganglionic sympathetic nerve endings and systemic release of epinephrine from the adrenal medulla. These endogenous pressors cause venoconstriction with increased return of blood to the heart, and tachycardia with increased inotropy, leading to an increase in cardiac output. They also cause potent arteriolar constriction, increasing the peripheral resistance in the vascular bed. The combination of increased cardiac output and increased peripheral resistance elevates or maintains a systemic blood pressure gradient to the vital organs, even with a 15-20% loss of circulating blood volume.

The central stimulation caused by pain also stimulates the respiratory center, increasing respiratory rate and depth, and thus increasing minute ventilation. Heightened arousal and anxiety usually are evident, enhancing volitional effort and insuring intact airway protective reflexes.

Overzealous administration of narcotic analgesics can easily eliminate these beneficial effects of pain. Systemic blood pressure can decrease precipitously with elimination of the painful stimulus and reduction of sympathetic nervous system activity. Hypovolemic patients are at high risk for this complication. In general, adequately hydrated patients in pain will exhibit hypertension. Analgesics should not be administered to normotensive or hypotensive patients in pain until further evaluation and hydration have been carried out. The side effects of some narcotic analgesics (e. g. , histamine release with morphine, bradycardia with fentanyl) can intensify the hypotensive response.

Narcotics also depress ventilation, both by a sedative effect and by direct depression of the respiratory center in the brainstem. Normally, the respiratory center adjusts ventilation and PCO_2 to keep central nervous system pH within the normal range. Narcotics suppress the response to pH changes in the central nervous system, and thus decrease minute ventilation. The depressant effects of narcotics can precipitate severe hypoventilation, apnea and respiratory arrest, especially in patients with marginal cerebral perfusion from hypotension. Also, the sedative effects of narcotics can induce unconsciousness and loss of airway protective reflexes, placing the patient at grave risk for aspiration. In general, confused, sleepy, or obtunded patients should not be given narcotic analgesics without close observation. Finally, it is often difficult to distinguish between discomfort due to pain and agitation due to severe respiratory acidosis or hypoxemia. Administration of analgesics for the latter condition can easily precipitate respiratory arrest.

B. NARCOTIC ANALGESIA

Narcotics should be administered in small incremental doses, aiming toward a desired analgesic effect rather than a fixed dosage. The intravenous route of administration is preferable to speed the therapeutic effect and to avoid unnecessary uptake problems from intramuscular, subcutaneous, or oral routes. This approach minimizes the incidence of undesirable side effects or overdosage, and usually results in a lower total dose, conserving valuable medication. The potency of intravenous narcotics is high, so observation of the patient is required. However, analgesic effects are reliable and reproducible.

When titrating incremental doses toward effect, it is important to allow sufficient time for peak drug action to occur (1-2 min for fentanyl, 5-10 min for morphine). Acceptable incremental dosage varies with patient condition and size. Safe starting doses would be approximately 0.05 mg/kg of morphine, 0.5 mg/kg of meperidine, or 0.5 μg/kg of fentanyl (e.g., for a 70 kg man, 3.5 mg morphine, 35 mg meperidine, 35 μg fentanyl.)

Intramuscular injections are especially dangerous in cold or hypotensive patients. The vasoconstriction resulting from increased sympathetic nervous system activity severely curtails muscle blood flow, and creates a nonmobilized depot of injected drug. If dosage is judged by effect, an inordinate amount of drug may be required to achieve modest analgesia. When warming or rehydration restores muscle blood flow, the drug depot will enter the circulation, and can result in overdosage. Narcotics are much more useful for analgesia than for sedation. If sedation alone is required, then sedatives such as diazepam (2.5 mg intravenous increments) are far more efficacious and safe.

C. GENERAL ANESTHESIA

1. _Narcotic._ Any level of analgesia can be achieved by the intravenous administration of narcotics. When choosing the desired level of analgesia, one must consider the side effects of the drug, the consequences of eliminating the painful stimulus, and the level of care the patient will require. In the field or disaster setting, if the administration of analgesic or anesthetic drugs renders a patient unresponsive to verbal stimuli, one should consider the patient as being under general anesthesia.

General anesthesia for emergency major surgical procedures will be very hazardous and difficult to administer without proper anesthetic equipment. The safe administration of general anesthesia requires a continuous intravenous infusion, as well as the availability of supplemental oxygen. Since all emergency trauma patients should be treated as if they had a full stomach, securing the airway with an endotracheal tube is mandatory. Equipment and personnel must be available to monitor and completely support ventilation and circulation should the need arise. Any type of general anesthetic is prohibitively dangerous in the absence of these basic capabilities. In the field, it may be necessary to perform emergency amputations, arterial explorations, repairs, etc. , with moderate intravenous narcotic analgesia, supplemental oxygen, and restraint, accepting a degree of awareness and pain on the part of the patient. Such an unpleasant experience is preferable to death from an unmanageable airway, aspiration, respiratory arrest, or cardiovascular collapse.

    2. <u>Ketamine</u>. Ketamine, a phencyclidine derivative, is a highly useful alternative to intravenous narcotic analgesia for emergency surgical procedures. This potent analgesic produces a dissociative state in that the patient is aware of his surroundings, but dissociated from the painful stimulus. Unfortunately, the effects of ketamine are unpredictable. A moderate intravenous dose of ketamine (0. 25-0. 5 mg/kg) alone will preserve airway reflexes and ventilatory drive. When administered with or after narcotics, however, ketamine is a potent respiratory depressant and often ablates the airway reflexes. Similarly, ketamine alone generally maintains heart rate and systemic blood pressure and is useful in hypovolemic trauma patients. However, in conjunction with other analgesics or anesthetics, ketamine can cause profound myocardial depression and hypotension. There is also a relatively high incidence of dysphoria, agitation, or combativeness after ketamine administration.

VI. SUMMARY

The choice of anesthesia and analgesia in a field or disaster setting will be affected by the availability of equipment, medication, and personnel, as well as by the clinical condition of the patient. Prior to the administration of analgesic or anesthetic medication, critical assessment of airway patency, ventilation, circulation, and history are essential. Anesthesia for superficial surgical procedures can be safely performed using infiltration of local anesthetic solution. More involved surgical procedures on the hands, feet, and chest wall may be performed by utilizing simple nerve blocks. Complex nerve blocks, spinal anesthesia, and epidural anesthesia should be avoided unless administered by experienced personnel equipped to deal with the serious complications inherent in these procedures.

Narcotic analgesia should be administered incrementally and
dosage should be titrated toward a desired effect. Close observation of the patient's ventilatory and cardiovascular status
are essential as the level of pain is diminished. The safe administration of general anesthesia in the field requires continuous venous access, endotracheal intubation, supplemental
oxygen, and the equipment necessary for the constant monitoring and support of ventilation and circulation by an experienced
individual. If these requisites cannot be met, the patient should
not be rendered unconscious by the use of analgesics or anesthetics.

SUGGESTED READING

Erickson, E. : Illustrated Handbook in Local Anaesthesia.
Philadelphia, W. B. Saunders, 1980.

Lebowitz, P. W. , and Clark, J. L. : Emergencies Complicating
Anesthesia. In Clinical Anesthesia Procedures of the
Massachusetts General Hospital. Lebowitz, P. W. , ed. Boston,
Little, Brown, and Company, 1978.

Loomis, J. C. : Shock. In Clinical Anesthesia Procedures of the
Massachusetts General Hospital. Lebowitz, P. W. , ed. Boston,
Little, Brown, and Company, 1978.

Moore, D. C. : Regional Block, Springfield, Ill. , Charles C
Thomas, 1981.

Stanley, T. H. : Pharmacology of Intravenous Narcotic Anesthetics. In Anesthesia. Miller, R. D. , ed. New York, Churchill-
Livingston, 1981.

Stoelting, R. K. : Endotracheal Intubation. In Anesthesia.
Miller, R. D. , ed. New York, Churchill-Livingston, 1981.

United States Government: Emergency War Surgery. Chp. XV.
Washington, D. C. , United States Government Printing Office,
1975.

Chapter 22

ORTHOPEDIC TRAUMA
Oscar M. Jardon, M.D.

I. INTRODUCTION

Skeletal injury is incurred in 60% of trauma cases. Patients with severe multiple injuries present a number of problems ranging from anesthesia to hypovolemic and triage considerations. Injury to the skeletal structures incurred in trauma may be closed fractures but are most often open in violent trauma. Closed injuries are not an emergent problem in any respect other than for care of associated trauma. They do require immediate splint application to allow safe and comfortable movement from the field. Any elective surgical work upon these cases is delayed until a few days to perhaps a few weeks later depending upon the availability of care facilities.

The open fracture or dislocation, penetrating joint injuries, fractures with associated vascular damage, or extensive soft tissue damage are true emergencies; and care begins immediately upon discovery. Once the patient has been assured of an airway, any hemorrhage is controlled, usually with digital pressure and occasionally with a tourniquet, only until an appropriate pressure point can be found and the bleeding tamponaded by pressure dressing. Tourniquets should not be used to control bleeding except for short periods while another control of hemorrhage is established. Pressure dressings imply point pressure over an artery to control bleeding. Controlling arterial hemorrhage in an injured extremity is usually simple, and fatal hemorrhage should be unnecessary and fairly rare. No vessel in an extremity is larger than an index finger and direct digital pressure can control it. A pressure dressing applied in the same area can continue to control it in most cases. If not, the finger should be kept in the dike.

The primary objective after control of hemorrhage becomes that of splinting a skeletal injury. The old adage of "splint 'em where they lie" meant to splint early and did not mean that the attendant should leave a fractured extremity in some grotesque position and splint it in such position.

An open fracture should be dressed with a sterile dressing if available. After that the extremity is pulled gently and steadily in its long axis to bring it into alignment; then the splintage is done (as will be described later in this chapter).

The next priority becomes prevention of infection and salvage of extremities—in that order. This requires rapid wound care, and in some instances, arterial repair and fasciotomy. Careful debridement and delayed wound closure (staged wound management) are the keys to infection prevention. Surgery is the prime prevention tool and antibiotics simply help in some cases. Deviation from staged wound management early in the care of these patients results in a horrible incidence of infection, death, and disability and cannot be tolerated.

Open wounds should be debrided and cleansed at the earliest possible moment and never closed. Wounds closed secondarily are histologically identical at 14-16 days to primarily closed wounds. Primary closure is never indicated in situations where definitive care will be delayed or in which gross contamination has occurred.

In summary, closed fractures alone are not an emergency as they do not threaten life. Emergent problems are:

A. Open fractures
B. Fractures with hemorrhage and arterial injury
C. Open dislocations
D. Penetrating joint injuries
E. Complete or partial amputations
F. Fractures associated with loss of circulation

Head and spinal injuries are discussed in another section of the text.

II. MANAGEMENT AT THE SITE OF INJURY

Immediate care consists of a rapid evaluation of the patient. Obstruction to airway is corrected if present. Hemorrhage, if present, is controlled by pressure directly over the artery followed by pressure dressing. A tourniquet is rarely ever needed. The wounds are then dressed and splintage is applied as described. Open fractures can be aligned and splinted after wound care and dressings have been applied. All fractures, open and closed, should be splinted before movement to prevent further injury. The patient is then ready for transport to the first definitive care facility. On occasion, well-trained medical personnel can begin resuscitation with fluids during or prior to transport.

A. SPLINTAGE

Volumes have been written on splintage and this, perhaps, has led to confusion. The objective of splintage is to reduce further damage to soft tissues and bone, and to reduce pain. Secondarily, it allows for less painful and easier transport of the injured. In most situations, elaborate splintage is not available and usually not really needed.

All fractures of the upper extremity can be adequately splinted by binding the arm and hand to the chest with a sling and swath (Valpeau) dressing. All fractures of the lower extremity can be adequately splinted by binding the injured limb to the uninjured limb. In instances where both are injured, they can be bound together with a well-padded splint between the extremities. All fractures of the spine can be splinted by fixation to a rigid litter or board.

When available, inflatable splints are useful, but are satisfactory only for those fractures below the knee or below the elbow. They are detrimental for humerus or thigh fractures because they provide a long lever arm which disrupts the fracture.

Humeral fractures should be splinted by sling and swath (Valpeau) dressing. Femoral fractures should be bound to the good leg or should be placed in a supportive traction splint (e. g. , Hare or similar half-ring traction splint) if it is available.

Fractures of the forearm and lower leg can also be splinted by cardboard splints, padded boards, blankets, or pillows bound over the extremity. Rigid, preformed, "fit everyone," splints fit no one and if used, should be used only over a previously applied pressure dressing. They must never be used unless a pressure dressing has been applied over the entire extremity prior to splint application; this can prevent bleb formation and skin damage which delay definitive surgery.

Rules for splint application are simple and sensible:

1. Assemble material and help after evaluation of the injury.
2. Cleanse and dress open wounds.
3. Protect normal bony prominences with adequate padding.
4. Pull gently in the long axis of the extremity to align.
5. Apply the splint or bandages to hold the fracture comfortably and support joints above and below fracture site.

The application of a traction splint incorporates these five principles but continues through seven more steps:

6. Continue traction, lifting the leg to position the splint.

7. Fix the splint with proximal strap firmly holding the splint against the ischial tuberosity as an anchor point.
8. Tie traction hitch to the ankle and foot and end of splint.
9. Apply windlass traction.
10. Release manual traction when windlass traction is effective.
11. Support leg and thigh with slings under the splint bars.
12. Elevate splint end to prevent heel pressure.

The properly splinted patient with dressed wounds and bleeding controlled is then ready for transport. Transport should be gentle and careful. Morphine or other strong narcotics are not usually necessary for a well-splinted patient and are used only for severe pain and in amounts only sufficient to relieve the pain. Most wounds are not extremely painful in the first few minutes post injury, and splintage properly applied will relieve most pain.

III. MANAGEMENT AT THE FIRST MEDICAL FACILITY

If splinting and first aid assistance have been proper, the next stage is a complete reassessment of damage and diagnosis. An examination is made of the entire body. The examiner is looking for multiple injuries, either bones or soft parts, including head, thorax, spine, pelvis, abdomen, and extremities. The only orthopedic injuries apt to give hypovolemic shock are pelvic fractures and femur fractures. These need blood and fluid replacement as well as monitoring of CVP and urinary output as described for hypovolemic shock. They rarely need emergency surgery unless the bowel or urinary tract is injured.

Open fractures are taken to surgery after stabilization and, with the patient under suitable anesthesia, are debrided according to the principles described under surgical care of open fractures. The examiner must know the amount of comminution, injury to the surrounding tissue, and presence of nerve and arterial damage, as well as whether other fractures exist. He/she must also determine whether dislocations are present.

These determinations are made by means of an inspection which assesses the amount and character of the deformity, swelling, ecchymosis, and obvious tissue damage. Palpation will disclose local tenderness, tenseness in some cases, pulsation over a closed arterial extravasation, and crepitance. The pulse, color, and skin temperature are assessed as indicators of circulatory changes. Motor and sensory assessment is done to detect nerve damage before and after any reduction. Biplane x-rays will aid in the diagnosis of fracture and the evaluation of reduction. Joint injuries may require additional oblique x-rays.

Closed fractures not complicated by other limb-threatening damage may be casted after reduction. Imperfect reduction can be corrected in a few days and time should not be wasted on attempting perfection in reduction. No internal fixation is used. Circular plaster casts are recommended to immobilize the joint above and below the fracture. These are bivalved (i. e. , cut both sides down to the skin) which allows space for swelling and easy access for evaluation. Spica casts must be kept narrow to fit litters and transportation doors. Elevation will reduce swelling.

Complication of fractures are frequently diagnosed by the patient's complaints. Increased, severe, local pain requires removal of the cast and reassessment to detect late arterial damage symptoms or compartment syndrome. Fat embolism can occur early in treatment and must be considered.

IV. STABILIZATION OF ORTHOPEDIC INJURIES

Exsanguinating hemorrhage is a possibility in relatively few fractures. Only some pelvic and some femoral shaft fractures are apt to result in hypovolemic shock. The vascular injuries associated with fractures and dislocations are a serious complication and far more apt to cause problems than the musculoskeletal injury itself.

Assessment of respiratory tract compromise is, therefore, a first priority. Correction of hypovolemia and control of hemorrhage are the next considerations. Assessment of motor and sensory function, pulses, and capillary filling are of great importance in musculoskeletal trauma and follow the other priorities.

The clinical findings of fracture are simple—tenderness, deformity, swelling, ecchymosis, abnormal motion, and crepitance are all indicative of this injury. Remember, fractures per se are not life-threatening and take a low priority in the triage schema. Uncomplicated splinted fractures and well-debrided, immobilized open fractures are delayed treatment cases.

Stabilization in the fracture victim is not generally a problem unless there is some other wound causing hypovolemia or respiratory management problems. The stabilization of these problems is discussed elsewhere in this text.

A. OPEN FRACTURE MANAGEMENT

The open fracture is essentially of immediate concern only as soft tissue wound. Hence, the priority is the prevention of

infection and the promotion of uncomplicated healing. Repair of
a wound is a continuous process from wounding to the point of
healing. This is determined by three variables: The time from
injury to initial surgery, the adequacy of the initial surgical
care, and systemic and local support to the wounded tissues.

The management of the open fracture is a three-stage process:

1. The wound is thoroughly explored and thorough sharp
   debridement is done.
2. There is delayed closure at 4-10 days after debridement
   in clean cases.
3. The fracture continues to be immobilized until it is
   healed or until any further necessary reconstructive
   surgery can be performed.

The initial exploration and debridement is done as soon as a
patient is at a site which permits such surgical cleanup. All
that is needed is:

1. A minimal field surgical kit
2. Irrigation solutions
3. Dressings
4. Some appropriate anesthesia
5. A physician experienced in debridement

Delayed closure and reconstruction are done much later.
Antibiotic therapy is only ancillary, and the real help is from
careful, sharp debridement and copious irrigation. Such irrigation may be saline with ordinary soap, betadine solution 25-
50% in saline or Ringer's solution, or if nothing else is available, clean water with soap.

The patient is prepared for debridement by x-rays in two
planes when available (more if joints are involved or if needed).
These help to show foreign bodies and the extent of skeletal
damage. Tetanus prophylaxis is given early, and antibiotics
with broad-spectrum coverage are given in full therapeutic
doses.

B. TECHNIQUE OF ORTHOPEDIC WOUND DEBRIDEMENT

After induction of anesthesia, the patient's wound is undressed
and surgically cleansed. A tourniquet is useful to control bleeding during debridement of the extremities and should exert
enough pressure to occlude arterial flow. Tourniquets should
not be left in place longer than 1-2 hrs for surgery.

Good exposure is the key to accurate and adequate debridement. Such incisions should be longitudinally oriented on an extremity and be capable of extension when needed. The incision is carried through the subcutaneous tissues and fascia; devitalized skin edges are sparingly debrided. When a joint is crossed, the incision should be s-shaped. Muscle and other tissues are gently separated to identify the wound tract. Any foreign matter is removed and the wound copiously irrigated to assist in debris removal.

Viable muscle tissue is recognized by color (light pink), good blood supply, and twitching when cut or pinched. Dead muscle is dark and does not bleed or contract. All dead muscle is removed with a sharp knife, staying just within viable muscle. Scissors tend to pinch and damage tissue; they offer poor control, and hence may damage a vital structure. Stained and shaggy connective tissues are removed. While complete excision of all devitalized muscle and other tissues is mandatory, nerves, blood vessels, large bone fragments, and skin are spared. Debridement should be done gently and with respect for tissues. Major vessels are repaired and covered with viable tissue. Nerves are not repaired but are also covered. Bone is covered if possible, but it is not mandatory. Tendons are not extensively debrided and are repaired later.

The wound is irrigated copiously and repeatedly, and all foreign matter removed. Upon completion of debridement, the tourniquet is released and hemostasis is meticulously obtained. A nonocclusive dressing is applied and if dependent drainage is not possible, a counter incision may be used to assure wound drainage. No occlusive packing is allowed. No closure is attempted—even in part. Wounds are left widely open. The wound is dressed; then the fracture is aligned as well as possible and casted. The cast is bivalved to accommodate later swelling and for ease of removal for wound inspection and secondary closure when appropriate. The cast is also dated. Findings of vessel and nerve damage as well as fracture type are documented. Once an open fracture is within clean, healed tissue, it is treated as any closed fracture would be; later reconstruction is done in a similar fashion.

V. PENETRATING WOUNDS OF THE JOINTS

Both civilian and military studies have pointed out the high potential for infection in joints penetrated by projectiles and other modalities. Over 50% of those with infection as a consequence of injury often end in amputation.

The following precepts are applicable to care of the penetrated joint:

1. The joint must be opened either by extension of the wound entrance or, on occasion, by an arthrotomy incision. In the knee, this is usually medial or lateral parapetellar in location, paralleling the long axis of the extremity. In other joints, a standard approach, which avoids nerves and vessels and allows thorough inspection of the joint, is used.

2. Anteroposterior (AP) and two oblique x-rays are helpful if available.

3. The open joint is copiously irrigated, as outlined in the care of open fractures; and small bony fragments, foreign material and clots are removed. The large bone fragments are left in place.

4. All recesses of the joint are explored and copiously irrigated.

5. Broad-spectrum antibiotics are given early and continued for 1-3 days; tetanus prophylaxis is also used early.

6. The wound is not closed. The synovium is closed only if you are absolutely certain of total cleansing of the joint. (Such certainty is a rarity.)

7. The wound is dressed with sterile dressings without packing the joint and casted as a fracture would be. The cast is bivalved.

8. The wound is closed secondarily at 4-10 days.

9. No reconstructive work is done until later.

VI. DISLOCATIONS

Dislocations of joints, if open, are attended as are open fractures. If closed, the joint is reduced as early as possible; it can often be done with analgesia rather than anesthesia. This is especially true of smaller joints or if the attempt is made very soon after injury.

Following reduction, the dislocation is immobilized in either a Valpeau dressing for the shoulder or slight traction in bed for the hip. Other dislocations are splinted or casted. There is not usually a surgical priority for the uncomplicated dislocation.

Two dislocations are notorious for vascular and neurological damage:

1. The shoulder should have verification of neurovascular status before and after reduction. Ligamentous damage may need late repair.

2. The completely dislocated knee often tears the popliteal artery and may need arterial repair. Failure to repair the artery will result in a 70-80% amputation rate. The ligamentous damage about a dislocated knee should be surgically attended within 8-10 days if possible.

VII. SPRAINS

Sprains are painful stretches to ligaments. These are common
injuries and, in the field situation, are best handled by compression dressings and analgesics; the patient may return to
duty unless the sprain is exceptionally severe in which case a
cast may be used. Sprains have no immediate major surgical
considerations and the majority will heal with minimal treatment. The most common are ankle, knee, and thumb sprains.

VIII. VASCULAR REPAIR IN EXTREMITIES

Many amputations can be prevented or a lower level accomplished by reanastomosis of an arterial injury. Often this can
be done in the field hospital situation. All that is needed are
some appropriately shod clamps or vascular clamps, vascular
suture, and a surgeon who understands the rudiments of arterial suturing. When done, they should be followed by fasciotomy
of major osteofascial compartments below the repair as described in the section on fasciotomy discussed in this chapter.
This is done to prevent a compartment syndrome.

The general condition of the patient must be such that repair
of the vasculature is warranted. Some will have other massive
injuries which require care to salvage life or the major vessels
will be in poor condition for repair. Often the question is whether the patient can survive the needed extra operating time.

Not all arterial injuries require emergency repair. Some
can be delayed for several days until evaluated by arteriography
and then treated by anastomosis of ligation. Pressure dressing
over a pulsating hematoma in a viable limb can often be treated
by delayed repair. Experience with lacerated axillary arteries,
as described by LaCroix in the Franco-Prussian War, has
shown that there is often collateral circulation sufficient to
maintain a viable limb for a period of time; therefore, these
can sometimes be treated in a delayed fashion. However, when
surgical capability is satisfactory and the patient is well enough,
one should elect immediate operative management of arterial
injury.

Surgical repair in most situations will be an end-to-end repair although autologous vein grafting will be an occasional procedure, as will lateral repair of a torn branch from an artery
or lateral repair of a short clean-cut laceration to the vessel.

If it is believed that repair can be effected and the surgical
skill is available to do the repair, it should be accomplished
early. In general, most surgeons being trained at present have
some expertise; however, the repair should only be done when

there is adequate help and when there are surgical facilities available.

Diagnosis of vascular injury can be difficult at times. A cold, pulseless, dusky extremity may be caused by unreduced fracture, dislocation, or crush injury. One should be suspicious of missile wounds in the vicinity of major vessels; this type of injury, which ranges from laceration or partial laceration with thrombosis to intimal damage with thrombosis, may be evident in such a wound.

Arterial damage is presumed in cases of cold, cyanotic limbs, those with absent pulses, or where a pulse was present and has subsequently disappeared. Pain on passive stretch, anesthesia, or pallor are suggestive. External hemorrhage is not an indicator as it may or may not be seen.

The timing of such repair is important and should be done at the earliest possible moment. As the time from wounding to the time of vascular repair lengthens, the rate of complication rises and success declines to such an extent that repair is rarely justified after 8-10 hrs. The ideal time lapse to restoration of blood flow is 4 hrs or less.

After an artery has been controlled from hemorrhage by pressure, tourniquet, or clamping, it is isolated and examined. On occasion, a small arteriotomy is done, and following clot removal by Fogarty catheters or other means, blood flow is reestablished and closure of the arteriotomy is sufficient.

Usually, however, damage to the vessel is present and the devitalized portion must be debrided to normal intima. Only the grossly damaged vessel is removed; conservatism in debridement is the rule.

Distal patency is evaluated by passage of a Fogarty balloon to remove the thrombus, backflow is also evaluated. The only true indicator of distal patency, however, is a successful reestablishment of a distal pulse. The artery is then sutured end-to-end (intima-to-intima) if possible, or, on occasion, a reversed vein graft is inserted.

End-to-end repair is done when tension is not excessive at the suture line. Most repairs are done with three or four carefully placed, running, synthetic vascular sutures which evert the edge of undamaged intima.

Any lacerated, major accompanying vein must be preserved if at all possible, and, occasionally, lateral repair of minor damage in large veins can be done. Ligation of major arteries is not a desired treatment and is accompanied by a high incidence of gangrene necessitating amputation. Even when viability is maintained, the extremity is often dysvascular and function is severely compromised. Studies in wartime surgery have shown an incidence of gangrene near 100% with severence at the popliteal artery; 90% at the common femoral; and about 50% at the brachial artery. Ligation is a last resort for use in patients in poor condition or when nothing else can be accomplished.

Fracture associated with arterial injury can be managed by splintage or, in instances of bone loss, traction can maintain length. Internal fixation in dirty, contaminated wounds under field conditions is not justified. Transverse pins and plaster or other external fixation may be indicated on very rare occasions.

Following vascular repair, fasciotomies should be done to relieve distal osteofascial compartments and the extremity is placed in neither an elevated nor a dependent position. Gangrene, Clostridial myositis, or severe, secondary hemorrhage in a field medicine setting are indications for amputation.

Partial gangrene can be allowed a day or two to demarcate a level and then amputation may be done. In the context of several hours' delay of treatment, there is no place for reimplantation surgery, and storage of amputated parts in ice and saline is not considered.

IX. NERVE INJURIES

Peripheral nerve injuries occur frequently in severe trauma and range from transient concussive injury, through contusions that require a protracted recovery time, to laceration or separation which must be repaired.

The initial, surgical care of wounds which involve nerves consists of an adequate and safe debridement sparing the nervous tissue. If a nerve is seen, its appearance and position should be recorded for future reference and care. Nerve injuries are not emergent alone and should be repaired only after healing of wounds is complete. No attempt is made at primary repair as the results are often poor. Elaborate surgery is often needed to effect repair and cannot be done as a primary nerve suture in field or mass casualty situation; it is frequently not even justified in a modern emergency hospital setting.

Surgical exploration of closed nerve injury is never indicated in an emergency situation. It is preferable to explore and repair these, if indicated, at 3 or 4 weeks after injury when the patient is set up for elective work.

Peripheral nerve injuries require no treatment other than preservation of substance and good wound debridement. At the most, the nerve ends in open wounds are placed under viable soft tissue for protection and later repair. Flail extremities require splinting in functional positions. Insensitive areas need protection from heat, cold, or pressure.

X. GUNSHOT WOUNDS IN THE EXTREMITIES

Injuries to arteries, nerves, and bones are covered under these headings. Fractures of bones in gunshot wounds are appropriately the concern of the orthopedic surgeon. Conservatism in removal of bone from wounds is critical as reconstruction of gaps in bone is apt to fail. Excision of all other devitalized tissue is essential to prevention of infection.

Antibiotics, such as penicillin, streptomycin, or cephalosporin, may seem to be indicated, but, in truth, there is little evidence that they are crucial to the outcome. In contrast, expert debridement and staged wound management, coupled with good immobilization and later reconstruction, have been proved to be the most effective deterrent to catastrophic complications.

Shotgun wounds have many of the characteristics of high velocity wounds due to a concentration of multiple fragments which carry tissue away from, and dirt into, the wound. Rocket and shell fragments can also be devastating and usually do severe soft tissue damage. These need open debridement and treatment similar to the high velocity wound.

Fractures associated with gunshot wounds are treated as is any open fracture. All wounds, low or high velocity, which involve a joint should be explored and cleansed of foreign material and small fragments. Wounds near large vessels should be studied by arteriography where feasible.

In summary, about the only gunshot wounds requiring minimal care are low velocity pistol and standard .22 rifle wounds. The remainder are specialized surgical problems of varied complexity. The interested reader is referred to K.G. Swan's excellent monograph on gunshot wounds. [8]

XI. AMPUTATIONS

There are two rules which must govern amputations:

1. Amputations should not be done unless indicated.
2. Maximal length must be preserved.

These two precepts, when heeded, will preserve maximal function.

A complete amputation in the context of massive wounding, multiple injuries, and field medicine where several hours are to elapse before definitive care requires only that the stump be revised, preserving maximal length, and delayed closure of the stump be done. The surgical techniques of amputations apply equally to partial and complete amputation and will be outlined later in this section.

The preservation of limbs is dependent upon three elements:

1. The general condition of the patient should be such that major arterial repair is feasible.
2. The condition of the limb should be such that it can be salvaged as a useful unit.
3. Surgical skill sufficient to repair the arterial flow and venous return must be available.

It is often wise for a surgeon to consider arterial repair in a proximal artery injury as an effort to achieve a longer amputated extremity (e. g. , femoral artery repair to remain below the knee or external iliac repair to allow a long above-knee, or perhaps even a below-knee, amputation). Often this will work well even when done under field hospital conditions if the surgeon is skilled.

The following are clear indications for an emergency amputation:

1. Massive destructive injury to the structures of an extremity which are clearly beyond repair and which obviously have nonviable tissues.
2. Overwhelming local infection which, despite adequate surgery and antibiotics, if life-threatening (not highly likely within 24-36 hrs).
3. Cases wherein loss of skin, muscle, nerves, and bones preclude any useful function.
4. Clostridial myositis (gas gangrene) is another indication for amputation, if generalized. If localized to one muscle group, wound excision is a better choice. This condition may develop in hours and is best prevented by adequate debridement and staged wound management.
5. Vascular injuries which have resulted in death (gangrene) of a limb are an indication for amputation. Amputation is never indicated when blood supply is merely doubtful; such measures as decompressive fasciotomy reduction, fracture, or dislocation can often restore circulation sufficient to maintain viability in doubtful cases.

A. TECHNIQUES OF AMPUTATION IN FIELD SITUATIONS

Remember that preservation of maximal length is the first priority and that prevention of infection is directly related to this priority. Thus, the level is at its lowest viable point. Viable

distal flaps of undamaged full-thickness skin, not longer than
1-1 1/2 times width, should be preserved when practical for
use in delayed closure.

The classical emergency amputation is the open circular or
guillotine amputation. This can be modified in some cases to
incorporate a skin and fascial flap or flaps of short extent
which can be closed secondarily. However, the most acceptable
amputation in field situations is the open circular; this is performed in the following manner:

1. The skin is incised circumferentially through the deep
fascia at the lowest possible level (large veins are ligated).
This is allowed to retract without any dissection.

2. With the retracted skin proximally as an indicator, each
muscle bundle is separated and divided sharply at that level.
Hemostasis is obtained on large vessels.

3. Large arteries are isolated and suture ligated after
clamping and cutting. Large veins are handled by ligation.

4. Nerves are pulled distally and transected and allowed to
retract.

5. The bone is now exposed. The periosteum is not stripped
or disturbed. The periosteum is incised circumferentially at
the level to which the muscles have retracted. This incision
line marks the cut for the amputation saw. Once the bone is
severed, the amputation is complete.

6. The tourniquet is released and meticulous hemostasis is
accomplished. A fluffy dressing is applied over the stump and
compressive wrapping is done with elastic bandages.

7. No stump is ever closed primarily in contaminated or
grossly septic situations. If a skin flap or flaps were preserved, these can be placed loosely over a thick layer of
dressing, and then the limb wrapped with a compressive dressing.

In a complete amputation, the technique is simplified in that
only nonviable, dirty tissues or those which leave the stump
irregular, are removed. Hemostasis and dressing are then
done as described. Skin traction of 4-5 lbs is applied.

Skin traction can be obtained by gluing stockinette to the
skin, just proximal to the stump dressing. This is then attached to a weight or a wire ladder splint, or a similar device
can serve to attach an elastic band for traction to the skin.

Closure is effected 5-7 days later if the stump is clean. In
some instances, skin traction can effect closure without revision when the amputation has been well done.

In summary, the following principles govern amputation
surgery:

1. An obviously useless or life-threatening limb should be amputated early.
2. Amputation is done to preserve the life of the patient.
3. All amputations are left open.
4. The ideal site for amputation in the field is that which preserves maximal length.
5. Frostbite is not an indication for early amputation.
6. Ideally, skin traction should be applied (4-5 lbs) to prevent excessive retraction of skin.
7. Closure is delayed until it is certain that the wound is uninfected.

XII. CRUSH INJURIES

These injuries usually happen from falling debris or vehicle accidents. If compression is maintained for 1 hr or more, the patient can develop what is known as the crush syndrome. This syndrome is typified by shock with crushed tissues. Upon pressure release, the crushed part swells rapidly from damaged capillaries and this may precipitate hypovolemic shock. Hypotension must be treated to help prevent renal complications. Muscle myoglobin, potassium, and lactic acid are liberated in large amounts and can increase renal damage in the hypovolemic patient.

Crush injuries should be splinted early and the extremities kept cool to reduce metabolic load. Excessive dressings are not advisable. A tense, swollen extremity should have decompressive fasciotomy performed as an emergent procedure. Amputation is done for gangrene and other indications (as described in the section on amputations) rather than simply because of the compression injury.

The crush injury patient needs plasma, blood, and fluid replacement to restore the circulatory volume. The patient should have central venous pressure maintained to prevent overhydration and a urinary catheter to monitor quality and quantity of urine. The urinary output should be kept in the range of 50 ml/hr or more. Some hydration can be by mouth. Sodium bicarbonate can be titrated to control lactic acidosis, and mannitol can be used to maintain the renal output while volume replacement is being accomplished.

The blood pressure and electrocardiogram should be monitored if at all possible. Cases with renal failure must have a marked reduction in fluid replacement and probably will need renal dialysis. This can be a triage consideration for the physician.

XIII. COMPARTMENT SYNDROME AND FASCIOTOMY

Surgical decompression is the only effective treatment for ischemia of muscles and nerves from compartment compression.
Compartment syndrome is defined as a pressure within a closed
osteofascial space in excess of perfusion pressure (27 mmHg).

Compartment syndromes challenge the best of physicians as
they can occur in a variety of situations (e. g. , trauma, ischemia, excessive exercise, postoperatively, drug and alcohol
abuse, crush injury, or blunt trauma). Diagnosis is not easy as
other conditions can produce similar signs.

The condition typically will give a tense, tight, painful compartment or extremity when compared with the normal. There
will be pain on passive stretch, later paralysis, and anesthesia
of the sensory distribution of any nerve passing through the affected compartment. Distal pulses will usually be present and
pallor is absent, as contrasted with arterial interruption.

The pathological problem is that the container is too tight;
treatment is enlargement of the container. Elevation is of no
use as it further reduces perfusion pressure. Ice only slows deterioration; compression dressings compound the problem. One
of the first acts indicated in suspected compartment syndrome
is to remove all constrictive dressings for examination, for
pressure measurement, and possibly for improvement in perfusion.

Tissue pressure can be measured and monitored through a
wick catheter (i. e. , a Jelco catheter with a wick of suture
through the lumen) or a split catheter placed into the compartment in question. The catheter is either attached to a continuous infusion-filled tube leading to a transducer for direct readout, or a partially-filled tube leaving a meniscus, which is attached to a syringe and three-way stopcock and another tube to
a common mercury sphygomanometer.

Pressures over 30 mmHg on direct readout or 40 mmHg
by the syringemanometer method are significant. If any of the
symptoms of pain, tenseness, passive stretch pain and paralysis, or anesthesia are present with a definite measured pressure elevation in the compartment, a fasciotomy is indicated.

XIV. TECHNIQUE OF FASCIOTOMY

A. LOWER EXTREMITY

In the lower extremity, the two-incision fasciotomy is recommended. Access to the anterolateral and anterior compartment
is through an incision just anterior to the fibula, centered at

midcalf, and about 8-10 cm in length. This is carried down to
the deep fascia. The fascia over the peroneal muscle is incised
with scissors in both directions to open this compartment. The
fascia over the tibialis anterior is opened in similar fashion.
Care is taken not to damage the common or deep peroneal
nerves.

The posterior compartments (superficial and deep) are relieved by a similar longitudinal incision just posterior to the
medial border of the tibia and the fascia, over the gastrocnemi-
us and soleus, opened proximally and distally. These muscles
will bulge through the cut fascia. The deep compartment with
tibialis posterior and flexor muscles is identified, and this
fascia is incised proximally and distally. A check for adequacy
can be done by repeating pressure readings. Do not close the
skin. The wounds are dressed and closed secondarily and rarely require skin grafting.

B. UPPER EXTREMITY

Fasciotomy of the forearm can be done by longitudinal incision
through the skin either volarly or dorsally or both, and the fascia over the superficial or deep muscle can be incised longitudinally to relieve pressure. Care is taken not to cut nerves or
large vessels. In the forearm, decompression of the volar compartment often decompresses the dorsal compartment and vice
versa. This is not the case in the lower extremity. If pressure
remains high within an unreleased forearm compartment after
fasciotomy of the other, it should be opened. The wounds are
handled as are those in the lower extremity. If fracture is
present, the limb is casted and the cast bivalved after dressing
the wounds. The wounds are redressed and checked as indicated
by pain, drainage, and progressive improvement; and they are
closed secondarily after all is stable and uninfected.

XV. FAT EMBOLISM

Fat embolism is a frequent early complication of the multiply-
injured patient. The syndrome is commonly associated with
femoral fracture and one other long bone fracture. The disease
is defined as an abnormal aggregation of fat globules in the
lungs, brain, and other organs.

Two theories of etiology prevail. One is traumatic release
of depot fat from a fracture; the other is that the disease is a
disturbance of phospholipid metabolism allowing aggregation of
fat into large chylomicra. The latter seems most tenable to
this author. Many causes other than trauma have been described,

including hemoglobinopathies, altitude decompression, collagen disease, burns, diabetes, infection, anesthesia, hepatitis, neoplasia, transfusion, renal infarct, and a number of other problems.

Fat embolism is a respiratory disease reported to have an incidence of 10% in multiple injuries during World War I. The incidence is probably higher and about the same in both civil and wartime multiple injuries.

Sixty-five percent of fat embolism cases left untreated will end in death. The condition does occur in children, according to a study in Montreal in the late 1970s. The effect is anoxia, secondary to fat aggregation, with the lung tissue. The disease is usually clinically manifested from 4 hrs to 3 days post injury. At 12 hrs there will be 25% of the expected cases manifested; 75% by 24-36 hrs; and 85% by 48 hrs. A lucid interval is always emphasized, but this is not always present. Brain trauma is the biggest differential diagnostic problem.

The early symptoms of the disease are confusion, unexplained urinary incontinence, tachypnea, fever, tachycardia, late coma, and central nervous system symptoms of a changing and vacillating nature. Petechiae of antigravity distribution on face, conjunctiva, and upper thorax are late signs.

Attempts at diagnosis by laboratory fat determination are not particularly helpful. A pO_2 decreased below 60 mmHg and a pCO_2 in the normal range are very helpful. The pathology is a shunting of blood flow in the lungs with decreased O_2 transport and microinfarcts of lung, brain, kidney, and retinal tissue; permanent brain damage is rare in survivors.

The most common injury combinations are fractures of multiple bones associated with intraabdominal, thoracic, intracranial, or major arterial injury.

Treatment is respiratory assistance. O_2 by mask is used (nasal catheter will not give sufficient O_2 partial pressure) and then pO_2 is checked. If it is above 65 mmHg, this is sufficient. If pO_2 is not maintained, then positive end pressure respiratory assistance is needed. This is usually successful. Tracheotomy is rarely ever needed as most cases are resolved within a week and a tube can be tolerated this long.

Heparin alcohol, dextrose, and cortisone are of no real use in therapy. The key is respiratory support and adequate hydration. Gentle handling of well-splinted patients appears to reduce the number of cases as does adequate early hydration.

XVI. TRIAGE CONSIDERATIONS IN ORTHOPEDIC SURGERY

1. As mentioned earlier, there are only two types of fracture which can exsanguinate the patient: those of the pelvis and

upper femur. Often this does not occur, but it is a potention problem. It is treated by blood fluid replacement and is not normally an emergent operative problem, hence is not a priority for surgery.

2. Fractures of and by themselves are not emergent problems and can be in a delayed treatment classification if they are closed.

3. Open fractures are a surgical priority, as are gunshot wounds to the extremity, and open penetrating joint injuries. Once debrided and immobilized, they need only redressing and debridement until clean enough for secondary closure at 4-10 days.

Thus, we see that the triage considerations in orthopedic injuries are those of the associated injuries rather than the musculoskeletal injury per se. Once this precept is thoroughly understood, the triage of fracture cases becomes a simple matter of classifying by severity of associated injury.

BIBLIOGRAPHY

U.S. Government: Emergency War Surgery. NATO Handbook, First U.S. Revision, 1975.

Gallagher, J.T., et al.: Post-traumatic pulmonary insufficiency, a treatable disease. South Med J 70:1308-1310, 1977.

McManus, J.: Brachial plexus lesion complicating anterior fracture-dislocation of the shoulder joint. Injury 8:63-66, 1976.

Meislin, H.W. (ed.): Priorities in Multiple Trauma. London, Aspen Publishers, 1980.

Markus, A., Blair, W., Shuck, J., and Omer, G.: Low velocity gunshot wounds to extremities. J Trauma 20:1061-1064, 1980.

Shea, J.D.: Surgical techniques for lower extremity amputation. Ortho Clin North Am 3, 2:287-301, 1972

Spak, I.: Humeral shaft fracture treatment with simple hand sling. Acta Orthop Scand 49:234-239, 1978.

Swan, K.G.: Gunshot Wounds—Pathophysiology and Management. Littleton, Massachusetts, PSG Publishing Co., 1980.

Chapter 23

ABDOMINAL AND PELVIC ORGAN TRAUMA
Valeriy Moysaenko, M. D.

I. INTRODUCTION

Abdominal trauma is usually assessed after the immediate
lethal problems are corrected, i. e. , airway, breathing, circulation. In the mass casualty situation, if immediate laparotomy
is required and it cannot be performed as a lifesaving procedure, the patient should be characterized as expectant, so as
not to consume limited resources and manpower. In the total
assessment of the patient, the sole decision to be made is
whether or not intraabdominal injury exists.

II. TYPES OF INJURY

A. The types of abdominal injury are:

    1. Penetrating
    2. Blunt

All penetrating abdominal trauma should be explored. In
blunt trauma, a decision must be made as to whether intraabdominal injury has occurred

B. RESULT OF ABDOMINAL TRAUMA

There are several conditions caused by trauma to the abdomen
which require surgery. They include:

    1. Bleeding
        a) Ruptured liver
        b) Ruptured spleen
        c) Ruptured blood vessels
        d) Ruptured kidney

Parenchymal injuries to liver, spleen, and kidney often
stop bleeding. Therefore, the patient who initially presents

with this type of injury and shock can be stabilized with expansion of intravascular volume. If the parenchymal injuries are severe, the patient will not stabilize readily. If immediate surgical capabilities exist, the patient may be saved; if none exist, the patient is expectant. Disruption of major abdominal vessels will usually preclude any successful resuscitation.

Patients with intraabdominal hemorrhage may present with external evidence of abdominal injury (e. g. , bruises, abrasions, lacerations and/or fractures of ribs and pelvis), abdominal distention, absence of bowel sounds, direct and rebound tenderness. If the injury is suspected but the above physical signs are absent, peritoneal lavage will often clarify the situation.

2. Spillage of Luminal Contents
   a) Biliary
   b) Pancreatic
   c) Bowel
   d) Bladder

The spillage of luminal contents after disruption of a hollow viscus may present very subtly. There may be external evidence of abdominal trauma (e. g. , bruising, abrasions, lacerations, fractures, etc.), but the abdomen in the acute situation may still be flat and relatively nontender with propulsive bowel sounds. The patient's vital signs may be stable. However, repeated examination may show increased abdominal pain, distention, and decreased bowel sounds. These signs and symptoms may evolve over 6 hrs. Again, if hollow viscus injury is strongly suspected or other injuries (e. g. , unconsciousness, regional fractures, or drugs) prevent accurate clinical evaluation, peritoneal lavage with recovery of bile, amylase, stool, or urine will confirm the intraabdominal injury and aid in planning therapy and priority for evacuation.

3. Evisceration

Evisceration may result in penetration of the eviscerated organ with spillage of aluminal contents, parenchymal injury of a solid organ or vascular compromise of the involved viscus.

III. EVALUATION OF ABDOMINAL INJURIES

For a proper evaluation of the abdomen, a logical sequence of physical examination should be followed.

A. Physical Exam

   1. Visualize abdomen front and back. Visualize perineum. Observe for:
     a) Penetration, evisceration
     b) Bruising, abrasions, contusions, lacerations
     c) Bloody urine

   2. Auscultate
     a) Bowel sounds absent: Abdominal injury is possible
     b) Bowel sounds present: Abdominal injury may still be present and bowel sounds will disappear later.

   3. Palpate
     a) Localized pain
     b) Rebound pain
     c) Referred pain
     d) Palpate pelvis, lower ribs
     e) Rectal exam (prostate, rectal wall)
     f) Bimanual pelvic exam in females

B. Recognition of Abdominal Trauma

   1. Clinical Appearance
     a) Distention
     b) Pain (direct, rebound)
     c) Absent bowel sounds
     d) Penetrating injury
     e) Evisceration
     f) Blood in rectum
     g) High riding prostate

   2. Peritoneal Lavage

If the physical exam is conclusive for intraabdominal injury, no other procedures need to be accomplished. However, if the patient is stable but intraabdominal injury is suspected yet not clinically certain, peritoneal lavage can aid in diagnosis. Peritoneal lavage will not detect retroperitoneal injury, but it is usually performed to help make an immediate surgical decision. In the mass casualty situation, when immediate surgical intervention is not possible, this procedure may assist you in making triage and evacuation decisions.

3. Radiographic Evaluation

X-ray studies, if available, may detect intraabdominal and retroperitoneal injuries. Useful studies include the following flat plate and upright abdominal x-rays:

a) Free air in abdomen
b) Contrast studies
   (1) IVP (renal or ureteral disruption)
   (2) Gastrograffin UGI (gastric, duodenal disruption)
   (3) Cystogram (bladder, urethra disruption)

IV. MANAGEMENT

All intraabdominal injuries require surgery; however, some may be stabilized and held because they are not immediately life-threatening. Definitive intervention can then be deferred for 6 hrs without change in surgical outcome. After 12 hrs, there will be no further increase in mortality even if the patients undergo appropriate surgery. Therefore, there is urgency to obtain surgical treatment for intraabdominal injury up to 6 hrs post injury; after a 12-hr delay, the urgency is lost. This information is useful for evacuation logistics. The appropriate supportive treatment is described below.

A. NASOGASTRIC SUCTION/DRAINAGE

1. Relieves abdominal distention
2. Prevents
   a) Aspiration
   b) Respiratory compromise secondary to abdominal distention
   c) Shock secondary to gastric distention

B. INTRAVENOUS FLUIDS

1. Resuscitation
2. Antibiotics

C. FOLEY CATHETER

1. Detect hematuria
2. Monitor effectiveness of fluid resuscitation

D. MOIST DRESSING OVER EVISCERATED ORGANS

No manual replacement of organs into abdominal cavity.

E. PELVIC INJURIES

Pelvic injuries present the problem of blood loss which can be managed with volume expansion. However, pelvic injuries may herald rectal and genitourinary injury and require careful evaluation. The bladder or rectal injury can be treated as the routine abdominal injury, but disruption of the urethra will require placement of a cystostomy catheter.

V. SUMMARY

An abdominal injury is not a mysterious lethal injury. Even in the mass casualty situations, when immediate surgical intervention is not available, patients with intraabdominal injuries can be salvaged. A significant percentage of parenchymal injuries, if not severe, will stop bleeding and the patient will survive with adequate supportive measures. About 50-60% of patients with hollow viscus injuries, if they are not severe, will survive even without surgical intervention although there may be high morbidity. The following facts will assist in treatment, triage, and evacuation decisions:

A. Penetrating abdominal injuries require surgery.
B. Luminal spillage requires surgery in 6-12 hrs; otherwise mortality is high. Up to 60% may survive with no surgical intervention.
C. Evisceration is equivalent to luminal spillage.
D. Rapid intraabdominal bleeding requires immediate life-saving laparotomy. If this is not possible, the patient is expectant.

BIBLIOGRAPHY

Walt, A. J., and Wilson, R. F.: Management of Trauma: Pitfalls and Practice. Philadelphia, Lea and Febiger, 1975.

Committee on Trauma, American College of Surgeons: Advanced Trauma Life Support. American College of Surgeons, 1981.

Swan, K. G., Swan, R. C., and Levine, M. G.: Management of gun shot wounds. Contemp Surg 17:11-36, 1980.

Lindsey, D. , and Silverstein, M. : Abdominal trauma: When to go in, when to stay out? Ariz Med 33(9):701-707, 1976.

Lindsey, D. : Teaching the initial management of major multiple system trauma. J Trauma 20(2):160-162, 1980.

Chapter 24

THORACIC TRAUMA
Kenneth L. Mattox, M.D.
David V. Feliciano, M.D.

I. DEFINITION

A. SCOPE OF THE PROBLEM

We derive much of our current knowledge about the treatment
of thoracic trauma from extensive experience collected during
past military conflicts. Sources as diverse as Homer, Pare,
Larrey, and reports of American casualties in the four major
conflicts of the last 80 years[1-7] provide excellent descriptions
of both penetrating and blunt thoracic injuries.

In recent years there have been increasing numbers of
civilian thoracic injuries secondary to urban violence and terrorism and to deceleration trauma in motor vehicle accidents.[8-10] At the present time, 25% of injuries occurring in
the general population involve the chest. Thoracic injuries account for 25% of all trauma deaths and are contributing factors
in another 25% of deaths.[11] During natural disasters or military mass casualty situations, patients with immediate life-
threatening thoracic injuries may die at the scene or during
transport to a medical treatment facility. Patients with potentially life-threatening emergencies may not survive the initial
triage when attention is directed to large masses of patients
with less severe injuries. Physicians can treat 85% of patients
with minor thoracic injuries secondary to penetration from low
velocity missiles or foreign bodies or secondary to general
blunt trauma with simple techniques such as tube thoracostomy,
pericardiocentresis, tracheostomy, and/or drainage of effusions and empyema.

Patients with more severe thoracic injuries, including destruction of the chest wall or extensive pulmonary or cardiac
disruption, require advanced techniques of resuscitation and
treatment. During a disaster the absence of trained personnel,
appropriate facilities, and adjuncts such as antibiotics and ventilation will cause more death in this group than would occur in
normal circumstances.

348

B. CATEGORIES OF THORACIC TRAUMA

Chest injuries and conditions which are usually nonlethal include:

1. Rib fractures
2. Simple pneumothorax
3. Simple hemothorax
4. Clotted hemothorax
5. Chylothorax
6. Pulmonary lacerations
7. Pulmonary hematoma
8. Sternal fractures
9. Traumatic asphyxia
10. Tracheobronchial aspiration
11. Mediastinal hematoma
12. Pneumomediastinum

Six potentially life-threatening thoracic injuries include:

1. Pulmonary contusion
2. Myocardial contusion
3. Aortic disruption
4. Tracheobronchial disruption
5. Esophageal disruption
6. Diaphragmatic disruption

Six immediate life-threatening thoracic conditions include:

1. Airway obstruction
2. Open pneumothorax
3. Tension pneumothorax
4. Flail chest
5. Massive hemothorax
6. Cardiac tamponade

II. FIELD EMERGENCY CARE FOR THORACIC TRAUMA

A. INITIAL ASSESSMENT AND RESUSCITATION

Recognizing that thoracic injuries can disrupt the airway, mechanics of ventilation, and central circulation, initial assessment of the patient with thoracic trauma must be accompanied by restoration of the ABCs of resuscitation (see Chapter 5). Once vital signs are improved, a secondary and more comprehensive evaluation of the injured patient should be performed.

If possible, radiographic investigation can then be completed.

A patient with a thoracic injury and a secure airway should be given supplemental oxygen. If present at all in the field, supplemental oxygen will be in cylinders which should be completely removed from the area when there is potential of fire. While supplemental oxygen should be humidified before being introduced in the trachea, this may not be possible. In such settings, oxygen catheters placed in the nose will allow for humidification via the turbinates. Adjuncts to proper control and management of the airway is covered in Chapter 5.

Once an adequate airway has been established, failure of the patient to start breathing or of a rescuer to ventilate the patient suggests some disruption of the thoracic bellows mechanism. Though many thoracic injuries may be responsible, a simple field treatment plan is again emphasized here:

1. Drain a closed pneumothorax, tension pneumothorax, or hemothorax.
2. Cover an open pneumothorax.
3. Stabilize a flail chest.

The above injuries are diagnosed in the field via inspection, palpation, percussion, and auscultation of the thorax. A closed pneumothorax is often present on the side of the chest where rib fractures are present. Inspection may reveal skin contusions; palpation may note bony crepitus or subcutaneous emphysema; percussion may reveal decreased tympany; and auscultation notes decreased breath sounds. Presentation of a tension pneumothorax is usually much more dramatic and generally involves severe air hunger, cyanosis, tracheal deviation away from the tension, hyperresonant percussion, and absent breath sounds. Signs of a hemothorax differ from those of a simple pneumothorax and include a dull percussion and perhaps signs of hypovolemia.

Evacuation of air, fluid, or blood from the pleural space is a skill which all individuals treating trauma patients must know. Providers able to perform these skills in mass casualty and disaster situations will save lives. Inserting a small catheter through the second or third interspace anteriorly and connecting the catheter to a one way valve will relieve a simple pneumothorax or a tension pneumothorax. For most patients, a lateral tube thoracostomy, using a #36 French tube at the midaxillary line, is preferable.

After local anesthesia is infiltrated at the fifth intercostal space, a small incision is made and a blunt dissection using the gloved finger is carried up to the superior margin of the fourth rib. The pleura is entered after the intercostal muscles have been separated with a large clamp. The presence or absence of pleural adhesions is ascertained and the initial hole is slightly enlarged. Using a clamp on a large chest tube, the physician should direct the tube posteriorly and superiorly (Figure 24-1), and then connect it to either an underwater seal, a Heimlich valve, an autotransfusion device, or a commercially available pleural collection bottle with a one way valve so that air is prevented from returning to the pleural space. If continuous accumulation of air, fluid, and blood is anticipated, the collection device should be connected to suction. If no further accumulation is anticipated, a simple underwater drainage seal is sufficient. Insertion of trocar chest tubes may produce further injury through penetration of intrathoracic or intraabdominal viscera and therefore should be avoided.

Open chest wounds, formerly called traumatic thoracotomies or sucking chest wounds, are common during field medical emergencies. This injury requires further debridement and closure in a medical treatment facility; however, in the field and during resuscitation, the sucking chest wound should be closed.

1. Ask the patient to cough. This will blow out as much clot as possible through the open wound.
2. Use occlusive dressing, such as vaseline gauze, plastic wrap, or other material, to close the open thoracotomy sucking wound.
3. Insert a chest tube through a separate incision and attach it to a one way valve or a field expedient chest decompressive catheter such as the McSwain dart. [11]

Bony crepitus, paradoxical respiration, and, frequently, severe respiratory distress secondary to an underlying pulmonary contusion with right-to-left vascular shunting characterizes a flail chest. Pressure in the bone segment may prevent the paradoxical respiration but will not alleviate respiratory distress. In a limited casualty situation, intercostal nerve blocks, good pulmonary toilet, and fluid restriction may be enough to relieve respiratory distress, even without endotracheal intubation. [12] With multiple casualties and few medical personnel, endotracheal intubation for internal pneumatic splinting of the flail segment may be necessary.

Once an airway and normal mechanisms of respiration are restored, hypotension in the patient with thoracic trauma suggests hypovolemia from massive hemothorax, from massive hemoperitoneum, or from a cardiac tamponade. Fluid

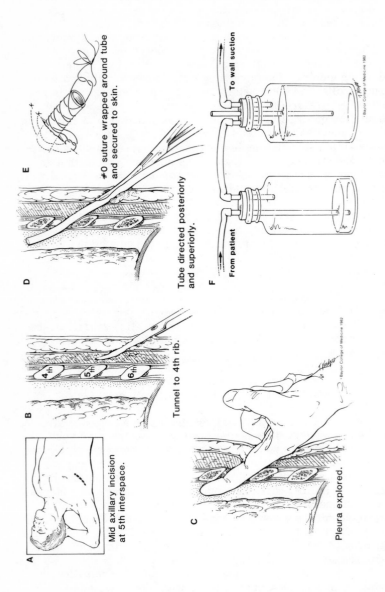

A — Mid axillary incision at 5th interspace.

B — Tunnel to 4th rib.

C — Pleura explored.

D — Tube directed posteriorly and superiorly.

E — #0 suture wrapped around tube and secured to skin.

F — From patient / To wall suction

Figure 24.1. Drawings depicting technique for lateral tube thoracostomy.

resuscitation through large bore intravenous lines is necessary
when blood loss is responsible for hypotension; however, certain precautions must be followed. Extensive lower neck or upper chest injury on one side may be accompanied by injury to
the jugular or subclavian veins on one side or to the superior
vena cava. In such patients, use of lower extremity intravenous
lines may be necessary. In penetrating trauma with hypovolemia, support of the patient through intravenous supplementa-
tion using crystalloid balanced salt solutions in a ratio of 3 cc
administered for every 1 cc anticipated or projected loss is
lifesaving up to severe losses of 30% or greater. In those instances, hemoglobin solutions which are capable of transporting hemoglobin (e. g. , blood, stoma-free hemoglobin, or fluoro-
carbons) should be considered. If the source of hemorrhage is
in the chest, tube thoracostomy with autotransfusion is indicated. Continued bleeding once 1000-1500 ml has been aspirated
from one pleural cavity means that the heart, a great vessel,
hilar lung, internal mammary artery, or an intercostal artery
is injured. If open chest surgery is not possible, these patients
probably will not survive and should be treated with this in
mind by triaging to expectant treatment area.

When the central venous pressure stays elevated in the face
of sudden hypotension and muffled heart sounds, treat the patient for a pericardial tamponade. In a field situation, needle
pericardiocentesis with a #16 gauge plastic sheathed needle,
inserted in a subxyphoid location and directed toward the right
shoulder, is indicated. If a medical treatment facility is distant, the needle or catheter is left in place and the cavity aspirated every few minutes to withdraw additionally accumulated
blood (Figure 24-2).

The secondary evaluation is based upon the priorities established during the initial evaluation. Secondary evaluation re-
establishes the presence or absence of the initial findings and
determines any alterations, improvements, or deteriorations.
Maintain a flow sheet showing circulatory activity including
heart rate, estimated cardiac output, urinary output, presence
or absence of breath sounds, and output from the chest tube.
During this secondary evaluation, a patient may profit from
thoracotomy, arteriography if at all available and indicated,
and perhaps a tube thoracostomy if not previously inserted. Patients with chest wall fractures may not initially manifest a
flail segment. As hypoxemia and/or excessive fluid hydration
occurs, respiratory embarrassment with paradoxical chest
wall movement can occur. In such instances, insertion of an
endotracheal tube may then be indicated.

In the field situation and in a disaster medical treatment

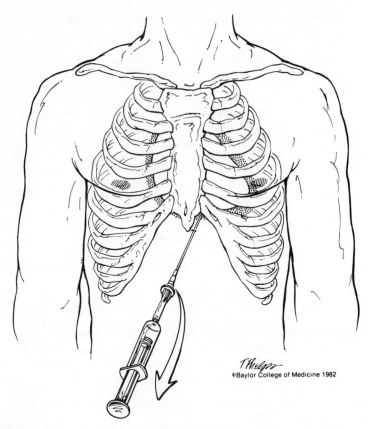

©Baylor College of Medicine 1982

Figure 24-2. Drawing depicting technique of pericardiocentesis.

facility, laboratory and radiographic evaluations are limited.
Helpful laboratory and radiographic determinations in chest
trauma patients include hemoglobin and/or hematocrit, arterial blood gases, urinalysis, and chest x-ray. The patient records, including x-rays and laboratory data, should be included
in packets accompanying the patient to subsequent treatment
facilities. In instances of mediastinal hematoma, arteriographic
contrast studies are indicated. If such arteriographic facilities
are available, contrast radiography is helpful when esophageal
or thoracic outlet injury is suspected. Concomitant with this
initial assessment and the establishment of treatment priorities
is obtaining a history of the mechanism of injury, time intervals
to initial evaluation, treatment previously administered, known
allergies, blood type (if known), and the amount of estimated
blood lost externally, into serous cavities or fracture sites.

B. TREATMENT OF SPECIFIC INJURIES

1. Nonlethal

a) <u>Rib Fractures</u>. Patients with first rib fractures generally require meticulous evaluation even if they do not appear seriously ill because of the high incidence of associated intracranial, intrathoracic, and intraabdominal injuries. [13] Intercostal nerve blocks may help patients with multiple rib fractures, since they can then inhale fully and cough, promoting good pulmonary toilet. Treat associated problems, such as blood loss and underlying pulmonary contusion, as necessary. Avoid circumferential binders which promote atelectasis. Give supplemental oxygen.

b) <u>Simple Pneumothorax/Simple Hemothorax</u>. Tube thoracostomy as previously discussed.

c) <u>Clotted Hemothorax</u>. Early evacuation by formal thoracostomy, especially if fever or empyema develop.

d) <u>Chylothorax/Pulmonary Laceration</u> (with Hemo- or Pneumothorax). Tube thoracostomy, as previously discussed.

e) <u>Pulmonary Hematoma</u>. Observation, fluid restriction, and ventilatory support if deterioration is noted.

f) <u>Sternal Fracture</u>. Early electrocardiogram to rule out myocardial contusion, serial chest x-rays to rule out widening of the mediastinum.

g) <u>Traumatic Asphyxia</u>. Support of respiration as indicated.

h) <u>Tracheobronchial Aspiration</u>. Early bronchoscopy (if available) with removal of large fragments, followed by saline lavage of major bronchi; consider broad-spectrum antibiotics and steroids.

i) <u>Mediastinal Hematoma</u>. Serial chest x-rays to rule out widening of mediastinum. Aortogram if possible.

2. Potentially Lethal

a) <u>Pulmonary Contusion</u>. Limit intravenous fluid to less than 1000 ml of crystalloid fluid for resuscitation. If hypovolemia exists, use colloid solutions. Early use of steroids and Lasix is controversial. [14]

b) <u>Myocardial Contusion</u>. Serial electrocardiograms and cardiac enzymes if available. In a field situation, restrict crystalloid administration. Use inotropic agents as necessary if congestive heart failure occurs. Expect cardiac arrhythmias.

c) <u>Aortic Disruption</u>. Major vascular injuries to the thoracic outlet or to the descending thoracic aorta are, in general, beyond the treatment scope in the field and in the initial triage treatment facility. Among the 10% of patients with this injury who reach a treatment facility alive, a smaller percent (5%) who remain untreated will develop a chronic traumatic aneurysm. Because of this possibility, at least one author has recommended this injury initially be treated with afterload reducing agents such as nitroprusside, trimethaphan camsylate, and reserpine. [14]

    d) <u>Tracheobronchial Disruption</u>. Major tracheobronchial disruption usually occurs within 1 cm of the carina. It is rare and most commonly is the result of blunt trauma, such as a motorcycle accident or direct blows to the midsternum. Associated fractures to the sternum and chest wall are common. Many patients with tracheobronchial disruption present with pneumothorax, pneumomediastinum and cervical emphysema. In others, tracheobronchial disruption will not be discovered until some time later, with the onset of atelectasis and pneumonia. In general, except for tube thoracostomy to treat the associated pneumothorax, tracheobronchial disruption should not be treated in the field or at the initial triage treatment facility. Acute tracheoesophageal fistula from blunt trauma to the thoracic outlet may occur 3-5 days postinjury.

    e) <u>Esophageal Disruption</u>. This injury is extremely rare and carries a 50% mortality. Treatment at a tertiary care center involves complex isolation techniques. [15]

    f) <u>Diaphragmatic Disruption</u>. Diagnosis of injury to the diaphragm is usually delayed until evaluation of the initial chest x-ray reveals abdominal contents, such as the stomach, herniated into the left pleural space. Do not place a chest tube unless a significant hemothorax is present. If you must insert a chest tube, carefully palpate for the spleen, stomach, colon, or omentum herniated into the left chest through the chest wall incision because this will confirm the diagnosis. Diaphragmatic disruption requires transabdominal surgical repair since concomitant intraabdominal injury is present in 80% of such injuries.

C. ROLE OF EARLY THORACOTOMY

Fifteen percent of patients require thoracotomy for control of thoracic injury. The decision to perform thoracotomy is based upon the following specific indications:

    Witnessed hypovolemic cardiorespiratory arrest
    Pericardial tamponade
    Mediastinal traverse by a missile with resultant refractory
       shock

Traumatic thoracotomy
Uncontrolled and/or continued hemothorax (greater than
   1500 ml)
Massive air leak
Radiographic or endoscopic evidence of tracheobronchial
   tears
Radiographic or endoscopic evidence of esophageal injury
Penetrating or blunt injury to the thoracic outlet
Radiographic evidence of great vessel injury
Bullet embolus to heart or pulmonary artery
Traumatic diaphragmatic injury
Industrial coal tar product injection into lung
Persistent chylothorax
Evacuation of clotted hemothorax
Removal of infected traumatic lung abscess

III.   PROBLEMS ASSOCIATED WITH DELAYED
TREATMENT OF THORACIC TRAUMA

Chronic traumatic conditions may develop in less than 15% of
survivors who do not receive initial definitive treatment for
life-threatening thoracic traumatic injury. These chronic conditions include:

1. Chronic false aneurysm
2. Chronic disruption of the trachea or bronchus
3. Pericardial effusion
4. Chronic diaphragmatic hernia
5. Healed chest wall fractures
6. Chronic arteriovenous fistula
7. Clotted hemothorax and fibrothorax
8. Chronic bronchopleural cutaneous fistula
9. Others

   Any one or combination of these conditions may result in
subsequent deterioration of the patient's status, such as a ruptured aneurysm; constrictive pericarditis and low cardiac output; strangulated abdominal contents through a chronic diaphragmatic hernia with gangrene, sepsis, and death; or pulmonary insufficiency from a fibrothorax. Should chronic empyema
occur, tube thoracostomy may be an ineffectual way of treating
a well established cavity. Placement of the largest chest tube
available and resection of a rib at the lowest level of the abscess cavity creates a cavernostomy or chronic draining sinus;
the resultant controlled chronic bronchopleural cutaneous fistula is compatible with life. Chest wall cutaneous infections

may be treated with frequent dressing changes soaked in
Dakin's (one-quarter strength Clorox), iodinated solution (such
as Betadine), or other solutions which encourage the development of granulation tissue. In the absence of constricting pericarditis, recurrent pericardial effusions may be treated with
recurrent pericardiocentesis. Chronic chylothorax should be
treated with a diet devoid of short chain fatty acids and triglyc-
erides as well as with a tube thoracostomy or repeated thoracentesis. As chyle is basically bacteriostatic, empyema is
rarely associated with chylothorax. Fluid restriction and respiratory support through supplemental humidified oxygen is
necessary for the patient with a contused or injured lung paren-
chyma. If hypoxemia is present, intubation and volume regu-
lated respiratory support or ventilatory support is indicated.

IV. TRIAGE CONSIDERATIONS IN THORACIC TRAUMA

Extrathoracic injuries, such as cranial, spinal, major abdominal, and major extremity fractures, carry a high morbidity
and involve prolonged hospitalization. Many patients with thoracic injuries possess a potential for recovery and early return
of function. Therefore, thoracic injury patients who survive
long enough to reach the first triage point should not a priori
be placed into an expectant category, but should receive stabilizing therapy.
    Casualties with the six immediately life-threatening thor-
acic conditions are ironically the group which will dramatically
respond to simple field maneuvers such as airway control,
pericardiocentesis, and tube thoracostomy. In the disaster
situation, patients with massive hemothorax and major heart
injuries may not reach a tertiary care facility. The patient with
a flail chest should be stabilized and evacuated if possible.
    Casualties with one of the 12 nonlethal conditions should be
expected to survive. Using relatively simple maneuvers, these
patients may be treated at the primary medical facility.
    Patients in a mass casualty situation who have one or more
of the six potentially life-threatening thoracic injuries pose
complex problems to the medical team. Such patients should be
evacuated to a thoracic surgery treatment facility as soon as
possible if such a facility exists. In the absence of any surgical
capabilities and with limited resources, the patients in this
category will have the highest mortality.
    All of this encouraging information about prognosis assumes
that the person who is initially responsible for providing evaluation and stabilization knows how to perform the simple motor
skills discussed in this chapter.

REFERENCES

1. Homer: The Iliad. Translated by Alexander Pope. New
   York, Heritage Press, 1934.
2. Hamby, W. B. : Ambroise Pare, Surgeon of the Renais-
   sance. St. Louis, Warren H. Green, Inc. , 1967.
3. Larrey, Baron Dominique-Jean: Memoirs of the Military
   Surgery and Campaigns of the French Armies. Translated
   from the French of D. J. Larrey by Richard Willmott Hall.
   Two vols. Baltimore, Joseph Cushing, 1814.
4. U. S. Government: The Medical and Surgical History of the
   War of the Rebellion. Surgical History. Pt I, Vol. II, pp.
   466-650. Washington, Government Printing Office, 1879.
5. Betts, R. H. : Initial surgery of thoracoabdominal injuries.
   J Thorac Surg 15:349, 1946.
6. U. S. Government: The Medical Department of the United
   States Army in the World War. Vol. XI, XV. Washington,
   Government Printing Office, 1925.
7. U. S. Government: The Medical Department of the United
   States Army Surgery in World War II—Thoracic Surgery.
   Vol. I. Washington, Office of the Surgeon General, Department of the Army, Government Printing Office, 1963.
8. Jones, K.W. : Thoracic trauma. Surg Clin North Am 60:
   957, 1980.
9. Reul, G. J. , Mattox, K. L. , Beall, A. C. , Jr. , et al. : Recent advances in the operative management of massive
   chest trauma. Ann Thorac Surg 16:52, 1973.
10. Wilson, R. F. , Murray, C. , and Antonenko, D. R. : Non-
    penetrating thoracic injuries. Surg Clin North Am 57:17,
    1977.
11. Wayne, M. A. , and McSwain, N. E. : Clinical evaluation of
    a new device for the treatment of tension pneumothorax.
    Ann Surg 197:760, 1980.
12. Trinkle, J. K. , Richardson, J. D. , Franx, J. L. , et al. :
    Management of flail chest without mechanical ventilation.
    Ann Thorac Surg 19:355, 1975.
13. Richardson, J. D. , McElvein, R. B. , and Trinkle, J. K. :
    First rib fracture: A hallmark of severe trauma. Ann Surg
    181:251, 1975.
14. Akins, C. W. , Buckley, M. J. , Daggett, W. , et al. : Acute
    traumatic disruption of the thoracic aorta: A ten-year ex-
    perience. Ann Thorac Surg 31:305, 1981.
15. Defore, W. W. , Jr. , Mattox, K. L. , Hansen, H. A. , et al. :
    Surgical management of penetrating injuries of the esopha-
    gus. Am J Surg 134:734, 1977.

Chapter 25

NEUROLOGICAL TRAUMA
Richard A. Pratt, M.D.

I. INTRODUCTION

The purpose of this chapter is to present information on the
sustained early management of multiple neurosurgical casualties in an isolated environment, including evaluation, prognosis, triage, evacuation, and treatment modalities of head and
spinal cord injuries. The chapter is intended to be as complete
and practical as possible, and to complement contributions already made.

II. HEAD INJURIES

Patients with head injuries can be lumped into one of two main
categories: those with transient loss of consciousness who have
an apparently complete recovery (concussion) and those with
persisting neurologic impairment. The second group includes
the delirious patient, the seizure patient, and the patient with
obvious penetrating or open wound. Neurologic injuries do not
occur in isolation. It is important to realize that injuries to the
nervous system must be placed in clinical perspective and that
patient airway, adequate respiration, and circulation are prerequisite to successful management. All too often, premature
clinical focus on the neurologic injury has delayed other diagnoses and has compromised management.

A. THE PATIENT WITH TRANSIENT LOSS OF
    CONSCIOUSNESS AND APPARENTLY
    COMPLETE RECOVERY (CONCUSSION)

In normal practice, some physicians admit and observe all patients with transient loss of consciousness. This practice gives
the physician the best opportunity to recognize complications
early and hopefully affords the patient the best chance for recovery. This policy should also be considered in mass trauma
situations as resources allow. Patients who have sustained

360

tangential head wounds have increased incidence of delayed intracranial hematoma and should always be observed and transferred to a larger facility. These patients have a high probability of developing a delayed intracranial hematoma. Patients who have had transient loss of consciousness by more traditional injuries, such as blows and falls, may need to be managed differently in a mass casualty situation. The clinical challenge is to select the patients who are most likely to develop complications and observe them, and to release those patients who have a very low chance of developing complications.

The history can be of great help in patient management. The duration of unconsciousness is generally correlated with the severity of the injury and the likelihood of complications. Complication is unlikely if the period of unconsciousness was brief (<1 min) provided the patient is alert and oriented 3-6 hrs later and denies difficulty with headache, impaired vision, unsteadiness, clouded thinking, motor weakness, or sensory change; the patient should also have a benign exam. These patients may be returned to duty or work with instructions to return if symptoms develop.

If the duration of unconsciousness is not known, the length of amnesia may assist the examiner in determining disposition. Generally, all patients who have lost consciousness will have amnesia including and following the event. This is called post-traumatic amnesia. Occasionally patients will have amnesia for events preceding the injury; this is called retrograde amnesia. It is probably safe to release a patient from mass casualty treatment if the total length of his amnesia is less than 10 min and he/she is alert and oriented, and denies neurologic symptoms; he/she should also have a normal neurologic exam and skull x-rays.

Neurologic examination should begin with assessment of the patient's vital signs and level of consciousness. This is conveniently and reliably done using the Glasgow Coma Scale. This scale assesses the patient's neurologic response in three areas: eye opening, verbal responses, and motor responses. These are individually scored and summed to a total of 3-16 points. The first area, eye opening, is scored 4 points if eyes open spontaneously, 3 points if they open to speech, 2 points if they open to pain, and 1 point if they do not open. The second area, verbal response, is scored 5 points if the patient is oriented, 4 points if he speaks appropriately but is confused, 3 points if he uses inappropriate words, 2 points for incomprehensible words, and 1 point for no speech. Motor responses, probably the most important area, are scored 6 points if the patient follows simple commands, 5 points if the examiner's hand is pushed away in response to localized pain (i. e. , supraorbital pressure), 4 points for general withdrawal from pain, 3 points for arm flexor posturing (decortication) to pain, 2 points for arm extensor posturing (decerebration) to pain, and 1 point for no motor response.

The scalp is inspected for injuries. The external auditory canals are inspected for both injury and leakage of cerebrospinal fluid (CSF). Subcutaneous blood surrounding the eyes or behind the ears indicates fracture and a demand for a more careful evaluation of hearing, sight, and the sense of smell. Pupillary size and reaction are recorded. Function of the cranial nerves, cervical spine, carotid arteries, motor and sensory responses of the extremities should be checked and recorded.

Not every patient with head injury requires skull x-rays. Only those patients with documented traumatic unconsciousness lasting more than one minute, possible skull penetration, palpable depression of the scalp, mastoid or periorbital ecchymosis, or discharge from the nose or ear should be considered for skull x-rays.

Patients who require continued observation in the triage area should be made npo. IVs are not always necessary. IV infusion, if elected, is best done with D5 1/2 NS, 50-60 cc/h for an average adult. If analgesics are indicated codeine, 30-60 mg q3h IM p. r. n. should be used initially. Codeine will control most symptoms of pain from neurologic injuries without altering the level of consciousness or pupillary reaction. Neurologic reassessment should be performed q 1-2 hrs depending on the degree of injury and the level of staffing. Glasgow Coma Scale checks should be continued. A change of 1 point is considered clinically significant, with lower scores suggesting complication and need for rapid reevaluation. Experienced trauma surgeons believe the most reliable sign of complication is a lowering of the motor response scores. Patients remaining stable for 24 hrs may be discharged.

B. MANAGEMENT OF THE PATIENT WITH PERSISTING
   NEUROLOGIC DEFICIT AFTER HEAD TRAUMA

It is important to reemphasize the need to place neurologic injuries into the clinical perspective. The airway needs to be secured and stabilized. The respiration must be adequate. The circulation must be supported. Fluids should be used as necessary for resuscitation of the circulation. Consideration of fluid restriction to prevent cerebral edema becomes secondary.

The neck should be stabilized, preferably by tape and sandbags, until x-rays have excluded a cervical fracture.

In mass casualty situations, the Glasgow Coma Scale is a valuable triage tool. Patients with arrival scores of 3-5 have a 15% chance of complete recovery. Scores 6-8 have a 35% chance of satisfactory results. Best results are seen in the patient whose admission score is 7 or above with a satisfactory result of 80%.

C. DISRUPTIVE PATIENTS

Patients with head injury and persisting neurologic deficits may be disruptive and delirious. Reassurance and compassion should be attempted to the extent that resources provide. Intramuscular Haldol is a valuable agent when sedation is needed. Haldol will control behavior without drastically impairing the ability to reassess the patient's level of consciousness or the Glasgow Coma Scale.

D. TRAUMATIC SEIZURES

Traumatic and posttraumatic seizures are commonly the generalized tonic, clonic type (grand mal). The airway should be protected and anticonvulsants given. Seizures are best treated with intravenous Dilantin, 1 g, at a rate of 50 mg/min for adults. Pediatric dose is 15 mg/kg, at a rate not to exceed 2 mg/min. If this fails, an additional infusion of Phenobarbital 500-1000 mg should be given for adults and 6-30 mg/kg for children. The Phenobarbital is given slowly, IV, with care given to signs of respiratory depression.

Patients with transient injuries described earlier never need prophylactic anticonvulsants. All patients with persisting neurologic deficits should be considered candidates for prophylactic anticonvulsants. Penetrating and open brain injuries should always receive prophylactic anticonvulsants. Dilantin is generally the best agent. Effective blood levels are achieved with 1 g IV or orally. Oral Dilantin loading dose is 400 mg followed by 300 mg 2 and 4 hrs later. Intramuscular Dilantin is not effective as the medication remains in the soft tissue for many years without effective absorption.

E. PERSISTING DEPRESSION IN LEVEL OF
CONSCIOUSNESS AFTER HEAD INJURY

These patients require the same general assessment and treatment as the three prior groups. Stabilization may require intubation, especially if the Glasgow Coma Scale remains 6 or below. Hyperventilation to achieve an arterial pCO_2 of 25-35 will produce prompt vasoconstriction (within 30 sec) and a decrease in intracranial pressure by shunting intravascular blood out to the skull. In a mass casualty situation where blood gas analysis is not available, ventilating at a rate of 18-21 times/min should achieve the expected pCO_2 level. Simply elevating the head of the patient's bed 45⁰ will also decrease intracranial pressure. Mannitol will further decrease intracranial pressure with a dose of 1/2-2 g/kg. It is best to reserve mannitol for the treatment of the rapidly deteriorating patient or the patient who has had a surgically treated mass lesion excluded. Furosemide (Lasix) given prior to mannitol may decrease ICP more rapidly than mannitol alone.

In isolated situations, prophylactic antibiotics should be given to all patients with open wounds or CSF leakage. Patients with CSF leakage should be treated with simple penicillin preparations. Penetrating injuries are best treated with antibiotics which are known to penetrate the brain substance (e. g. , methicillin and chloromycetin).

Corticosteroids have been used for several years in the treatment of head trauma patients. Recent studies have failed to find conclusive evidence that these drugs are effective and many neurosurgeons have discontinued their use.

The goal of treatment is to stabilize the patient and transport him/her to other facilities where better resources are available. All efforts should be directed toward maintaining vital signs and preserving neurologic functions. The patient must be protected from climatic environment (see Chapter 12).

If time and resources allow, additional tests may be obtained. Tests, however, should never delay the transfer of the patient.

F. EMERGENCY SURGICAL TREATMENT OF LIFESAVING LIMITED CRANIOTOMY UNDER ISOLATED CONDITIONS

Under exceptional circumstances, limited craniotomy for possible intracranial hematoma may be justified. If surgical resources are available, a patient who has shown signs of neurologic deterioration by the Glasgow Coma Scale either with or without focal neurologic signs (i. e. , pupillary dilation or hemiparesis) will warrant emergency craniotomy.

What equipment is needed?

1. One Hudson brace
2. One d'Errico cranial perforator
3. Two mastoid retractors

4. One Leksell rongeur
5. Two Adson retractors
6. Cautery
7. Suction
8. Hemostatic agents

What is the goal of the surgery? The surgeon should take limited measures to exclude an epidural hematoma. This is best
accomplished by exposing the skull at the site where the hematoma is highly probable, perforating the skull, and removing
additional bone to expose the dura. As a general rule, the dura
should not be opened by relatively inexperienced surgeons as
there is generally little to be offered to the patient with sub-
dural hematoma or intracranial hematoma. Exploratory surgery for these conditions in isolated or primitive conditions is
only likely to aggravate the patient's condition, expend limited
resources, and offer little to the patient. Naturally, a more
thoroughly trained surgeon must use clinical judgment and do
what he feels is best under triage circumstances.

When should emergency transfer be considered? If the patient
can be on the operating table at a better equipped and staffed
facility in less than 4 hrs, transfer is recommended. It is essential that the decision to operate or transfer be made in conjunction with a neurosurgeon, if possible. During transfer
mannitol should be infused and the patient hyperventilated. The
operation should be done on those patients who are likely to die
but may be saved with simple, limited surgery which requires
only a modest amount of neurosurgical skill.

Where do you operate? The scalp is incised, and retracted and
the skull is exposed. Burr holes are placed 1 inch off the midline and 1 inch anterior to the coronal suture. Another is
placed 1 inch above and behind the external ear, and the last is
placed in the temporal fossa. If an epidural collection is encountered, the burr hole is enlarged with the Leksell rongeur;
and the blood clot is removed. If any bleeding point is encountered, it is controlled by cautery or hemostatic agent. Bone
fragments are not replaced. A drain may be left in the epidural
space, and the scalp is closed with sterile dressings applied.
If there is pupillary inequality, the first hole should be placed
on the side of the larger pupil. The patient should be draped so
that the head may be easily turned to facilitate surgery on the
opposite side (Figure 25-1).

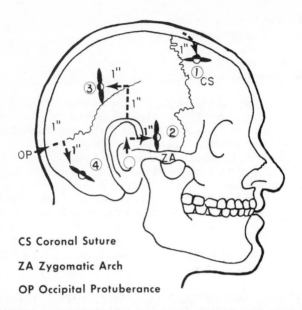

CS Coronal Suture

ZA Zygomatic Arch

OP Occipital Protuberance

Figure 25-1. Diagram of the skull showing sites of expiratory burr holes. (1) Incision 1 inch lateral to the midline and just anterior to the coronal suture. (2) Incision 1 inch above the external auditory meatus and 1 inch anterior to it. The lowermost point of the incision lies on the zygomatic arch. (3) Incision one inch above and one inch behind the ear. The lowermost point of the incision should be at the level of the top of the ear. (4) The suboccipital incision should lie 1 inch lateral to the external occipital protuberance and begin at a point 1 inch below the lateral sinus. (From Kahn, E. A. (ed.): Correlative Neurosurgery, 2nd ed. Courtesy of Charles C Thomas, Publishers, Springfield, Illinois.)

G. OPEN OR PENETRATING INJURIES

Impaired level of consciousness may be complicated by skull injury or penetration. These include depressed skull fracture, high velocity penetration, low velocity injury, stab wounds, and CSF leakage from nose or ear.

It is important to understand that a depressed skull fracture is a broken bone which may or may not be associated with a neurologic injury. If there is no abnormality on the neurologic examination, elevating the depressed skull fracture is elective. There is no increase in morbidity or mortality associated with a 24 hr delay in elevating a depressed skull fracture, even if

open. While the need for definitive surgical care is elective
and can be deferred, the patient must continue to be observed,
with rapid reevaluation if complications occur. Immediate local
care to scalp injuries should not be deferred.

Gun shot wounds are divided into low and high velocity categories (see Chapter 18). Low velocity injuries are caused by
small caliber hand guns found in civilian life. High velocity injuries are the result of military small arms. In general, low
velocity injuries can be observed. Bullet and fragment wounds
to the brain require meticulous debridement and dural closure
and should be undertaken at larger facilities. Detailed removal
of all bone and metal fragments is no longer considered necessary. Debridement should be tempered with good judgment as
more damage can be caused by debridement near critical centers.

Tangential wounds of the head may exert considerable kinetic energy displaced inward. Patients with these wounds, despite lack of an unconscious period, must be admitted and observed.

Leakage of CSF from the nose or ear is commonly seen.
Patients should be treated with rest and limited position
changes, and should not be allowed to smoke. They should be
started on antibiotics (e. g. , simple penicillin or sulfa).

H. STAB WOUNDS OF SKULL

Patients may present with a knife or a piece of metal shrapnel
embedded in the skull and brain. The foreign object may provide a tamponade effect to active bleeding. These patients will
require transfer with the object left in place.

III. THE EVALUATION AND MANAGEMENT OF THE
PATIENT WITH POTENTIAL SPINAL CORD INJURY

Preliminary evaluation of the patient's arm and leg movement
should be made early. Cervical spine x-rays are obtained as
early as possible. The cross table lateral film is the most
helpful, and, if taken with a large cassette, it will be possible
to view the lateral skull and neck on a single film. If there is
extreme respiratory compromise and it is either unsafe or impossible to insert an endotrachial tube, a cricothyroidotomy
should be performed before x-rays are taken. Ideally the cross
table lateral x-ray should visualize all seven cervical vertebra.
Drawing the shoulders down may aid in viewing the lower cervical spine. Occasionally even this technique will fail to reveal
all seven cervical vertebrae. A reasonable compromise is to

see the top 1/2 of the C-7 vertebra. This will be adequate under multiple trauma situations since fractures between C-7 and T-1 are unlikely. Time lost with repeated x-rays may compromise treatment. The cervical spine film should be systematically analyzed. The soft tissue shadow just anterior to the cervical vertebra should be assessed for thickness. It is normally less than one-third the sagittal diameter of the vertebral bodies in the upper cervical spine. If this shadow is thicker, it indicates that a significant amount of trauma occurred to the cervical spine and that a fracture is likely. The lateral cervical spine film should be further analyzed for signs of dislocation of the anterior and posterior margins of the vertebral bodies. The facets should be aligned above and behind each other.

If a cervical fracture or dislocation is revealed, then stabilization is indicated. If further evacuation is indicated, this is best done with sandbags on the side of the head and with wide adhesive tape securing the head across the forehead and the chin. Belts are utilized across the body to secure the patient firmly to a back board or stretcher. Cervical collars should be avoided as they can promote a false sense of security, possibly compromise the airway, or mask expanding lesions in the neck.

If a neurologic deficit is present, both a urinary catheter and nasogastric tube should be inserted. The patient is best transported in a slightly head down, supine position to improve circulation and respiration. IV fluid should be administered to maintain vital signs. Some authorities believe that large doses of corticosteroids (e. g. , Decadron or Solu-Medrol) are of benefit if given early.

If transfer is not possible, stabilization should be made with cervical tongs. Several varieties are available. Gardner Wells tongs are preferred for their simplicity. Placement is facilitated by locating the lateral mass of the first cervical vertebra and the external auditory meatus and by extending the line on the skull to just below the insertion of the temporalis muscle to the skull. Hair should be removed. A large bolus of local anesthetic should be administered to control pain of insertion. Final torque adjustment is made by following the instructions engraved on the tongs. A pulley arrangement with suspended weights should be used. The amount of weight depends on the level of the injury. This is determined by multiplying the number of the injured vertebral body by 5 and suspend that weight in pounds. For example, if there is a fracture at cervical 4, suspend 20 pounds (approximately 10 kg). If no tongs are available, a halter may be improvised with cord and ABD pads.

The patient should be placed on a turning frame if available. Such frames can be improvised using two field canvas stretchers with holes cut to accommodate the face, Foley catheter, and buttocks. The patient can be sandwiched and secured between these stretchers for turning. Ideally, turning should be done every 2 hrs to prevent pressure sores. The heels should not touch the stretcher or frame. Due to risk of ileus, feeding should be delayed for 48-72 hrs. Periodic x-rays should be obtained to check cervical alignment.

The majority of spinal injuries will be symmetrical, with consistent motor and sensory levels. A simplified system to determine the motor level is as follows:

Paralysis of finger adduction indicates a lesion at T-1.
Paralysis of grip indicates lesion at C-8.
Paralysis of finger extension indicates a lesion at C-7.
Paralysis of wrist extension indicates a lesion at C-6.
Paralysis of shoulder adduction indicates a lesion at C-5.

There are other less common lesions which may be seen. The Brown-Secquard syndrome represents a hemitransection of the spinal cord and is characterized by motor paralysis and loss of position sense below the lesion, ipsilateral with contralateral loss of pain and temperature sensation. Management is fundamentally the same as the complete and symmetric lesions.

The central cord syndrome is uncommon. This lesion is generally seen with hyperextension injury of the spine. It is characterized clinically by weakness of finger and hand function and loss of pain and temperature modalities in the hands and arms. Management remains fundamentally the same as above.

The anterior cord syndrome is unique in that these patients may benefit from prompt surgical intervention and they should be considered for urgent transfer if circumstances permit. These patients may appear to be identical to the complete lesion first described. However, they generally have preserved appreciation of joint position sense in the lower extremities. The decision for prompt evacuation should be made in conjunction with the receiving neurosurgeon.

IV. GENERAL TRIAGE PRINCIPLES
IN NEUROLOGICAL TRAUMA

Neurologic casualties are common in most mass civilian or military disasters. Triage decisions must be based on clinical information as sophisticated diagnostic studies will not be available.

The triage physician must stabilize and evacuate his casualties. The first group of neurologic casualties evacuated should be those who can be helped. More specifically, those patients who have had minimal injuries and are deteriorating are the most likely to be helped. Some of these patients may need emergency limited craniotomy when first seen. Patients with depressed levels of consciousness should then be transferred according to their ability to be helped at the next facility. Patients who require sustained skilled neurosurgical care should be the last to be evacuated.

BIBLIOGRAPHY

Gurdjian, E. : The treatment of penetrating wounds of the brain sustained in warfare. J Neurosurg 39:157-166, 1974.

Jennett, B. : Infection after depressed fracture of the skull. J Neurosurg 39:333-339, 1972.

Meirowsky, A. : Neurological Surgery of Trauma. Office of the Surgeon General, Department of the Army, Washington, D. C. , 1965.

McNealy, D. , and Plum, F. : Brainstem dysfunction with supratentorial mass lesions. Arch Neurol 7:26-45, 1962.

Pitts, L. , and Martin, N. : Head injuries. Surg Clin North Am 62:47-60, 1982.

van Dellen, J. : Stab wounds of the brain. Surg Neurol 10:110-114, 1978.

Youmans, J. : Neurological Surgery. Vol. 4. Philadelphia, W. B. Saunders Co. , 1982.

Young, B. : Early prediction of outcome in head-injured patients. J Neurosurg 54:300-303, 1981.